Advances in
Immunopathology

From a symposium sponsored by
Scripps Clinic and Research Foundation
La Jolla, California

Advances in Immunopathology

William O. Weigle, Ph. D.
Editor

Member and Chairman
Department of Immunopathology
Scripps Clinic and Research Foundation
La Jolla, California

Published by

Symposia Specialists Inc.

MEDICAL 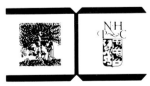 BOOKS

Distributed by

ELSEVIER/NORTH-HOLLAND
NEW YORK • AMSTERDAM • OXFORD

Published by:

Symposia Specialists, Inc.
1470 N.E. 129th Street, Miami, Florida 33161

Distributed in U.S.A. and Canada by:

Elsevier North Holland, Inc.
52 Vanderbilt Avenue, New York, New York 10017

Sole distributors outside U.S.A. and Canada:

Edward Arnold (Publishers) Limited
41 Bedford Square
London WC1B 3DQ
England

Library of Congress Catalog Card Number: 81-51627
International Standard Book Number: 0-444-00598-6

Manufactured in the United States of America

Contents

IMMUNOBIOLOGY:
BASIC CELLULAR AND BIOLOGICAL PROBLEMS

David H. Katz, M.D.
Department of Molecular Immunology
Scripps Clinic and Research Foundation
La Jolla, Calif.

Howard M. Grey, M.D., Robert W. Chesnut, Ph.D.
and Ralph T. Kubo, Ph.D.
Department of Medicine
National Jewish Hospital and Research Center/
 National Asthma Center; and
University of Colorado Health Sciences Center
Denver

Norman R. Klinman, M.D., Ph.D., Dwane E. Wylie, Ph.D.
and Judy M. Teale, Ph.D.
Department of Immunopathology, and
Department of Cellular and Developmental Immunology
Scripps Clinic and Research Foundation
La Jolla, Calif.

William O. Weigle, Ph.D., Edward L. Morgan, Ph.D.
and Marilyn L. Thoman, Ph.D.
Department of Immunopathology
Scripps Clinic and Research Foundation
La Jolla, Calif.

APPLICATION OF BASIC IMMUNOBIOLOGY
TO IMMUNOPATHOLOGY

Charles G. Cochrane, M.D.
    Department of Immunopathology
    Scripps Clinic and Research Foundation
    La Jolla, Calif.

Thomas S. Edgington, M.D., Gary A. Levy, M.D.,
Bradford S. Schwartz, M.D. and Daryl S. Fair, Ph.D.
    Department of Molecular Immunology
    Scripps Clinic and Research Foundation
    La Jolla, Calif.

Frank J. Dixon, M.D.
    Department of Immunopathology
    Scripps Clinic and Research Foundation
    La Jolla, Calif.

Curtis B. Wilson, M.D.
    Department of Immunopathology
    Scripps Clinic and Research Foundation
    La Jolla, Calif.

Peter A. Ward, M.D. and Kent J. Johnson, M.D.
    Department of Pathology
    University of Michigan Medical School
    Ann Arbor

Michael B. A. Oldstone, M.D.
    Department of Immunopathology
    Scripps Clinic and Research Foundation
    La Jolla, Calif.

INDEXES

Acknowledgments

This book resulted from a course presented during dedication of the new Immunology Laboratories Building, Scripps Clinnic and Research Foundation, on October 22, 1980. The course was supported entirely by Miles Laboratories, Incorporated, Elkhart, Indiana. The dedication also marked the twentieth year of immunology research programs at Scripps under the direction of Frank J. Dixon. The papers presented are contributed by supporters and former colleagues of F. J. Dixon and his present staff, all of whom have been in the development of this program.

Preface

During the past decade considerable, important information has accrued for all facets of the immune response. During this period, research has generated enormous insight into interactions between T and B lymphocytes and macrophages, identification of cell surface antigens involved in triggering these cells, molecular and biochemical consequences of triggering events, genetic restrictions governing the activation and interaction of lymphocytes, and mechanisms responsible for the regulation of cellular and subcellular events of immune responses, once initiated. Most significantly, these recent advances are now being used by experimentalists to further understand cellular and biochemical activities leading to the initiation and regulation of autoimmunity and other in vivo consequences of antibody-antigen interactions. Thus, we are now beginning to understand the initiating factors responsible for immunologically associated diseases, the accompanying tissue damage and the regulating mechanisms leading to their exacerbation and remission. Similarly, this vast amount of information delineating the basis of immunity has improved our understanding of the cellular, molecular and genetic rationale for the containment of tumor progression as well as viral and parasitic infections.

The first half of this book is concerned with cellular events responsible for the interaction and triggering of cells involved in various aspects of the immune response. This portion also deals with the nature of cell surface receptors for both antigen and antibody and the role of their modulation in lymphocyte inactivation. The manner in which these events are regulated is considered on both cellular and biochemical bases. The first paper by David Katz gives a basic overview encompassing the collaboratory activities of T and B lymphocyte activation, their genetic restrictions and the role of major histocompatibility complex products in lymphocyte triggering. He also discusses both the genetic and regulatory events responsible for controlling the immune response. Howard Grey and co-workers present enlightening data on the structure and function of membrane immunoglobulins of the B lymphocyte and compare their structure with those secreted into the body fluids. Norman Klinman's contribution deals with the activation of B cells through these immunoglobulin receptors. He describes the B cell repertoire, diversification, selection and generation followed by control of B cell expression. This theme is extended by William Weigle and co-workers, who treat the subject of specific cellular events in the activation of B lymphocytes through Fc receptors. These authors also cover cellular requirements in the induction, maintenance and termination of immunological tolerance in both T and B lymphocytes. The activation of specific helper T cells is addressed by DeFreitas and co-workers in terms of lymphocyte interactions. They take advantage of the T cell growth-enhancing factors to propagate clones of antigen-specific helper T cells. Such clones are used to define further the mechanisms of helper T cell activation and function. Characterization and development of specific cytotoxic lymphocyte clones are the subjects Jean-Charles Cerottini and co-workers explore. They define methods used in the generation and propagation of such clones and discuss T cell factors (lymphokines) as influences in the cloning of cytotoxic T lymphocytes. They have determined the frequency of such clones specific for antigens of the H-2 complex. Rolf Zinkernagel is working with immunoregulatory genes in respect to these cytotoxic T cells, and his paper is devoted to the major histocompatibility gene complex's part in T cell restriction during cytotoxic attact on viral-infected cells. Data on the participation of Fc receptors in modulation of lymphocytes and their activation constitute Hans Spiegelberg's presentation. He reports on the expression of Fc receptors specific for particular immunoglobulin classes and subclasses on lymphocytes and monocytes and the possible consequences of receptor/immuno-globulin interaction. Special emphasis is placed on the inter-action between IgE and its Fc_ϵ receptor in the context of such receptors' function in allergic disorders.

The activation of the complement pathways by the immune system is one of the main events leading to both inflammatory responses and host defense mechanisms. Hans Müller-Eberhard addresses this point in his discussion of the function and structure of the C3 component of complement. The structure of the active site of C3 is treated in relation to its activation and subsequent formation of biologically active factors.

The second portion of this book contains research results on the cellular, molecular and genetic events involved in auto-immunity and tissue injury resulting from in vivo interactions between antibody and either endogenous or exogenous anti-gens. In many instances, biochemical mediators resulting from interactions between antibody and antigen in vivo subsequently provoke tissue damage. Several of the contributions in this section concern the pathogenesis of inflammatory lesions. Charles Cochrane discusses a mechanism of inflammatory injury in which lipopolysaccharide of gram-negative bacteria is the activator of biochemical events that generate a sequence of injurious mediators. Thomas Edgington describes the triggering of T cells that results in induction of a cell membrane-associated procoagulant monokine. After defining the pathway of this reaction, he suggests its role in the pathogenesis of inflamma-tory lesions.

These two papers set the stage for discussion of specific disease models that are, in part, manifested by immunologic tissue damage and inflammatory lesions. One model is murine systemic lupus erythematosus, which Frank Dixon explains in terms of several murine strains that are genetically prone to this antoimmune disease. He theorizes that the hyperreactivity of their B lymphocytes is a major component of their autoimmune syndrome. After indicating the roles of intrinsic and extrinsic accelerating factors, he considers the pathogenic consequences of circulating immune complexes and their deposition in the tissues of these mice. Along similar lines, Curtis Wilson describes various mechanisms involved in renal injury. In addition to immune complex-induced glomerulonephritis, nephritogenic reactions resulting from direct binding of antibodies to glomeru-lar capillary wall antigens are the focus of his attention. Peter Ward and Kent Johnson also report on mechanisms of inflam-matory lesions, but in another target organ, the lung. In an experimental model of interstitial inflammatory disease of the lung, they have quantitated immune complexes, defined their nature and specified their sites of deposition.

Two papers are devoted to the subject of immunopathology associated with microbial infection; lymphocytic chorio-meningitis and measles viruses and protozoa are the experimental models. In Michael Oldstone's presentation of the immunopathology of tissue injury resulting from viral infections, he emphasizes the mechanisms of viral persistence, the manner in which viruses can elude an immune attack, the structural organization of viral polypeptides on the surfaces of infected cells and these molecules' relationship to the major histocompatibility complex. Paul Lambert and L. M. Rose then offer additional insight into the immunopathology of protozoan infections. They discuss the role of host responses in the pathological expression of these infections and give particular attention to tissue damage resulting from immune complexes formed between the parasite and specific antibody. That is, after parasitic infection effects an immune response, the parasite, in turn, determines the outcome of the immune response on infection. Their insight into the polyclonal activation of B cells and subsequent perturbation of the idiotypic network is particularly interesting.

The basic elements of immune responses to both artificial antigens and infectious agents are also applicable to tumor antigens. The biological significance of human myeloma-associated antigens is the topic contributed by A. C. Morgan and Ralph Reisfeld, who used specific antisera for the immunologic definition and characterization of these tumor-associated antigens. These investigators suggest that changes in the expression of these antigens or their glycosylation may be associated with transformational events. Joseph Feldman and Eduardo Fernandez-Cruz then present data on immunotherapy for virally and chemically induced transplantable syngeneic carcinomas. Their area of interest is the role of T cells generated in vitro by such tumors and the ability of rats transplanted with these sensitized T cells to reject established syngeneic carcinomas.

William O. Weigle, Ph.D.

Immunobiology: Basic Cellular and Biological Problems

Cellular and Molecular Interactions Regulating Immune Responses

David H. Katz, M.D.

The immune system is one of the most intricate of all the bodily systems, paralleling in many respects the endocrine system, in terms of the multiplicity of functions required of it for maintaining both homeostasis and the integrity of each individual's health. Both systems exert control over discrete functions at great distances within the body by virtue of circulating components capable of performing their roles at sites quite remote from their point of origin. In that sense, they display a level of versatility not found in most other multicellular organ systems. Accordingly, the complexity of the immune system has evolved from an intriguing communications network established between the components of the system, designed in such a manner as to permit a multiplicity of effects to arise from relatively few distinct cell types. This has been accomplished by the development of sophisticated regulatory mechanisms allowing either enormous amplification or contraction of a given response, depending upon the individual's needs. Under normal circumstances, the system functions remarkably well to maintain effective defenses against foreign agents or abnormal native cells which may have undergone neoplastic transformation. These events, of course, occur either as a

David H. Katz, M.D., Member, Department of Molecular Immunology, Scripps Clinic and Research Foundation, La Jolla, Calif.

This is publication #209 from the Department of Cellular and Developmental Immunology and publication #2308 from the Department of Immunology, Scripps Clinic and Research Foundation. The author's work was supported by NIH grants AI 13781 and AI 13874.

3

consequence of normal random mutational events or secondary to outside oncogenic influences.

Many other circumstances exist, however, in which abnormalities in one or more components of the immune system result in some form of breakdown in the network. This is manifested clinically in various ways and levels of severity. In this presentation I shall give an overview of the immune system, with particular emphasis upon the regulatory mechanisms involved in the responses developed by the system and the genetic control of such regulatory mechanisms. One of the remarkable features of the immune system is that its cellular and molecular components are so enormously complex that evolution has built into the system an incredible degree of flexibility. Rarely has the system created a single pathway to an end with no alternative avenue to take when a biological detour becomes advantageous.

The intricacies of the immune system stem from the remarkable communications network established between the main components of the system. These components are essentially the genes, molecules and cells that make it up. The interplay between them is reciprocal and circumscribed, thus laying the foundations of the regulatory mechanism controlling the system. A similar reciprocal and circumscribed relationship exists between the major cellular components of the system.

The major cellular components of the immune system are the macrophages and the lymphocytes. These cells also interact in a reciprocal and circumscribed manner. Macrophages are themselves extremely versatile in the functions they perform in a variety of immune responses, and although they themselves are not specific for any given antigen, they perform a very crucial role in concentrating and presenting antigens to lymphocytes. In particular, they appear to determine whether and which T lymphocytes will be induced to stimulation and function by various antigens. Moreover, macrophages secrete several very important, biologically active mediators capable of regulating the type and magnitude of lymphocyte responses by either enhancing or suppressing cell division or differentiation. All of this, of course, is in addition to their functional capabilities as the major phagocytic cells of the reticular endothelial system, clearing the system of debris, including molecular aggregates, foreign bacteria and dead cells.

The lymphocytes represent, of course, the specific cellular components of the system, specificity being conferred upon such cells by virtue of the existence on their surface of antigen-specific receptors. The nature of the receptor specificity is highly specialized in that each different clone of lymphocytes expresses its own unique specificity. The origin of such specialization has been very actively investigated for many years, and recent advances in molecular biology point to very interesting and sophisticated genetic mechanisms that lead to antigenic diversity.

The nature of the antigen receptors on the two major classes appears to differ in that the B cell clearly has surface immunoglobulin as its major receptor, whereas the nature of the receptor on the T cell is not yet totally defined, although there is reasonable evidence in recent years that they may use the same variable region genes for encoding the antigen-combining site. There are obviously a large number of genes and molecules that are important in the immune system. Here, I shall only highlight selected ones of major significance.

Immunoglobulin Genes and Molecules

The immunoglobulin gene system is genetically unique in that it is the only one known to involve participation of at least two discrete structural genes in the production of a single polypeptide chain. Thus, there is a structural gene for the variable, or V, region, which is that region containing the specific antigen-combining site; and this gene integrates with another structural gene for the constant, or C, region of the molecule, which is that region that determines the biological function of the molecule, such as the capacity of IgE to bind to mast cells. This results in a single polypeptide chain comprised of V and C regions — each intact immunoglobulin molecule consisting of four chains, two identical light, or L, chains and two identical heavy, or H, chains. Thus, there are VL and VH as well as CL and CH genes. Putting these together in proper fashion to make a functional immunoglobulin molecule in itself is a very complex affair.

Each immunoglobulin molecule has a unique antigen-combining site determined by the primary structure of the VL and VH genes comprising the molecule. The combining site possesses unique antigenic structures known as idiotypes. Recently, it has become increasingly clear that an individual can develop anti-idiotypic responses against his or her own unique combining sites on immunoglobulin molecules, and that these anti-idiotypic responses appear to perform in certain instances an important regulatory function in determining the magnitude and duration of antibody production to a given antigen.

As stated earlier, the conventional immunoglobulin molecules serve as antigen-specific receptors on the surface of B cells, in addition to performing their biological role as the secretory products of plasma cells which have differentiated from precursor B cells. With the exception of IgD, which appears to serve mainly as a cell-bound receptor, all of the classes of immunoglobulin ultimately circulate in the serum and, hence, operate at great distances from their points of origin. This in itself is an enormously efficient amplification process, particularly when one considers that a given cell can produce hundreds of thousands of immunoglobulin molecules.

Another gene family, as well as the molecules derived from it, that plays a very crucial role in the immune system is that concerned with the histocompatibility complex. In man and in mouse, where this system has been most thoroughly studied, the major histocompatibility gene complexes (MHC) are known as *HLA* and *H-2*, respectively. Both *HLA* and *H-2* have been shown to consist of several distinct regions, the genes of which are responsible for distinct functions. The *H-2* complex, which is located in a small segment of chromosome 17 of the mouse, consists of nine regions and subregions, the biological functions of which are summarized below.

The *I* region genes and molecules thus far have been shown to be the most versatile in terms of their functional relationships to immune responses. Contained within one or more of the five subregions of the *I* region, for example, are cell interaction, or *CI* genes that regulate interaction between macrophages, T cells and B cells; immune response, or *Ir*, genes that determine an individual's capacity to respond or not respond to various antigens, including different viruses and, hence, the susceptibility of an individual to certain diseases; genes encoding Ia antigens, which serve as the major antigens responsible for mixed lymphocyte reactions and graft-vs.-host reactions. There are genes involved in the synthesis of certain biologically active mediators that are produced by and active on T cells, B cells and macrophages. Finally, there are genes determining disease susceptibility, such as to allergic and autoimmune diseases, and resistance to certain viruses. It is not yet established whether distinct genes are responsible for the various functions just discussed, or whether such functions are controlled by relatively few genes.

Similar functional distinctions, such as those that have been shown in the mouse *H-2* complex, have also been assigned to different regions and subregions of the *HLA* gene complex in man. Other regions of the MHC which are immunologically important consist of the *H-2K* and the *H-2D* distal regions on either end of the complex, which contain the genes reponsible for the major transplantation antigens present on essentially all cells, and these are readily detectable with appropriate antibodies. The *K* and *D* genes are also the major antigens against which cytotoxic T lymphocytes are directed in graft rejection responses following tissue transplantation. Furthermore, it has been shown that the products of the *K* and the *D* genes interact with cytopathogenic viruses in a manner yet to be precisely determined, but which allows the most efficient recognition by cytotoxic T cells capable of eliminating virus-infected target cells from the individual.

Differentiation Antigens or Genes

Now let us discuss selective examples of differentiation antigens or genes in the molecules of differentiation stages which are prominently associated with distinct immunologic functions. The Ly antigens represent a family of cell surface antigenic determinants which are differentially expressed on T lymphocytes (known as Lyt) and on B lymphocytes (known as Lyb). The Lyt antigens are differentially expressed on distinct functional subpopulations of T lymphocytes. An analogous situation appears also to be true for the Lyb antigens on B cells. Fc receptors have been shown to exist on both classes of lymphocytes as well as macrophages and, of course, are detected by their ability to bind specifically to the Fc regions of either aggregated or antigen-complexed immunoglobulin molecules. Certain Fc receptors appear to be specific for IgG molecules — these are known as FcR_γ — whereas others are specific for Fc determinants on IgM — known as FcR_μ; IgE — known as FcR_ϵ; and, most recently, for IgA. Essentially, every heavy-chain class of circulating immunoglobulin has a corresponding Fc receptor displayed on lymphocytes as well as macrophages. Finally, receptor molecules capable of binding certain of the complement components, notably C3b and C3d, exist on certain populations of B and T lymphocytes, although the precise functional significance of these complement receptors is still not totally clear. What is important about the various molecules summarized here is that their appearance correlates in time with ontogenic development of the various lymphocyte classes and macrophages on which they appear; hence their designation as differentiation molecules.

Genetic Control of Immune Responses

I would like to turn now to a consideration of the control of immune responsiveness that is exerted by genes of the major histocompatibility complex. As stated earlier, the most important genes in this regard appear to reside in one or more regions of the *I* region of the *H-2* complex. There are cell interaction, or *CI*, genes which function to control the most effective cell-cell interactions in the immune system. It has been demonstrated that the interactions between macrophages and T cells and between T cells and B cells, and most recently, between macrophages and B cells, involve cell surface molecules called cell interaction molecules, the synthesis of which is controlled by the *CI* genes located in the *I* region of the *H-2* complex of the mouse or the *D* region of the *HLA* complex of man. As their name implies, these genes control the most effective macrophage-lymphocyte interactions and the most effective T-T or T-B lymphocyte interactions. In addition, cell interaction genes control the synthesis of several different biologically active molecules that are derived from lymphocytes and macrophages and which are capable in some instances of enhancing and in other instances of suppressing immune response. Some of these molecules show specificity for antigen, whereas others are nonspecific in their biological function. It is not yet known whether the genes that are responsible for encoding these biologically active molecules and the cell interaction genes controlling the most effective cell-cell interactions are identical or distinct. Finally, there are cell inter-action genes located in the *K* and *D* regions of the *H-2* complex which control the most effective lysis of virus-infected and neoplastic target cells by killer T lymphocytes.

Another area of genetically controlled immune responsive-ness concerns the function of specific immune response, or *Ir*, and immune suppression, or *Is*, genes. Indeed, the discovery of *Ir* genes represented the very first association between the major histocompatibility complex and regulation of immune respon-siveness. *Ir* genes have been found in essentially all species, including man, and appear to determine the ability of an individual to respond to a given antigenic determinant. They are inherited in a simple mendelian fashion as autosomal dominant traits. In certain select cases, it has recently been shown that two genes are responsible for permitting responses to develop to a given antigen. In these cases, absence of either one of the genes or both genes results in an inability of the individual to respond to the antigen in question. It has also been discovered that genes present in the *I* region also govern the development of specific suppressor T cells. These immune suppression, or *Is*, genes control specific stimulation of such suppressor T cells. Although considerable work has been conducted in these areas, it is still true that we do not yet know either the precise mechanism or the structural nature of *Ir* and *Is* genes. Moreover, further investigation is still needed to determine whether these genes are distinct from, or identical to, the cell interaction genes.

Now I would like to briefly discuss the various functional subpopulations of lymphocytes so I can more easily discuss the regulatory interactions between them. The two classes of T and B cells have very distinct functional capabilities. T lymphocytes do not themselves produce circulating antibodies, nor do they give rise to antibody-secreting cells. They can be subdivided into two major functional categories. Actually, they can be sub-divided into many more than that, if one has a tendency to be more complex, but I think this is the simplest and most easily digested way to do it. The first category I like to call regulatory T lymphocytes. Those are the cells that function to either facilitate, in which case they are helper cells, or suppress, naturally known as suppressor cells, the responses of other T lymphocytes or of B lymphocytes. These functions are mediated by distinct subpopulations of T cells, as evidenced by the fact that helper T cells are generally of the Lyt 1 phenotype, whereas suppressor T cells generally express the Lyt 2,3 phenotype. Effector T lymphocytes, the second broad category, are those cells that are responsible for cell-mediated immune reactions, such as delayed-type hypersensitivity responses, rejection of foreign tissue grafts and tumors, and elimination of virus-infected target cells. The last two responses, namely graft and tumor rejection and elimination of virus-infected target cells, involve the participation of cytotoxic T lymphocytes (CTL), commonly referred to as "killer" cells. Also involved in responses to foreign tissues are T cells which undergo rapid proliferation in mixed lymphocyte reactions (MLR). These cells can be distinguished from one another also by their Lyt phenotype. The MLR and the delayed-type hypersensitivity T cells are of the Lyt 1 phenotype; and CTL are of the Lyt 2,3 phenotype.

Categorization of functional subpopulations of B lymphocytes is quite easily done on the basis of the different immunoglobulin classes they synthesize. B lymphocytes give rise to cells synthesizing and secreting all of the classes of circulating immunoglobulin, namely IgM, IgG, IgA and IgE. The respective B cell precursors for these antibody-forming cells are B_μ, B_γ, B_α and B_ϵ. Memory B cells are functionally important, of course, for the development of very rapid secondary or anamnestic antibody responses upon subsequent antigenic exposure. These cells can be distinguished from primary or unprimed B cells by several features, including their tissue distribution, their size, their migratory properties and certain surface antigen differences. There is no hard evidence for the existence of regulatory B lymphocytes analogous in function to regulatory T cells, although the discovery of such cells in the near future would not be surprising.

Regulatory Interactions in Immune Responses

Basically, when one considers regulation in the immune system, as elsewhere, one is really dealing with processes of communication, the way cells are able to talk to one another and to listen to one another. This, of course, takes place via the molecules, specific molecules designated for this purpose, that these cells display. One of the major breakthroughs, in fact, in our understanding of the immune system in the last 15 years has been the discovery of this intricate network of regulatory interactions, stemming largely from the work done in the mid-1960s which was initiated in Denver by Henry Claman and his colleagues and which pointed out the requirement for T-B cell interactions for the successful development of antibody responses. Our perspective in this regard has been greatly enlarged so that today we can view such regulatory interactions as reflecting a dynamic interplay between all of the various genes, molecules and cells of the immune system. The genes and molecules provide, first, the specific antigen receptors on lymphocyte surface membranes, the circulating antibodies which perform effector functions and exert feedback regulation, crucial regulatory effects on various cell-cell interactions necessary for normal immunological homeostasis, and, finally, the biologically active molecules which are capable of enhancing or suppressing T cell and B cell functions.

It is now very clear that the cells of the system are interdependent upon one another so that the development of either a cell-mediated immune response, such as the delayed-type hypersensitivity or "killer" cell reactions, or humoral (antibody production) immunity is regulated by a program of essential interactions between T cells, macrophages and B cells. The net effects of these regulatory interactions between the genes, molecules and cells of the immune system span an entire spectrum, ranging from enhancement at one end to suppression at the other end. The qualitative and quantitative response that occurs at any given time reflects the net effect of this extremely dynamic interplay among these components.

Figure 1 summarizes current knowledge of regulatory cell-cell interactions necessary for the development of a normal antibody response. The example here represents the induction of an antibody response in the IgE class but is equally applicable to antibody responses from all other immunoglobulin classes. The antigen here is a classical hapten-carrier conjugate in which the antigen is picked up by the macrophage and presented to the T cell, the precursor of the helper T cell, and is able to stimulate that cell by virtue of its specific antigen receptor recognizing the carrier and a second interaction involving the cell interaction molecules which the T cell can

THE IgE ANTIBODY-PRODUCING APPARATUS

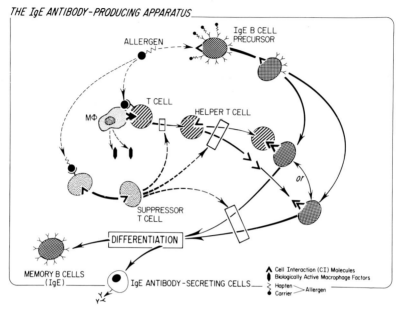

FIG. 1. Summary of the T lymphocyte regulatory influences in the immune system. (Reprinted, with permission, from Fudenberg, H.H. et al (eds.): Basic and Clinical Immunology, ed. 3, ©1980 Lange Medical Publications, Los Altos, Calif.)

recognize specifically on the surface of the macrophage membrane. This, together with perhaps the participation of biologically active molecules secreted by the macrophage, induces this precursor cell into a functional helper T cell now poised and able to effectively transmit the necessary signals to whatever partner cell is in need of them. In this case, it is a B cell which has surface immunoglobulin on its membrane. This B cell picks up antigen as well by virtue of its immunoglobulin receptor specific for the hapten in question. Following a series of events, part of which involves capping, endocytosis of the immunoglobulin receptor and the antigen attached to it, this B cell now becomes a poised partner cell to receive signals that will be transmitted by the helper T cell. Although the precise mechanism by which this interaction takes place is still ill-defined, it is clear that the T cell and the B cell must recognize one another through the specific cell interaction molecules that are also displayed on the cell surface. In any case, this occurs, I believe, by membrane-membrane contact, perhaps together with released soluble cell interaction molecules that can react directly with the B cell in close proximity. The consequence of this communication is the drive of this B cell to differentiate into its final, fully mature, secretory plasma cell progeny or along a pathway as a memory B cell which will be poised and ready to receive antigenic signals at a subsequent time in a qualitatively more rapid and quantitatively larger fashion than its native virginal ancestor.

Into this equation of the positive arm of the response comes the suppressor T cell. The suppressor T cell, of course, does the opposite of the helper T cell. It down-regulates the response. This cell, activated by antigen, in which case it would be an antigen-specific suppressor T cell, is able to do that in one of at least three ways. It is able to interfere with the differentiation of the precursor helper T cell into its functional, mature descendant. It is able to interfere even later by blocking the ability of the helper T cell to provide signals for the partner B cell. Lastly, some suppressor T cells are able to be called into the response and down-regulated by preventing the final differentiation steps of the B cell even after it has received all of its necessary differentiation-triggering signals. So the net consequence of this type of interaction is a very effective positive pathway to follow when the response calls for it and a very nice negative feedback pathway when it is unnecessary to have the response continue.

Figure 2 summarizes what is currently known about the T lymphocyte regulatory influences on the immune system. On the far left is depicted the helper T cell which has the surface phenotype Lyt 1. This T cell is genetically restricted in its functional activity by cell interaction genes located in the *I-A* region of the *H-2* complex or the *HLA-D* region of the *HLA* complex in man. These cells are capable of exerting positive regulatory effects on B cells, as depicted by the upper portion of this figure, stimulating their differentiation into fully mature, antibody-secreting plasma cells. As shown in the lower portion of the figure, this same cell, the helper T cell, is similarly able to exert positive regulatory influences on precursors of T cells that are ultimately destined to become cytotoxic T lymphocytes (CTL).

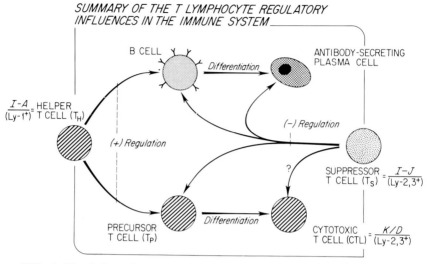

SUMMARY OF THE T LYMPHOCYTE REGULATORY
INFLUENCES IN THE IMMUNE SYSTEM

FIG. 2. The IgE antibody-producing apparatus. (Reprinted, with permission, from Fudenberg, H.H. et al (eds.): Basic and Clinical Immunology, ed. 3, ©1980 Lange Medical Publications, Los Altos, Calif.)

CTLs have the surface phenotype Lyt 2,3 and are genetically restricted in their cytolytic function by cell interaction genes located in the *K* or *D* regions of the *H-2* complex. Shown on the far right in Figure 2 is the suppressor T cell; again, as a reminder, the suppressor T cell has the surface phenotype Lyt 2,3, and these cells in general are genetically restricted by cell interaction genes that are located in the *I-J*, as opposed to *I-A*, region of *H-2*. As shown, suppressor T cells can exert their negative regulatory effects on differentiation events of B lymphocytes or precursors of cytotoxic T cells, either by acting directly on such cells or by interfering with the positive activity of helper T cells that would normally facilitate differentiation of their appropriate partners.

Figure 3 illustrates how all of these interactions at the genetic, molecular and cellular level actually operate in control of a given immune response system, in this case the IgE antibody system. One can break down the participants in this system into the immunologic components and the nonimmunologic components. In terms of the response that is going to generate IgE antibody production, genes involved in the control of this response are related to the histocompatibility system.

COMPONENTS OF THE ALLERGIC RESPONSE

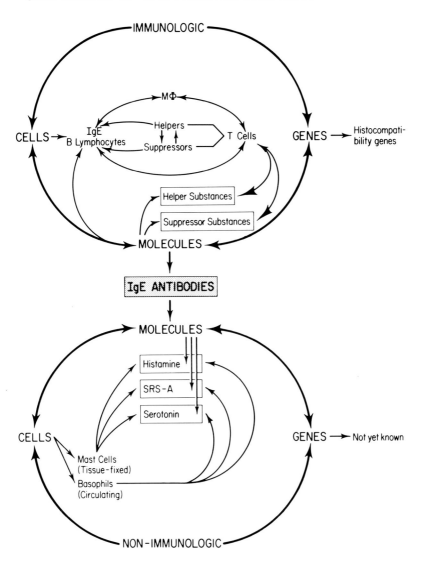

FIGURE 3.

The cells will be the IgE precursor B lymphocytes; macrophages, which of course will trigger helper T cells; and the helper T cells, which are able to stimulate the IgE precursor cell into an IgE-secreting plasma cell. There are also suppressor cells that down-regulate this positive arm; but once the IgE-B cells are stimulated, perhaps with the participation of helper substances, they secrete the relevant molecules, the IgE antibodies, which now leave the immunologic component of the system and exert their effector function at the level of the nonimmunologic component. These will be the cells that bind the IgE molecules specifically on their cell surfaces — mast cells, for example, which are tissue-fixed, or circulating basophils, which, upon appropriate cross-linking, will lead to the release of a number of pharmacologically active mediators, which can in turn exert the vasomotor effects that lead to both the defense mechanism and sometimes the unwanted and unpleasant deleterious side effects of IgE.

In summary, I hope I have provided a glimpse of what is a beautifully complex and sophisticated system which generates a very effective defense mechanism through the use of the dynamic interplay between the basic components of the system — the genes, molecules and cells — by means of specific recognition processes in which cells talk to each other, molecules talk to cells and, of course, genes control all of this as the very basic element.

Structure and Function of Membrane Immunoglobulins

Howard M. Grey, M.D., Robert W. Chesnut, Ph.D.
and Ralph T. Kubo, Ph.D.

The existence of immunoglobulin on the surface of B lymphocytes has been known for about 15 years. However, many aspects of its structure, its synthesis and its function have yet to be elucidated. This paper presents a progress report from our laboratory on these subjects.

Structure of Membrane Immunoglobulin

The major issue that has been addressed by ourselves and others interested in the structure of membrane immunoglobulin is whether there are differences between membrane and serum immunoglobulin that can account for the localization of B cell surface immunoglobulin in the plasma membrane. Prior to, and during the course of our studies there have been a few reports suggesting physicochemical differences between membrane and serum IgM. Differences in mobility of μ-chains on SDS gels [1] and differences in detergent-binding characteristics [2-4] have been reported. We decided to investigate the carboxy-terminal end of membrane immunoglobulin heavy chain in search of differences in primary structure. Such an investigation was prompted by antigenic studies on membrane Ig [5] and structural studies on other membrane proteins [6, 7] which

Howard M. Grey, M.D., Robert W. Chesnut, Ph.D. and Ralph T. Kubo, Ph.D., Division of Basic Immunology, Department of Medicine, National Jewish Hospital and Research Center/National Asthma Center; and University of Colorado Health Sciences Center, Denver.

This work was supported in part by USPHS grants AI-09758 and CA-21825.

suggested that the carboxy-terminal portions of these molecules were most likely involved in their anchorage to the plasma membrane. For this purpose the IgM synthesized by the human B cell line, Daudi, was studied. Previous investigations on this cell line have shown that it has a relatively large amount of membrane IgM but lacks the capacity to secrete IgM [8].

The strategy employed to obtain a comparative analysis of the C-terminus of Daudi μ-chains with that of secreted IgM was (1) to analyze the release of amino acids after carboxypeptidase A (CPA) digestion of μ-chains that had been internally labeled with radioactive amino acids, and (2) to determine whether the C-terminal octapeptide generated after CNBr cleavage of serum μ-chains could be identified after CNBr cleavage of Daudi μ-chains.

The μ-chains from Daudi and a secreted human IgM, Ram, that had been labeled with different amino acids were eluted from SDS gels and digested with CPA for varying periods of time. The radioactivity associated with a given residue was calculated from the counts of a particular amino acid and the number of residues of that amino acid present in μ-chain [9]. The release of amino acids by CPA was determined by analyzing the supernatant radioactivity recovered, after ethanol precipitation to stop CPA digestion, on an amino acid analyzer. The quantity of an amino acid released by CPA was calculated from the radioactivity eluted at the position of the amino acid in question. When CPA digestion was performed on secreted Ram μ-chains biosynthetically labeled with ^{3}H-Tyr, 0.95 to 1.05 residues of Tyr were released by the enzyme within 30 minutes. Since Tyr is the C-terminal residue of serum μ-chains, these results indicated the validity of the methodology used to analyze the carboxy-terminal residues of Daudi μ-chains. Sufficient incorporation into μ-chains of the following amino acids was obtained to allow for their analysis after CPA digestion: His, Trp, Ser, Thr, Ala, Val, Leu, Met, Ile, Phe, Tyr, Cys. The results obtained are shown in Table 1. After 60 minutes of digestion relatively high release of only three residues was observed: Val, Leu and Phe. Questionably significant release (0.14 to 0.22 residues) of Tyr, Ile and Thr was obtained, and essentially no release ($\leqslant 0.05$ residues) of the remaining six amino acids tested was observed.

Table 1. One-Hour Carboxypeptidase A Digestion of
Internally Labeled Daudi μ-Chains

Amino Acid	Residue Released	Amino Acid	Residue Released
^{3}H-Leu	0.55	^{35}S-Met	0.05
^{3}H-Val	0.53	^{3}H-Ser	0.05
^{3}H-Phe	0.44	^{35}S-Cys	0.02
^{3}H-Tyr	0.22	^{3}H-His	<0.01
^{3}H-Ile	0.21	^{3}H-Trp	<0.01
^{3}H-Thr	0.14	^{3}H-Ala	<0.01

(Reprinted from Williams et al [13], ©1978 Williams & Wilkins Co., Baltimore.)

Because of the importance of determining whether Tyr was C-terminal or not, the rates of release of Val and Tyr were compared. These data, shown in Figure 1, indicate that Val is released more rapidly and to a greater extent than Tyr when both residues are measured in the same digest, thereby indicating that Val is located closer to the C-terminus than Tyr. For comparative purposes, the kinetics of Tyr release from

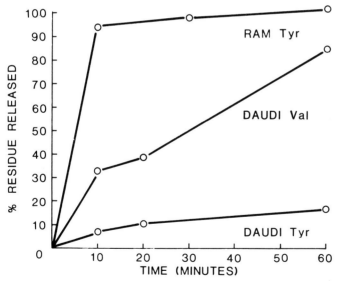

FIG. 1. Kinetics of release of amino acids following carboxypeptidase A digestion of internally labeled Daudi and Ram μ-chains. (Reprinted from Williams et al [13], © 1978 Williams & Wilkins Co., Baltimore.)

Ram-secreted μ-chains is also shown. Of equal significance to this finding of the release of Val, Phe and Leu from Daudi μ-chains is the lack of significant release of Cys since this residue is found in the penultimate position immediately adjacent to the C-terminal Tyr residue of secreted μ-chains (Fig. 2).

In order to evaluate the presence of the CNBr-generated C-terminal octapeptide in Daudi μ-chains, conditions for the isolation of the octapeptide were established by using unlabeled myeloma μ-chains as well as ^{35}S-Cys-labeled Ram-secreted μ-chains. It was found that a two-step procedure involving Sephadex G-50 gel filtration in 1 M formic acid followed by high-voltage electrophoresis at pH 1.6 was adequate to obtain purification of the octapeptide. Thus, octapeptides isolated from myeloma μ-chains, when subjected to amino acid analysis, yielded the expected amino acid composition. When a similar isolation procedure was applied to ^{35}S-Cys-labeled Ram μ-chains, a radioactive peak was obtained in essentially identical positions after Sephadex G-50 gel filtration and high-voltage electrophoresis (Table 2). However, when these same procedures were used to analyze the CNBr-treated Daudi μ-chains, quite different results were obtained. First, the low-molecular weight peptides eluted from the G-50 column were in a somewhat smaller elution volume than that expected for the C-terminal octapeptide (0.79 Rf vs. 0.85 Rf). Second, when these small ^{35}S-Cys-labeled peptides of Daudi were analyzed by high-voltage electrophoresis, no radioactivity was found in the region where the C-terminal octapeptide should be located. All of the radioactivity was recovered in and around the point of application of the sample. Similar results were obtained with the CNBr peptides from ^{3}H-Ser-labeled Daudi μ-chains.

Studies on the C-terminal structure of membrane IgM using other sources of cells have been performed in other laboratories.

(Met)-Ser-Asp-Thr-Ala-Gly-Thr-Cys-Tyr-COOH

FIG. 2. Amino acid sequence of the carboxy-terminal octapeptide generated by cyanogen bromide cleavage of serum μ-chains. (Reprinted from Williams et al [13], © 1978 Williams & Wilkins Co., Baltimore.)

Table 2. Analysis of Low-Molecular Weight μ-Chain
Cyanogen Bromide Peptides

	Rf G-50*	Rf HVE†
Myeloma peptides	0.85	0.30
35S-Cys-Ram peptides	0.84	0.31
3H-Ser-Daudi peptides	0.79	<0.05‡
35S-Cys-Daudi peptides	0.79	<0.05

*Sephadex G-50 fine (100 × 1.5 cm) equilibrated in 1 M formic acid. Rf calculated from the formula: Vx − Vo/Vt − Vo.

†Relative to methyl green marker.

‡No radioactivity fround at an Rf of 0.3; <0.05 indicates that all radioactivity remained at the origin.

(Reprinted from Williams et al [13], ©1978 Williams & Wilkins Co., Baltimore.)

Although results conflicting with those presented above were initially reported [10-12], it is generally agreed at present that our results [13] with Daudi μ-chains are representative of membrane μ-chains, whereas the conflicting data were obtained in stituations where contamination with secreted IgM might have been a contributing factor.

Recently, the conclusion that membrane and secreted μ-chains have different C-termini was substantiated and markedly extended by analyses of the DNA and mRNA that code for membrane and secreted IgM. Two discrete mRNAs have been described: a 2.4-kb mRNA that codes for secreted μ-chains and a 2.7-kb mRNA that codes for membrane μ-chains [14, 15]. This finding eliminated the possibility that there was a precursor-product relationship between membrane and secreted μ-chains. Nucleotide sequence analysis of cDNA and germ line DNA [15, 16] indicated that:

1. Membrane μ-chains are identical with secreted μ-chains up to the final 20 residues, at which point their sequences differ markedly. Furthermore, membrane μ-chains contain an extension of an additional 21 residues beyond residue 572, the C-terminus of secreted μ-chains.

2. The resultant C-terminal amino acid sequence of membrane μ-chains predicted from the nucleotide sequence is fully compatible with the results obtained with Daudi μ-chains, i.e. the presence of valine, phenylalanine and

leucine near the C-terminus; the absence of tyrosine; and the absence of a cyanogen bromide-generated C-terminal octapeptide.

3. The predicted sequence is similar to certain other integral membrane proteins such as glycophorin, having highly charged hydrophilic regions flanking a trans-membrane stretch of about 25 residues which is very hydrophobic.

4. The DNA segment that codes for the secreted C-terminal 20 residues is separated from the coding sequences for the membrane μ C-terminus by an intron of 1.8 kb. This finding has suggested two mechanisms by which the synthesis of membrane and secreted μ-chains is regulated:

   (a) An RNA-splicing event which would splice out the RNA segment that codes for the secreted C-terminus and bring the membrane coding segment in contiguity with the mRNA coding for the remainder of the μ-chain.

   (b) Regulation dictated by whether poly(A) addition occurs prior to or following transcription of the membrane encoding segment or not.

Although these transcriptional and RNA processing events will undoubtedly prove to be very important in regulating Ig expression, they may not be the only regulatory mechanisms. Recent studies from our laboratory suggest that there are instances in which posttranslational control of Ig expression is very important. For instance, we have shown that certain hybridomas that resemble pre-B cells phenotypically [17], synthesize large amounts of secreted-type μ-chains, but no secretion takes place. Similarly in the Daudi cell line, which also fails to secrete IgM, secreted-type IgM is made in an amount similar to that of membrane IgM, but this IgM appears to be rapidly catabolized rather than being transported out of the cells (Kubo and Grey, unpublished observations). The post-translational regulatory mechanisms responsible for these results are at present unknown but may involve the vesicle system, which transports secreted and membrane proteins to the cell surface [18].

Function of Membrane Immunoglobulin

Although somewhat controversial in the past, it is generally agreed that antigen binding to membrane immunoglobulin can result in the stimulation of B cells to proliferate and that in the case of T-dependent antigens, another signal provided by helper T cells is necessary to stimulate B cells to secrete antibody [19]. The studies to be described are concerned with testing the hypothesis that another function of membrane Ig is to focus large amounts of antigen onto antigen-specific B cells which can subsequently process and present antigen to antigen-specific T helper cells. The attractiveness of this hypothesis emanates from the body of evidence which indicates that antigen-specific T helper cells and B cells recognize the same antigen in quite different ways. Native and denatured forms of the same protein are highly cross-reactive antigens as recognized by helper and proliferating T cells, whereas they are completely non-cross-reactive at the B cell level [20-22]. Furthermore, while B cells can readily be shown to bind conventional soluble antigens [23], helper T cells cannot [24, 25]; however, following antigen processing by syngeneic Ia-positive macrophages, antigen-dependent binding of helper T cells to macrophages has been demonstrated [26, 27]. Data such as these have led to the postulation that B cells recognize intact, unprocessed antigen, whereas helper T cells recognize processed antigen presented in the context of macrophage Ia antigens. This postulate presents some difficulties for how T-B collaboration works, especially if antigen is important in bridging the two cell types as has been proposed in the hapten-carrier system first described by Mitchison [28]. The mechanism of T-B collaboration via antigen bridging proposed above involves the processing of antigen by antigen-specific B cells and subsequent presentation of the antigen, in the context of the B cell Ia, to antigen-specific helper T cells [29].

We have tested this hypothesis using a mouse T cell proliferation assay. Rabbit IgG was chosen as the antigen and the capacity of B cells to present this antigen to T cells was tested by determining the ability of rabbit anti-mouse Ig (RAMIG) (which can bind to all B cells via their membrane Ig) to stimulate T cell proliferation when B cells were used as accessory cells. The data indicate that B cells can indeed present antigen to T cells in this system.

Macrophages were extensively depleted from both the antigen-presenting B cell compartment (MDSC) and the responding T cell compartment by a combination of plastic, Sephadex G-10 and nylon wool adherence. Normal rabbit γ-globulin (NRGG), an antigen which would bind to only a very few antigen-specific B cells, and rabbit anti-mouse Ig (RAMIG), an antigen which could bind to all B cells via their membrane Ig, were compared for their capacity to stimulate a T cell proliferative response when B cells or macrophages were used as the source of antigen-presenting cells. The data from four representative experiments are shown in Table 3. When macrophages were pulsed with NRGG or RAMIG, nearly equivalent T cell proliferation was observed in response to either antigen. In contrast to this, when MDSC were pulsed with the same antigen preparations, RAMIG consistently stimulated a significant response but NRGG failed to elicit T cell proliferation.

The fact that NRGG failed to stimulate any proliferative response indicates that contaminating macrophages in the B cell population were not responsible for the capacity of this population to present antigen. This was further strengthened by

Table 3. Presentation of Rabbit Anti-Mouse Immunoglobulin to Rabbit IgG-Primed T Cells by Macrophages and Macrophage-Depleted Spleen Cells (MDSC)

Antigen-Presenting Cells	Antigen*	^3H-Thymidine Incorporation $(E - C, CPM \times 10^{-3})$† Experiment Number			
		1	*2*	*3*	*4*
Macrophage	NRGG	124	234	121	142
Macrophage	RAMIG	99	186	103	144
MDSC	NRGG	0	0	4	0.5
MDSC	RAMIG	169	68	148	32

*MDSC were pulsed with 1 mg RAMIG or NRGG/2×10^6 cells for one hour at 37°C; macrophages were pulsed with 250 μg/well of RAMIG or NRGG for four hours at 37°C.

† ^{3}H-Thymidine incorporation expressed as experimental (E) cpm minus unstimulated control (C) cpm.

(Reprinted from Chesnut and Grey [30], ©1981 William & Wilkins Co., Baltimore.)

experiments in which the proliferative capacity of ovalbumin-primed T cells was tested with antigen presented by the same type of B cell population. In no case have we observed an OVA-specific response when B cells were used as antigen-presenting cells.

If there were significant numbers of macrophages contaminating our T cell preparations, it could be possible that RAMIG-pulsed B cells served simply as passive carriers of the antigen to that population of macrophages. To evaluate this possibility, two types of experiments were performed. In the first, after the B cells were pulsed with RAMIG they were killed or inactivated by freeze-thawing or ultraviolet irradiation, prior to their addition to T cells. We reasoned that if contaminating macrophages present in the T cell population were taking up RAMIG-Ig immune complexes and thus were responsible for the T cell triggering, then inactivation of the B cells following antigen pulsing should have no effect on that stimulation. Figure 3 shows that both freeze-thaw lysis and UV irradiation of the RAMIG-pulsed B cells completely eliminated the T cell proliferative response.

The second type of experiment involved testing the importance of the genetic background of the antigen-presenting B cells. If B cells can process and present antigen in a manner analogous to macrophages, it would be anticipated that this capacity would show genetic restriction. If, on the other hand, B cells were acting as passive carriers of antigen to macrophages present in the T cell preparation, then the genotype of the B cell should not be a determining factor. To test for genetic restriction, NRGG-sensitized BDF_1 T cells were assayed for their capacity to respond to RAMIG-pulsed MDSC that were either syngeneic or allogeneic to the BDF_1 T cells. The results of one such experiment are shown in Table 4. RAMIG-pulsed BDF_1 MDSC induced an excellent proliferative response, whereas MDSC from two allogeneic strains, B10.S and B10.M, induced much weaker, albeit significant, responses. In this experiment the response induced by syngeneic MDSC was 10- to 30-fold greater than that induced by allogeneic MDSC.

In conclusion, these results suggest an additional and somewhat novel role for membrane Ig on B cells: to focus antigen onto B cells so that they can process and present antigen, in the context of B cell Ia, to antigen-specific T cells.

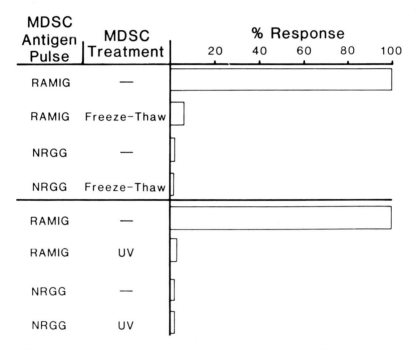

FIG. 3. T cell activation following freeze-thaw lysis or UV irradiation of antigen-pulsed MDSC. MDSC were pulsed with NRGG or RAMIG (1 mg/2 × 10^6 cells) and then freeze-thawed three times or exposed to UV light. The treated cell suspension was then added, as the source of antigen, to NRGG-primed T cells. (Reprinted from Chesnut and Grey [30], © 1981 Williams & Wilkins Co., Baltimore.)

Table 4. Genetic Restriction of the Response of BDF_1
T Cells to RAMIG-Pulsed MDSC

MDSC*	Antigen Pulse†	^3H-Thymidine Incorporation $(E - C, CPM \times 10^{-3})$‡
BDF$_1$	—	0
	RAMIG	112
	NRGG	0
B10.S	—	0
	RAMIG	10
	NRGG	0
B10.M	—	0
	RAMIG	4
	NRGG	0

*Cells were prepared from BDF$_1$ (H-$2^{b/d}$), B10.S (H-2^s) and B10.M (H-2^f) mice.

†MDSC were pulsed with 1 mg RAMIG (Fab$'_2$) or NRGG (Fab$'_2$)/2 × 10^6 cells for one hour at 37°C.

‡ ^3H-Thymidine incorporation expressed as experimental (E) cpm minus T cell control (C) cpm.

(Reprinted from Chesnut and Grey [3], © 1981 Williams and Wilkins Co., Baltimore.)

This provides a mechanism of antigen-specific, MHC-restricted cell-cell interaction in which T and B cells may interact with one another via an antigen bridge despite the fact that the two cells react with quite different forms of the same antigen.

Acknowledgments

The authors would like to thank Michele Pelanne and Patricia Cain for their excellent technical assistance and Edna Squillante for superb secretarial assistance.

References

1. Melcher, U. and Uhr, J.W.: Cell surface immunoglobulin. XVI. Polypeptide chain structure of mouse IgM and IgD-like molecule. J. Immunol. 116:409, 1976.
2. Melcher, U. and Uhr, J.W.: Density differences between membrane and secreted immunoglobulins of murine splenocytes. Biochemistry 16:145, 1977.

3. Vassalli, P., Tedghi, R., Lisowska-Bernstein, B. et al: Evidence for hydrophobic region within heavy chains of mouse B lymphocyte membrane-bound IgM. Proc. Natl. Acad. Sci. U.S.A. 76:5515, 1979.

4. Parkhouse, R.M.E., Lifter, J. and Choi, Y.S.: Chemical characterization of the Fab and Fc fragment from surface immunoglobulin. Nature 284:280, 1980.

5. Fu, S.M. and Kunkel, H.G.: Membrane immunoglobulins of B lymphocytes. Inability to detect certain characteristic IgM and IgG antigens. J. Exp. Med. 140:895, 1974.

6. Tomita, M. and Marchesi, V.T.: Amino-acid sequence and oligosaccharide attachment sites of human erythrocyte glycophorin. Proc. Natl. Acad. Sci. U.S.A. 72:2964, 1975.

7. Snell, D.T. and Offord, R.E.: The amino acid sequence of the B-protein of bacteriophage ZJ-2. Biochem. J. 127:167, 1972.

8. Klein, E., Klein, G., Nadkarni, J.S. et al: Surface IgM-kappa specificity on a Burkitt lymphoma cell in vivo and in derived culture lines. Cancer Res. 28:1300, 1968.

9. Putnam, F.W., Florent, G., Paul, C. et al: Complete amino acid sequence of the mu heavy chain of a human IgM immunoglobulin. Science 182:287, 1973.

10. McIlhinney, R.A.J., Richardson, N.E. and Feinstein, A.: Evidence for a C-terminal tyrosine residue in human and mouse B-lymphocyte membrane μ-chains. Nature 272:555, 1978.

11. Bergman, Y. and Haimovich, J.: B lymphocytes contain three species of μ-chains. Eur. J. Immunol. 8:876, 1978.

12. Vassalli, P., Jaton, J.C. and Tartakoff, A.: Comparison of the biosynthesis and structure of secreted and membrane mouse polyclonal IgM molcules. In Cooper, M., Mosier, D.E., Sher, I. and Vitetta, E. (eds.): B Lymphocytes in the Immune Response. New York: Elsevier/North-Holland, 1979, vol. 3, p. 3.

13. Williams, P.B., Kubo, R.T. and Grey, H.M.: μ-Chains from a nonsecretor B cell line differ from secreted μ-chains at the C-terminal end. J. Immunol. 121:2435, 1978.

14. Alt, F.W., Bothwell, A.L.M., Knapp, M. et al: Synthesis of secreted and membrane-bound immunoglobulin μ heavy chains is directed by mRNAs that differ at their 3' ends. Cell 20:293, 1980.

15. Rogers, J., Early, P., Carter, C. et al: Two mRNAs with different 3' ends encode membrane bound and secreted forms of immunoglobulin mu chain. Cell 20:303, 1980.

16. Early, P., Rogers, J., Davis, M. et al: Two mRNAs can be produced from a single immunoglobulin μ gene by alternative RNA processing pathways. Cell 20:313, 1980.

17. Kloppel, T.M., Kubo, R.T., Cain, P.S. et al: Structural analysis of the μ chains synthesized by fetal liver hybridomas. J. Immunol. (In press.)

18. Rothman, J.E. and Fine, R.E.: Coated vesicle transports newly synthesized membrane glycoproteins from endoplasmic reticulum to plasma membrane in two successive stages. Proc. Natl. Acad. Sci. U.S.A. 77:780, 1980.

19. Parker, D.C.: Induction and suppression of polyclonal antibody responses by anti-Ig reagents and antigen-nonspecific helper factors. Immunol. Rev. 52:115, 1980.
20. Chesnut, R.W., Endres R.O. and Grey, H.M.: Antigen recognition by T cells and B cells: Recognition of cross-reactivity between native and denatured forms of globular antigens. Clin. Immunol. Immunopathol. 15:397, 1980.
21. Schirrmacher, V. and Wigzell, H.: Immune responses against native and chemically modified albumins in mice. I. Analysis of non-thymus-processed (B) and thymus-processed (T) cell responses against methylated bovine serum albumin. J. Exp. Med. 136:1616, 1972.
22. Ishizaka, K., Okudaira, H. and King, T.P.: Immunogenic properties of modified antigen E. II. Ability of urea-denatured antigen and α-polypeptide chain to prime T cells specific for antigen E. J. Immunol. 114:110, 1975.
23. Wigzell, H., Sundqvist, K.G. and Yoshida, T.O.: Separation of cells according to surface antigens by the use of antibody-coated columns. Fractionation of cells carrying immunoglobulins and blood group antigen. Scand. J. Immunol. 1:75, 1972.
24. Basten, A., Miller, J.F.A.P. and Abraham, R.: Relationship between Fc receptors, antigen-binding sites on T and B cells, and H-2 complex-associated determinants. J. Exp. Med. 141:547, 1975.
25. Lamelin, J.P., Lisowska-Bernstein, B., Matter, A. et al: Mouse thymus-independent and thymus-derived lymphoid cells. J. Exp. Med. 136:984, 1972.
26. Lipsky, P.E. and Rosenthal, A.S.: Macrophage-lymphocyte interaction. II. Antigen-mediated physical interactions between immune guinea pig lymph node lymphocytes and syngeneic macrophages. J. Exp. Med. 141:138, 1975.
27. Swierkosz, J.E., Rock, K., Marrack, P. and Kappler, J.W.: The role of H-2-linked genes in helper T-cell function. II. Isolation on antigen-pulsed macrophages of two separate populations of F1 helper T cells each specific for antigen and one set of parental H-2 products. J. Exp. Med. 147:554, 1978.
28. Mitchison, N.A.: The carrier effect in the secondary response to hapten protein conjugates. II. Cell cooperation. Eur. J. Immunol. 1:18, 1971.
29. Benacerraf, B.: A hypothesis to relate the specificity of T lymphocytes and the activity of I region-specific Ir genes in macrophages and B lymphocytes. J. Immunol. 120:1809, 1978.
30. Chesnut, R.W. and Grey, H.M.: Studies on the capacity of B cells to serve as antigen presenting cells. J. Immunol., vol. 126. (In press.)

B Cell Expression and Stimulation

Norman R. Klinman, M.D., Ph.D., Dwane E. Wylie, Ph.D.
and Judy M. Teale, Ph.D.

Introduction

In this presentation we will present evidence for the thesis that the basis of the exquisite specificity of the immune system and its capacity to discriminate among the enormous array of environmental antigens rests primarily on three basic elements. First, the repertoire of uniquely specific B cells is enormous. Indeed, as will be seen, far more specificities exist in an inbred murine strain than can be reasonably assessed experimentally. Second, the mode of antigenic stimulation of these cells must be exquisitely specific so that any two cells in that vast repertoire, even those with quite similar recognition sites, can be discriminated by virtue of their recognition of antigen. Third, this vast and diverse repertoire and the selection upon it are the product not of random phenomena, but rather of highly specific, and highly conserved and reproducible mechanisms both at the level of repertoire generation and at the level of control of repertoire expression.

The Life History of B-Cell Clones

If one follows the life history of a single B cell clone, it must be presumed that such a clone initiates as a relatively undifferentiated stem cell. This postulated stem cell would contain the genetically inherited elements which ultimately could give rise to the vast repertoire of antibody clonotypes.

Norman R. Klinman, M.D., Ph.D., Member, Department of Immunopathology; Dwane E. Wylie, Ph.D., Research Fellow; and Judy M. Teale, Ph.D., Research Associate, Department of Cellular and Developmental Immunology, Scripps Clinic and Research Foundation, La Jolla, Calif.

This work was supported by USPHS Grant #AI 15797.

31

During the differentiated history of this cell, the progeny of such a cell undergo a series of highly complex molecular events which ultimately lead to their commitment to a single antibody clonotype. These events are in the process of being clearly defined at the molecular level, and the findings to date have been summarized in several recent reviews [1-3]. In summary, it would appear that each individual inherits hundreds of genes encoding the N-terminal portion of the variable region of both heavy chains and light chains. During the differentiation of a given lymphoid cell precursor, one such variable region for the heavy and one for the light chain are selected and juxtaposed at the DNA level to other gene elements responsible for encoding the more C-terminal regions of these variable regions. For the κ light chain in the mouse this juxtaposition is to one of several J region encoding segments, whereas for many heavy chains, a D region appears to be inserted between the variable and J regions. Each of these processes has built into it the capability of generating a considerable degree of sequence diversity. Thus, in addition to the hundreds of variable region genes available for selection, diversity is created by the selection and combinatorial association of any given variable region with a given D or J region [4]. Additional diversity is created at the junction between these gene segments, depending on the exact position at which they are joined. Given all of these processes, it has been calculated that at least 10^4 κ light-chain variable region sequences and 10 to 100 times more heavy-chain variable region sequences could be generated. Thus, by combinatorial association of heavy and light chains, it would be relatively simple to account for the 10^7 to 10^8 clonotypes estimated to constitute the mature mouse clonotype repertoire.

It is not yet known at which precise stage in the lifetime of a B-cell clone that the cells have reached a stage in which they are committed to either a given heavy-chain sequence or a given light-chain sequence. At the earliest detectable maturational stage the B cell precursors express the selected clonotype in the form of μ cytoplasmic heavy chains [5, 6]. At this stage, the clone of developing B cells is considered to be at the pre-B cell stage. Although no precursor-product relationship has been established, it appears that the pre-B cells, after several division cycles, begin to express immunoglobulin on their surface and in so doing can be either stimulated or tolerized by antigens [7].

Thus, they are considered B cells. In the mature animal, the major part of this developmental process apparently occurs in the bone marrow, with the more mature B cells exiting the bone marrow and seeding the peripheral lymphoid organs such as the spleen [8].

Several important points can be made about the above processes involved in inheriting the immune repertoire. First, the molecular mechanisms just described could readily accommodate an enormously diverse repertoire without having to superimpose totally random mechanisms such as mutation. Thus, although it is possible that the selecting and joining processes may have random elements, and that mutations found within the variable regions occur somatically [9], the role that such random processes play in repertoire establishment remains questionable. Second, B cell clones continue to be generated throughout the lifetime of an individual. Thus, the processes described above are presumably not limited to fetal or neonatal development, but rather are ongoing processes which are being reiterated time and again within the generative cell pool of mature individuals [10]. Third, the entire lifetime of a B cell clone from the stage where pre-B cells can first be identified through total expansion and maturation and ultimate cell death probably represents only a few weeks [8]. Therefore, the representation of a clone in the repertoire waxes and then wanes only to be replaced by new clones which themselves wax and wane. This eventuates into a repertoire that is always in a state of flux and consists of B cell clones at various stages in their life history. Finally, it appears that at the time a B cell matures to the stage where it acquires its immunoglobulin receptor (or very soon thereafter), B cell clones cease to expand [8, 11]. Thus, the bulk of clonal expansion antedates receptor acquisition. Since environmental influences such as tolerance or anti-idiotypic suppression can only operate subsequent to receptor acquisition, such processes must act at the level of expanded clones.

Repertoire Diversity and Immunologic Specificity

The aforementioned processes depict a B cell repertoire which is not only being continually generated and continually changed but is also extraordinarily diverse. It is this diversity that provides the first cornerstone of immunologic specificity. While it is impossible to estimate the total number of antigenic determinants which can be discriminated by the antibody repertoire, a simple calculation can provide an insight into both the specificity of humoral responses and their potential discriminatory power. If an individual has only ten antibody clonotypes, then any antigen entering the system could select among cells bearing these ten clonotypes. If it is assumed that such an antigen would either turn one or several such cells on or not turn them on, then the maximum number of possible different responses would be two raised to the tenth power, or approximately 1000. Thus, the antibodies formed from such a clonotype composite would have an extremely limited resolution power (every 1000 antigens giving exactly the same response), and the discriminatory power within those responses would be highly limited since a great deal of cross reactivity would exist. The larger the clonotype repertoire, however, the larger the total number of possible clonotype sets for any given response and the greater the potential for resolution. Thus, given calculations (see below) which indicate that the repertoire of a given murine strain exceeds 10^7 clonotypes, then the total number of antigenic determinants which could be discriminated from one another would exceed 2 to the 10^7 power, an extraordinarily large number. Therefore, the chances that any two different determinants would stimulate precisely the same set of clonotypes, and thus be totally cross reactive, would be very, very small. For this reason, the size of the repertoire in absolute numbers becomes crucial.

Most efforts to estimate repertoire size have chosen a similar strategy. Since it is impossible to fully characterize all of the components of the repertoire, investigators have attempted to determine how many clonotypes make up a given response and the frequency of B cells which constitute that response. If the examined response is typical for immune responses, and if the clonotypes measured are representative of the B cell population as a whole, then the answers to these two questions should provide an estimate of the average occurrence of any given clonotype within the repertoire, and by extrapolation, the total number of clonotypes which comprise the repertoire. As an example of such investigations, we have estimated that approximately 1 in 10^5 B cells can respond to the hemagglutinin glycoprotein of the influenza virus PR8 (PR8-HA) [12]. By using a panel of closely related viral hemagglutinins, we have been able to extrapolate that BALB/c mice express between 10^2 and 10^3 clonotypes which can recognize this antigen. Thus, any given PR8-HA-specific clonotype represents between 1 in 10^7 to 10^8 of the B cells of the entire repertoire, giving a repertoire estimate of 10^7 to 10^8 specificities. Studies of either similar antigens or quite distinct antigens by a number of laboratories have yielded approximately the same estimate [13-15]. Thus, it is likely that the repertoire of inbred murine strains is comprised of greater than 10^7 individual clonotypes. Recently, the same conclusion has been drawn by an analysis of responses to antigens for which quite restricted clonotype responses are characteristic. It was found that although the majority of such responses are comprised of a family of very similar clonotypes, each representative clonotype within such families is also extremely rare, yielding a clonotype repertoire estimate similar to those of the above-mentioned studies [16-18].

Stimulation Selectivity and Immunologic Specificity

Given the extraordinary diversity of the available B cell repertoire, the second and equally important requisite for the exquisite specificity of the immune system is that the selection by antigens from that repertoire must be highly selective. For example, even given an extremely diverse repertoire, if each antigen had the capacity to stimulate between 5% and 10% of all B cells, the final discriminatory capacity of the system as a whole would be greatly limited and the number of cross reactivities would be enormous. This example is not far-fetched since it has been the assumption of many investigators and has been indicated by the results of certain types of experiments. Thus, if one estimates the frequency of B cells which recognize a given antigenic determinant by enumerating those cells which can bind that antigen, it would appear that 1% to 10% of all B cells may recognize a particular antigen via their immunogobulin receptors [19-21]. Importantly, the measured number of antigen-binding cells for most antigens is directly dependent on the antigen concentration used in the binding assays. Therefore, it is likely that the seemingly high number of antigen-recognizing cells is an experimental phenomenon which plays on the nature of antigen-antibody interactions, and as such it is difficult to predict its relevance physiologically.

The binding of antigen by antibody is a reversible interaction with a measurable association constant. By the law of mass action, therefore, the higher the antigen concentration, the greater the proportion of antibody sites that will be occupied even when absolute affinities are relatively low. This is particularly true when multivalent binding can be achieved in which affinities between antibodies and antigens, or cell receptors and antigens, can be markedly exaggerated [22]. Since most proteins bind almost all ligands with some affinity, the cut-off of such binding measurements can be made to be totally dependent on the sensitivity of the experimental mode utilized to measure the binding. Thus, if one simply measures the antigen bound multivalently to a given cell at high antigen concentrations, the affinity cut-off may be exceedingly low, and many, if not most, B cells might be able to bind almost any antigen. Likewise, if one stimulates cells polyclonally with mitogens and assesses the number of cells producing antibody specific for a given antigen, using a binding or plaque assay technique with a low affinity cut-off, a large proportion of cells may again appear to be specific [23, 24]. The findings from such studies by many laboratories have led to the impression that the responsiveness of B cells is relatively nonspecific and that a large proportion of B cells can recognize and respond to any particular antigen. Under these circumstances it would be hard to imagine how the immune response, itself, could be highly specific and that phenomena such as tolerance to self molecules could play a meaningful role. That is, even if tolerance were highly specific, it would have little effect on the overall responsiveness to antigens if the stimulation of B cells were as nonspecific as antigen binding. Also, if tolerance itself displayed such a degree of nonspecificity, then recognition of the vast array of self antigens would eliminate the repertoire many times over.

Our own studies have come to precisely the opposite conclusion. Several years ago, we carried out a comparison of the effect of antigen concentration on the frequency of antigen-binding cells vs. the frequency of cells which would respond in a T-dependent fashion to give rise to clones of antibody-producing cells [25, 26]. Table 1 presents a summary of the data obtained. It can be seen that as the concentration of a polyvalent antigen increases, the frequency of antigen-binding cells increases until several percent of the B cells can be shown to bind the 2,4-dinitrophenol (DNP) determinant. On the other hand, when one measures the frequency of B cells which are stimulated by antigen over the same range of antigen concentrations, it can be seen that only at low antigen concentrations is there an increase in the frequency of primary B cell responses with increasing antigen concentrations, and at 5×10^{-7} M antigen, a plateau is reached at which approximately 1 in 5000 B cells will respond to DNP. Increasing antigen concentrations above that level, while markedly increasing the number of antigen-binding cells, does not increase the frequency of B cells which can be stimulated by antigen. These data have been interpreted as indicating that antigen binding per se is not sufficient for the stimulation of B cells, but rather only those cells whose receptors exceed a given threshold affinity for a particular antigen can be triggered by that antigen. Thus, once a sufficient concentration of antigen is present to bind to all cells whose receptors exceed this threshold affinity, the binding of antigen to additional cells, whose receptor affinity is lower than the triggering threshold, does not recruit new cells into the response. This conclusion is confirmed by the finding that the average affinity of the monoclonal antibodies produced by

Table 1. Evidence for Affinity Dependence of the Stimulation Trigger

Molar Antigen Determinant Concentration (DNP on DNP-Hy)	Number of Clones/ 10^6 Transferred Spleen cells*	Ko $7^\circ C$ $\times 10^6$ l/m†	A B C/10^6 Spleen Cells (estimated)‡
10^{-5}	2.3	1.8	4×10^4 (4%)
10^{-6}	3.8	2.0	2×10^4 (2%)
5×10^{-7}	4.1	1.8	1×10^4 (1%)
10^{-7}	2.9	3.0	2×10^3 (0.2%)
10^{-9}	1.9	7.2	$<1 \times 10^3$ (<0.1%)
10^{-11}	1.3	10.1	

*Detected in the splenic focus assay.
†Association constant of monoclonal antibodies obtained in the splenic focus assay.
‡Number of antigen-binding cells (DNP)/10^6 spleen cells.

stimulated B cells also reaches a plateau at 5×10^{-7} M antigen. If increasing antigen concentrations were to recruit B cells of lower affinity, then one would have expected to see a lower average affinity of responses at antigen concentrations higher than 5×10^{-7} M. Thus, only 1 in 5000 B cells appears to be capable of responding to a determinant such as DNP, which would be consistent with a highly specific, affinity-dependent triggering event.

Since it can be shown that B cells which recognize the closely related haptenic determinant 2,4,6-trinitrophenyl (TNP) will bind DNP at high antigen concentrations, it was of interest to ask whether DNP could stimulate TNP-specific cells. Additivity experiments were carried out using DNP- and TNP-coupled antigens, alone or in combination. The results of this study indicated that there was no detectable stimulation of TNP-specific cells [27]. Again, this demonstrated the extreme specificity of the triggering event and the fact that the triggering process is much more discriminatory than simple antigen binding to cell surface receptors. The frequency of B cells responsive in the splenic focus system has been measured for a large variety of antigens. In general, the frequencies for haptenic determinants range between 1 in 5,000 to 1 in 100,000 B cells, whereas the frequencies for complex carbohydrates and protein determinants range from 1 in 20,000 to 1 in 200,000 [15]. Thus, for a broad range of antigenic determinants, the triggering mechanism appears to be exquisitely specific and highly discriminatory.

Tolerance Selectivity and Immunologic Specificity

If our arguments stated above concerning the basis of the specificity of humoral responsiveness are correct, then not only stimulation but also tolerance induction should be extremely specific. If tolerance induction is specific, then it would be easy to see how the highly selective elimination of clones whose receptors exceed the triggering threshold affinity for self antigens could be specifically accomplished without affecting the vast bulk of the repertoire whose receptors do not recognize the self antigenic determinants, or whose affinity for such determinants is lower than the necessary threshold for triggering. It is assumed that the latter cells would not normally constitute a danger in terms of potential autoimmunity since under normal circumstances they would not be triggered by self antigenic determinants.

Several years ago we described a tolerance phenomenon which appeared applicable only to B cells during a short time in their development [28, 29]. In the introduction we delineated the presumptive developmental stages in the maturation of a B cell clone. In that discussion we described a stage in which clones appear to be considerably expanded but have not as yet acquired their immunoglobulin receptors.

It is now clear from both in vivo and in vitro studies that for the brief period of time during which these B cell clones are acquiring their immunoglobulin receptors, they pass through a transition phase in which they are exquisitely susceptible to tolerance induction. Before this phase, prior to the acquisition of immunoglobulin receptors, they are impervious to antigen contact either in terms of stimulation or tolerance. Beyond this stage they are susceptible to stimulation but become extraordinarily resistant to tolerance induction. Within this transition phase, however, they can either be stimulated if the antigen is presented in a T-dependent form in the presence of helper T cell function, or tolerized if the antigen is presented multivalently but in the absence of potential T cell help. This tolerance induction appears to be extremely specific, relatively independent of the carrier moiety, and operational over a very wide range of antigen concentrations.

Recently, we have carried out a series of experiments designed to define carefully the requisites for the tolerance induction of immature B cells [30]. The experimental procedure is to place the immature, tolerance-susceptible B cells in culture in the presence of tolerogen and in the presence or absence of a potential inhibitor of tolerance induction. After removal of the tolerogen and inhibitor, the cells are then stimulated and the effects of the inhibitor on tolerance induction are assessed by the frequency of the remaining responsive B cells. In our first series of studies, it was demonstrated that tolerance induction could be prohibited by the inhibition of energy metabolism or protein biosynthesis. These findings were interpreted as indicating that the tolerance of immature B cells is a true triggering event.

Figure 1 presents the data obtained when tolerance of DNP-specific B cells by DNP coupled to ovalbumin (OVA) was analyzed for its capacity to be inhibited by various monovalent or polyvalent cross-reacting determinants. It can be seen in this figure that the homologous haptenic determinant DNP-lysine readily blocks tolerance induction of DNP-specific B cells by DNP-OVA even at relatively low concentrations. This finding demonstrates that the haptenic determinant can bind to the receptor moicty with sufficient affinity to block the binding of the polyvalent tolerogen but does not itself induce tolerance. This finding serves as formal evidence that multivalent binding is necessary for the tolerance trigger. Figure 1 also shows that the cross-reacting haptenic determinant TNP-lysine can block tolerance induction of DNP-specific B cells by DNP-OVA but requires a higher concentration to accomplish this than was

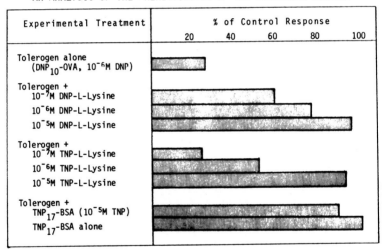

AN ANALYSIS OF THE PREREQUISITES OF THE TOLERANCE TRIGGER

FIG. 1. Neonatal spleen cells were transferred to carrier-primed recipients (4 to 6×10^6 donor cells per recipient). Fragment cultures were incubated for 18 hours in the presence or absence of the inhibitor. The tolerogen and/or inhibitor was/were washed out after 18 hours and stimulated for three days with DNP-Hy (10^{-6} M DNP). Supernates were collected at days 10, 13 and 17, and the frequency of anti-DNP-secreting clones was detected by radioimmunoassay. Data are expressed as percent of control response. (Data abstracted from Teale and Klinman [30].)

necessary for DNP-lysine. This finding demonstrates the affinity dependence of the blocking phenomenon in addition to demonstrating that the DNP receptors can bind TNP. That the binding of TNP by receptors of DNP-specific B cells is not of sufficient affinity to trigger those cells is demonstrated in Figure 1 by the inhibition of tolerance induction of DNP-specific B cells by the addition of TNP-bovine serum albumin (BSA). Thus, TNP presented in a polyvalent fashion can bind to DNP-specific B cells in such a way as to block the binding of DNP-OVA and prohibit tolerance induction. TNP-BSA itself, however, is not capable of tolerizing the DNP-specific B cells whose receptors it occupies.

These findings confirm and extend the earlier studies for the T-dependent stimulation trigger and demonstrate unambiguously that antigen binding to a cell's receptors is not sufficient for triggering that cell. Such binding must be multivalent and of sufficient affinity in order for triggering, either stimulation or tolerance, to ensue. Thus, not only is an extremely diverse array of clonotype specificities available for response to the antigenic universe, but both the stimulation and tolerance of clonotypes within this array are exquisitely specific and extremely discriminatory. This, then, is clearly the basis for the remarkable specificity of the immune response.

The Reproducibility of Repertoire Expression

The final segment of this presentation will address the question of whether this extraordinarily specific and elegant mechanism is the product of random accidental events which accumulate in a stochastic fashion, or whether it is the product of highly conserved, evolutionary and genetically predetermined mechanisms which give rise in a highly consistent and reproducible fashion to a vast repertoire that can then be selected by equally specific and reproducible mechanisms. In order to approach this question, one must attempt to define fully the repertoire in a given individual to an extent compatible with meaningful comparisons between genetically identical and nonidentical individuals. As mentioned earlier, the adult mammalian repertoire is so diverse as to preclude fully defining even a segment of the repertoire of any given individual, thus eliminating the possibility of meaningful comparisons. In order to circumvent this difficulty, various laboratories have adopted a variety of strategies. Some laboratories have chosen to study lower vertebrates such as the frog, where the entire repertoire is limited [31]. In these studies, it has been found that genetically identical individuals appear to share much, if not all, of their repertoires specific for a variety of antigens. Other investigators have analyzed the repertoire of genetically similar or identical chickens in which diversity has been truncated by early bursectomy [32]. Again, when the repertoire responsive to a given antigen was limited, genetically identical individuals appeared to share large portions of their repertoire.

This laboratory has chosen the approach of analyzing the repertoire of mice at a stage in their postnatal development when the repertoire is still sufficiently limited to allow a comprehensive definition. Several years ago we found that at birth or soon after, the entire repertoire of an inbred murine strain, as determined by the analysis of several antigenic determinants, was dominated by approximately 10^4 clonotypes, as opposed to greater than 10^7 in mature adults [33]. Additionally, it was found that identifiable clonotypes first appeared in the repertoire during the first week of postnatal development in a highly reproducible fashion [34]. Recently, in collaboration with Drs. Michael Cancro and Walter Gerhard, we have carried out a comprehensive analysis of the repertoire of two-week-old inbred murine strains specific for the PR8-HA antigenic determinant [35]. The findings revealed that, rather than the hundreds of clonotypes specific for this antigen available to mature BALB/c mice, neonatal (two-week-old) BALB/c mice express fewer than ten clonotypes. On the average, each of these clonotypes appears to represent approximately 1 in 10^6 B cells. Furthermore, statistical analyses indicate that at this stage in development, all BALB/c mice share essentially the same PR8-HA-specific clonotypes. Thus, at a time in development when individuals and the strain as a whole express approximately 10^6 specificities, all mice appear to share precisely the same clonotypes. These studies and those mentioned above in other species imply that repertoire acquisition and expression is not the product of haphazard random or stochastic processes, but rather the product of genetically predetermined and highly reproducible events.

It should be pointed out that each of the cited studies analyzed primarily mature B cells. Even though the individuals were neonates, the B cells themselves were representative of clones which had developed quite early and, therefore, were at a stage of full maturation. Thus, the reproducibility of the expressed repertoire represented an extraordinarily reproducible generative process, and any selective processes, such as tolerance to self antigens or anti-idiotypic selection of specificities, were also highly reproducible. This conclusion is further exemplified by findings obtained by analyses of the PR8-HA-specific repertoire of neonates of other murine strains [36]. These findings are consistent with the findings of the BALB/c neonatal repertoire in that individual neonates expressed only a very few clonotypes, and all neonates within a strain appeared to express precisely the same clonotypes. However, the repertoire expressed by neonates of other strains, B10.D2 for example, contains PR8-HA-specific clonotypes which are different from those expressed in the BALB/c neonates. Thus, there seems to be polymorphism at the level of expression of clonotypes between two different murine strains. An analysis was also carried out on F_1 mice constructed between BALB/c and B10.D2 parents. These studies revealed that the repertoire of such F_1 neonates did not contain all of the clonotypes expressed by either parent and, in fact, expressed clonotypes not seen in either parental strain. Since clonotypic composition was also extremely limited and highly consistent within the F_1 individuals, these findings may serve as evidence not only of the extreme complexity of the molecular events in repertoire generation described earlier, but also of the extreme reproducibility of whatever selective events may be playing a role in the establishment of the repertoire.

It should be noted that none of the aforementioned studies can actually delineate between control of repertoire expression exhibited at the level of the molecular events which lead to variable region diversification and control of those events which fashion the repertoire at the level of environmental selection on B cell clones as they express their immunoglobulin receptors. Indeed, it is likely that definitive answers to the questions and postulates posted in this presentation will only be obtained when a comprehensive understanding of the role of each of these two levels of control of repertoire generation and expression is gained. In order to approach such an analysis, we have initiated a series of studies which represents an effort to compare the repertoire of B cells as expressed prior to environmental contact (thus the result solely of molecular mechanisms for variable region diversification) with the repertoire as expressed in the mature B cell pool (thus the composite of both molecular and environmental controlling mechanisms). The strategy we have chosen is to isolate, from the bone marrow of adult individuals, cells which represent the stage in maturation where the clones have already expanded but have not, as yet, matured to the stage at which they express their immunoglobulin receptors. This is accomplished by eliminating immunoglobulin-bearing cells from bone marrow cell populations [37]. These Ig-negative cells in toto represent approximately 20% to 25% of all bone marrow B cells which can respond to antigenic stimulation in the splenic focus system. It has been found that the majority of these cells can be tolerized and consequently represent the bulk of tolerizable bone marrow B cells [7, 38]. Furthermore, the antibody-producing cell clones emanating from these B cells cannot give rise to IgG antibodies, a phenomenon characteristic of the most immature population of stimulatable B cells. Finally, in collaboration with Dr. David Katz, it has been shown that this B cell subpopulation remains intact, even in animals which have been rendered profoundly tolerant by a month of treatment with a potent tolerogen, DNP coupled to the copolymer of D-glutamic acid and D-lysine (DNP-DGL) [7]. In the bone marrow of such animals, few immunoglobulin-bearing B cells can be found which can respond to the DNP haptenic determinant coupled to hemocyanin. Yet, among the immature B cells, which by definition have not yet acquired their immunoglobulin receptors, there is no diminution in responsive B cells. Thus, it seems that we can indeed analyze the population of B cells which represents clones in the stage of development at which they have acquired their clonotypic specificity but have not yet interfaced with the environment.

Preliminary studies of this B cell subpopulation have enabled the following conclusions. First, the PR8-HA-specific repertoire of these prereceptor B cells from mature animals is highly diverse and quite distinct from the neonatal PR8-HA-specific repertoire [11, 39]. Thus, a considerable degree of diversification must take place prior to the acquisition of immunoglobulin receptors. Second, as mentioned earlier, individuals appear to have multiple representatives of cells of each clonotype, indicating that clones have expanded prior to their acquisition of immunoglobulin receptors.

As studies of these B cells progress, it should be possible to determine how this B cell population compares with the mature B cell population of the same animals. Such comparisons may eventually enable us to define fully the role in repertoire expression of molecular diversification of variable regions, and the effect of environmental selection upon the generated clonotypes. Such analyses should ultimately lead to a more comprehensive understanding of the biological mechanisms which, in a highly reproducible fashion, provide a defense mechanism elegant in both its diversity and its specificity.

References

1. Adams, J.M.: The organization and expression of immunoglobulin genes. Immunol. Today 1:10, 1980.
2. Hood, L. and Early, P.: Organization and rearrangements of heavy chain variable region genes. *In* Battisto, J.R. and Knight, K.L. (eds.): Immunoglobulin Genes and B Cell Differentiation. Amsterdam: Elsevier/North Holland, 1980, pp. 7-15.
3. Seidman, J.G., Max, E.E., Norman, B. et al: The sources of kappa light chain diversity: A review. *In* Battisto, J.R. and Knight, K.L. (eds.): Immunoglobulin Genes and B Cell Differentiation. Amsterdam:Elsevier/North Holland, 1980, pp. 35-49.
4. Early, P.W., Huang, H.V., Davis, M.M. et al: An immunoglobulin heavy chain variable region gene is generated from three segments of DNA: V_H, D, and J_H. Cell 19:981, 1980.
5. Levitt, D. and Cooper, M.D.: Mouse pre-B cells synthesize and secrete μ heavy chains but not light chains. Cell 19:617, 1980.
6. Siden, E.J., Baltimore, D., Clark, D. and Rosenberg, N.E.: Immunoglobulin synthesis by lymphoid cells transformed *in vitro* by Abelson murine leukemia virus. Cell 16:389, 1979.
7. Klinman, N.R., Schrater, A.F. and Katz, D.H.: Immature B cells as the targets for *in vivo* tolerance induction. J. Immunol. (In press.)
8. Osmond, D.G.: Production and differentiation of B lymphocytes in the bone marrow. *In* Battisto, J.R. and Knight, K.L. (eds.): Immunoglobulin Genes and B Cell Differentiation. Amsterdam: Elsevier/North Holland, 1980, pp. 135-154.
9. Weigert, M., Perty, R., Kelly, D. et al: The joining of V and J gene segments creates antibody diversity. Nature 283:497, 1980.

10. Metcalf, E.S., Sigal, N.H., Pickard, A.R. and Klinman, N.R.: V_H diversification and tolerance marker. Prog. Immunol. 111:162, 1977.
11. Wylie, D.E. and Klinman, N.R.: Assessing repertoire diversity in precursors to mature B cells. In Klinman, N.R., Mosier, D., Scher, I. and Vitetta, E. (eds.): Proceedings of the Second International Conference on B Lymphocytes in the Immune Response. New York:Elsevier/North-Holland, 1981, p. 63.
12. Cancro, M.P., Gerhard, W. and Klinman, N.R.: Diversity of the primary influenza specific B cell repertoire in BALB/c mice. J. Exp. Med. 147:776, 1978.
13. Kreth, H.W. and Williamson, A.R.: The extent of diversity of anti-hapten antibodies in inbred mice: (4-Hydroxy-5-iodo-3-nitro-phenacetyl) antibodies in CBA/H mice. Eur. J. Immunol. 3:141, 1973.
14. Kohler, G.: Frequency of precursor cells against the enzyme β-galacto-sidase. An estimate of the BALB/c strain antibody repertoire. Eur. J. Immunol. 6:340, 1976.
15. Sigal, N.H. and Klinman, N.R.: The B cell clonotype repertoire. Adv. Immunol. 26:255, 1978.
16. Schilling, J., Clevinger, B., Davie, J.M. and Hood, L.: Amino acid sequence of homogeneous antibodies to dextran and DNA rearrange-ments in heavy chain V-region gene segments. Nature 283:35, 1980.
17. Marshak-Rothestein, A., Beneditto, J.D. and Gefter, M.L.: Unique determinants associated with Hybridoma proteins expressing a cross-reactive idiotype: Frequency among individual immune sera. J. Immunol. 125:1987, 1980.
18. Stashenko, P. and Klinman, N.R.: Analysis of the primary anti(4-hydroxy-3-nitrophenyl) acetyl (NP) and responsive B cells in BALB/c and B10.D2 mice. J. Immunol. 125:531, 1980.
19. D'Eustachio, P. and Edelman, G.M.: Frequency and avidity of specific antigen-binding cells in developing mice. J. Exp. Med. 142:1078, 1975.
20. DeLuca, D., Miller, A. and Sercarz, E.: Antigen binding to lymphoid cells from unimmunized mice. IV. Shedding and reappearance of multiple antigen binding Ig receptors of T and B lymphocytes. Cell. Immunol. 18:286, 1975.
21. Weigle, W.O., Chiller, J.M. and Louis, J.A.: Tolerance: Central unresponsiveness or peripheral inhibition. In Brent, L. and Holborow, J. (eds.): Progress in Immunology II, Biological Aspects II. New York:Elsevier/North Holland, 1974, vol. 3, p. 187.
22. Klinman, N.R. and Karush, F.: Equine anti-hapten antibody. V. The non-precipitability of bivalent antibody. Immunochemistry 4:387, 1967.
23. Eichmann, K., Coutinho, A. and Melchers, F.: Absolute frequencies of lipopolysaccharide-reactive B cells producing A5A idiotype in un-primed streptococal A carbohydrate-primed anti-A5A idiotype-sensitized and anti-A5A idiotype-suppressed A/J mice. J. Exp. Med. 146:1436, 1977.

24. Moller, G.: Mechanism of B cell activation and self non self discrimination. Cold Spring Harbor Symp. Quant. Biol. 41:217, 1976.
25. Klinman, N.R.: The mechanism of antigenic stimulation of primary and secondary precursor cells. J. Exp. Med. 136:241, 1972.
26. Klinman, N.R., Pickard, A.R., Sigal, N.H. et al: Assessing B cell diversification of antigen receptor and precursor cell analysis. Ann. Immunol. 127:489, 1976.
27. Klinman, N.R., Press, J.L. and Segal, G.: Overlap stimulation of primary and secondary B cells by cross reacting determinants. J. Exp. Med. 138:1276, 1973.
28. Metcalf, E.S. and Klinman, N.R.: *In vitro* tolerance induction of neonatal B cells. J. Exp. Med. 143:1327, 1976.
29. Teale, J.M., Layton, J.E. and Nossal, G.J.V.: *In vitro* model for natural tolerance to self antigens. J. Exp. Med. 150:205, 1979.
30. Teale, J.M. and Klinman, N.R.: Tolerance as an active process. Nature 288:385, 1980.
31. Dupasquier, L. and Wabl, M.R.: Antibody diversity in amphibians. Inheritance of isoelectric focusing antibody patterns in isogenic frogs. Eur. J. Immunol. 8:428, 1978.
32. Huang, H.V. and Dreyer, W.J.: Bursectomy *in ovo* blocks the generation of immunoglobulin diversity. J. Immunol. 121:1738, 1978.
33. Klinman, N.R. and Press, J.L.: The characterization of the B cell repertoire specific for the DNP and TNP determinants in neonatal BALB/c mice. J. Exp. Med. 141:1133, 1975.
34. Sigal, N.H., Cancro, M.P. and Klinman, N.R.: The significance of minor clonotypes in the dissection of B cell diversification. *In* Sercarz, E.E., Herzenberg, L.A. and Fox, C.F. (eds.): ICN-UCLA Symposia on Molecular and Cellular Biology. Vol. VI. Immune System: Genetics and Regulations. New York:Academic Press, 1977, p. 217.
35. Cancro, M.P., Wylie, D.E., Gerhard, W. and Klinman, N.R.: Patterned acquisition of the antibody repertoire: Diversity of the hemagglutinin specific B cell repertoire in neonatal BALB/c mice. Proc. Natl. Acad. Sci. U.S.A. 76:6577, 1979.
36. Cancro, M.P. and Klinman, N.R.: B cell repertoire ontogeny: Heritable but dissimilar development of parental and F_1 repertoires. J. Immunol. 126:1160, 1981.
37. Wysocki, L.J. and Sato, V.L.: "Panning" for lymphocytes: A method for cell selection. Proc. Natl. Acad. Sci. U.S.A. 75:2844, 1978.
38. Metcalf, E.S. and Klinman, N.R.: In vitro tolerance induction of neonatal and adult bone marrow cells as a probe for the study of B cell diversification. J. Immunol. 118:2111, 1977.
39. Klinman, N.R., Wylie, D.E. and Cancro, M.P.: Mechanisms that govern repertoire expression. *In* Fougereau, M. and Dausset, I. (eds.): Immunology 1980 — Progress in Immunology IV. London:Academic Press, 1980, p. 123.

Activation of Lymphocytes in Immunity and Tolerance

William O. Weigle, Ph.D., Edward L. Morgan, Ph.D.
and Marilyn L. Thoman, Ph.D.

Introduction

When cells involved in the immune response come in contact with antigen in an appropriate manner, a variety of cellular and subcellular events can take place which lead to various parameters of immunity. As a result of primary contact with antigen, helper T cells and/or B cells may be activated. Whether B cells alone or both T and B cells are activated depends on the nature of the antigen. With thymus-dependent antigens, both helper T cells and B cells can be activated and macrophages are required, whereas with thymus-independent antigens, only the B cells are activated and macrophages may or may not be required [reviewed in 1]. In thymus-dependent responses, helper T cells may be activated with suboptimal concentrations of antigens which do not result in antibody production. In this case, the second contact with antigen results in an enhanced antibody response. Another population of T cells of the same phenotype as helper T cells (Lyt 1) can be activated to give delayed-type hypersensitivity [2-4]. A third

William O. Weigle, Ph.D., Member and Chairman; Edward L. Morgan, Ph.D. and Marilyn L. Thoman, Ph.D., Research Fellows, Department of Immunopathology, Scripps Clinic and Research Foundation, La Jolla, Calif.

This is publication No. 2339 from the Department of Immuno-pathology, Scripps Clinic and Research Foundation. This work was supported in part by USPHS grants AI07007 and AI15761, American Cancer Society Grant IM-42J and Biomedical Research Support Grant RRO-5514. E.L.M. is the recipient of USPHS National Research Service Award AI105813 and M.L.T. is the recipient of USPHS National Research Service Award AI106085.

49

population of T cells of a different phenotype (Lyt 2) can be activated and in the presence of yet another subpopulation of T cells (also Lyt 1) are cytotoxic [reviewed in 5]. Once these various responses are initiated, they are accompanied by a cascade of events in the T cell compartment that is responsible for the regulation of the immune response. Under selected conditions the antigen can be given in such a manner that none of the above events takes place, and the host fails to respond to the antigen when it is given under conditions which usually lead to an immune response. This immunological tolerance may mimic the tolerance that animals enjoy to their own body components.

Regulation of the Immune Response via Fc Receptors

In addition to the circuit of regulatory T cells, which include feedback-inhibitory cells, suppressor cells, inducer cells [reviewed in 6, 7], contrasuppressor cells [8] and their suppressive and enhancing factors, the immune response is regulated by both antigen and antibody. The kinetics of the induction of the immune response and its waning depends on, among other factors, the nature of the antigen and its in vivo behavior.

It is also well established that antibody produced as a result of the immune response can itself cause feedback regulation [reviewed in 9]. A number of investigators have shown that passive antibody given either with or shortly before antigen results in either suppression or enhancement of the immune response [reviewed in 9-11]. In suppression, the mechanism responsible is determined by the quantity of antibody given. With large amounts of antigen, suppression is independent of the Fc region of the antibody molecule since suppression can be achieved with intact antibody, the Fab or the $F(ab')_2$ subfragments [12, 13]; in this case suppression is apparently the result of masking the antigenic determinants in such a manner that the antigen is ineffective in triggering competent lymphocytes. On the other hand, the suppression of the immune response with small amounts of antibody, involving an active process, is dependent on the Fc region of the antibody molecule [14-18]. Enhancement with preformed antigen-antibody complexes also has been reported to require the Fc portion of immunoglobulin (Ig) [18]. Whether the response is suppressed [19] or enhanced [20, 21] appears to depend on the ratio between the antibody and antigen.

Modulation by Fc Fragments

Lymphocyte Proliferation. It is well known that the Fc portion of the immunoglobulin molecule is responsible for a variety of biological functions that the immunoglobulin molecule posseses [reviewed in 11]. It has also been shown more recently that Fc fragments prepared by enzymatic cleavage are capable of stimulating cells possessing Fc receptors [22-25]. Fc fragments prepared by digestion of Ig with papain were found to cause an in vitro proliferative response in murine B lymphocytes [22]. This mitogenic activity of the Fc fragment was first found with Fc fragments prepared from a commercial batch of human gamma globulin (HGG). It has since been shown that Fc fragments prepared from human IgG1, IgG2, IgG3, IgG4, IgD, IgM and IgA, as well as Fc fragments prepared from goat and mouse immunoglobulins, are effective in inducing a proliferative response in murine B cells [11, 26]. This proliferative response is specific for Fc fragments in that it cannot be induced by intact Ig or Fab or $F(ab')_2$ fragments. The addition of 10 to 15 μg of Fc fragments per culture results in maximal incorporation of tritiated thymidine (Fig. 1). Although similar concentrations of aggregated HGG result in a significant proliferative response in mouse spleen cells, only a questionable response is obtained with intact HGG and no response is seen with deaggregated preparations of HGG or with the $F(ab')_2$ and Fab fragments.

The cell type responsible for the proliferative response is the B cell. Splenic cells from the athymic (nude) mouse give an optimal response to 10 μg of Fc fragments, although these cells do not respond to the T cell mitogen, concanavalin A (Table 1). In related experiments it was shown that B cells derived from mouse spleen cells treated with anti-thymocyte serum plus complement also give a proliferative response in the presence of Fc fragments that is equivalent to, if not greater than, that seen with intact spleen cells. On the other hand, populations of T cells prepared by passage over nylon wool columns do not proliferate in response to the Fc fragment. Deletion of either Ig^+ or μ^+ cells removes the ability of mouse spleen cells to

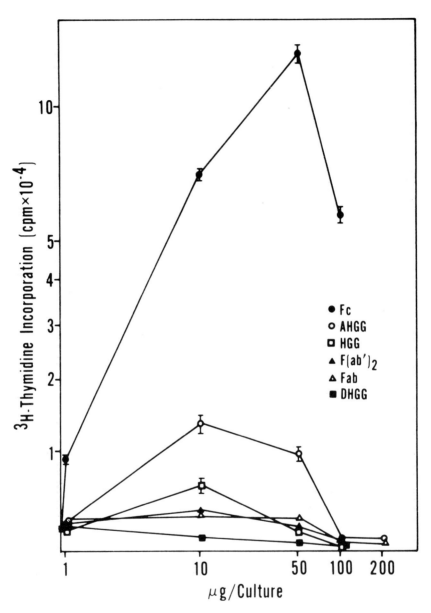

FIG. 1. Response of mouse spleen cells to HGG and HGG fragments. (Reprinted from Berman and Weigle [22].)

Table 1. Response of Athymic (Nude) Mice to Fc Fragments

| | Counts/Min ^3H-Thymidine (Uptake Day 2-3) | | |
	Con A	LPS	Fc
BALB/c nu/+	154,997	35,707	35,254
BALB/c nu/nu	2,815	36,025	38,610

Concanavalin A 0.5 μg, LPS 10 μg and Fc 10 μg.
(Reprinted in part from Berman and Weigle [22].)

proliferate to the Fc fragments [27]. The depletion of Ia^+ cells by treatment with anti-Ia sera plus complement markedly diminished the ability of splenic cells to proliferate. Further-more, depletion of spleen cells containing receptors for the third component of complement (CR^+) removes the ability of the cells to respond. Thus, the responsive cell is a Fc^+, Ia^+, Ig^+ and CR^+ B cell [11, 27].

The proliferative response of B cells to Fc fragments requires a population of adherent accessory cells [23]. Passage of mouse spleen cells over a Sephadex G-10 column removed the ability of these cells to give a proliferative response to Fc fragments, but did not alter their ability to respond to LPS (Fig. 2). Less than 0.1% esterase-positive cells remained in the passed

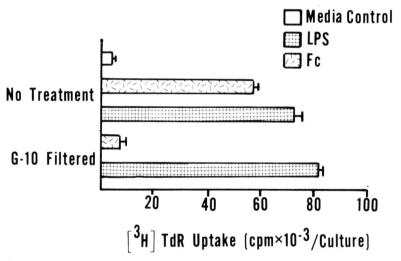

FIG. 2. The proliferative response of Sephadex G-10-filtered mouse spleen cells. LPS was used at a concentration of 50 μg/ml and Fc at 250 μg/ml. (Reprinted from Morgan and Weigle [23].)

cell population. Adherent cells appear to be macrophages since they adhere to plastic, phagocytize carbonyl iron, are esterase positive and irradiation resistant, and are not susceptible to lysis by anti-thymus serum and complement [28]. The macrophage populations are prepared by irradiating mouse spleen cells, allowing them to adhere to plastic for 30 minutes at 37°C and then washing out the nonadherent cells (Fig. 3). Anti-thymus serum plus complement is added to the adherent cells in order to deplete persisting T cells. After washing, these cells are used as the preparations of enriched macrophages. Macrophage-depleted spleen cells are prepared by passing spleen cells over a Sephadex G-10 column. These latter cells when added directly to the macrophages in the presence of Fc fragments give a proliferative response, whereas the G-10-passed cells not reconstituted with macrophages fail to respond (Fig. 4). The macrophages themselves do not give a proliferative response to the Fc fragments.

When Fc fragments are added to macrophages in the absence of B cells, active supernatants are obtained which cause proliferation of spleen cells. The active supernatant is generated

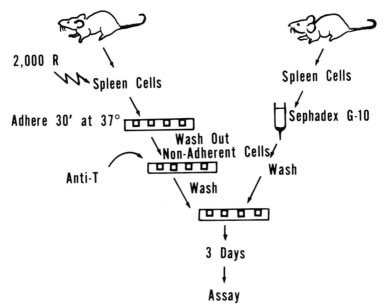

FIG. 3. Procedures for preparing enriched populations of adherent and nonadherent spleen cells.

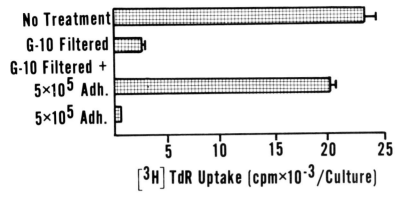

FIG. 4. Restoration of the Sephadex G-10-filtered spleen cell proliferative response to Fc with splenic plastic-adherent cells. Fc was used at a concentration of 250 µg/ml. (Reprinted from Morgan and Weigle [23].)

within ten minutes after addition of Fc fragments to the cultures (Fig. 5). The activity of the macrophage supernatant is not due to the presence of Fc fragments since these supernatants are able to activate B cells in the absence of macrophages [22]. As mentioned above, Fc fragments are unable to cause a proliferative response in macrophage-depleted spleen cells (Sephadex G-10 filtered). It is important to note here that supernatants obtained from untreated macrophages do not result in a proliferative response when added to the G-10-filtered spleen cells. It appears that the active substance in the macrophage-Fc fragment supernatant is related to the Fc fragment itself. Passage of the macrophage-Fc fragment supernatant over an anti-Fc column removes the ability of these supernatants to cause a B cell proliferative response [28]. On the other hand, passage of the supernatants over an anti-bovine serum albumin column has no effect on their ability to activate B cells (Table 2). That the active substance in the supernatant is a subfragment of the Fc fragment was shown by sizing the active material on a G-50 Sephadex column (Fig. 6). The elution of the active material from this column in relation to that of protein markers of known molecular weight (MW) indicates that the active subfragment has a MW of approximately 14,000. Since the digestion of intact immunoglobulin with plasmin yields a subfragment composed of the third domain, which is active in B cell proliferation [29], it is

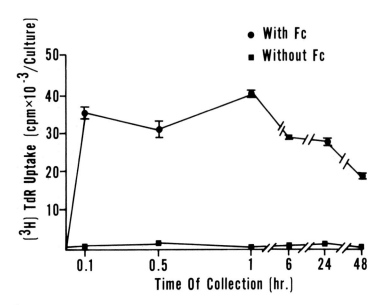

FIG. 5. Adherent cell supernates were collected from 0.1 to 48.0 hours after addition of either 1 mg Fc fragments (•) or media without Fc fragments (■) to the adherent cells; 100 μl of the supernatant material was added to cultures of Sephadex G-10-filtered spleen cells and proliferation was assayed on day 3. (Reprinted from Morgan and Weigle [28].)

Table 2. The Ability of Anti-Fc Column to Remove
the Mitogenic Activity from the Adherent Cell Supernatant

Supernatant Source	Treatment	cpm ± SE	% Reduction
Fc adherent*	None	39,813 ± 822	—
Fc adherent	Anti-Fc (1×)†	12,393 ± 548	69
	Anti-Fc (2×)	3,229 ± 781	92
Fc adherent	Anti-BSA (1×)	37,166 ± 1,089	7
	Anti-BSA (2×)	44,119 ± 3,334	0

*The 14,000-MW fraction from the Sephadex G-50 chromatographic separation of Fc adherent cell supernate.
†1× = filtered once; 2× = filtered twice.
(Reprinted from Morgan and Weigle [28].)

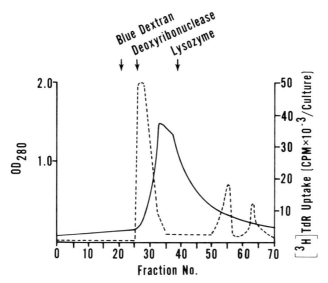

FIG. 6. Sephadex G-50 superfine chromatographic separation of Fc-adherent cell supernate. Each column fraction was assayed for protein content by OD and for mitogenic activity. the MW of the standards were: blue dextran, >50,000: deoxyribonuclease, 31,000; and lysozyme, 14,300. OD_{280} (----), mitogenic activity (———). (Reprinted from Morgan and Weigle [28].)

tempting to speculate that the active 14,000-MW subfragment is one half of the third domain.

Polyclonal Response. In addition to the B cell proliferative response, the addition of Fc fragment to intact spleen cells results in a polyclonal response (Table 3). Thus, spleen cells cultured with Fc fragments show a markedly enhanced polyclonal response, as evidenced by an increased appearance of plaque-forming cells (PFC) to TNP [30]. In contrast to the proliferative response, T cells are required for the polyclonal response. Fc fragments added to athymic (nude) spleen cells give a proliferative but not a polyclonal response, whereas the addition of Fc fragments to normal littermate spleen cells results in both a proliferative and polyclonal response. Similarly, Fc fragments give a proliferative response, but not a polyclonal response, when added to spleen cells depleted of T cells by treatment with anti-thymus serum plus complement. On the other hand, B cells from either athymic mice or B cells prepared by treatment of spleen cells from conventional mice

Table 3. The Ability of Fc Fragments to Induce
a Polyclonal Antibody Response

Stimulator*	Cpm ± SE	Anti-TNP PFC/10^6 Cultured Cells ± SE†
None	<2,000	10 ± 2
Fc fragments	42,500 ± 2,062	190 ± 15
LPS	80,720 ± 816	479 ± 48

*100 μg Fc fragment and 20 μg LPS/culture.
†Direct PFC response.
(Reprinted from Morgan and Weigle [30], © 1980 Williams & Wilkins Co.,
Baltimore.)

with anti-thymus serum and complement show both proliferative and polyclonal responses in the presence of lipopolysaccharide (LPS). The requirement of macrophages for the
polyclonal response to Fc fragments is shown by the elimination of this response after passage of spleen cells over Sephadex
G-10 columns (Table 4). Depletion of macrophages in this
manner abolishes the ability of the remaining cells to mount a
polyclonal response to Fc fragments, but does not diminish
their ability to respond to LPS.

It is of interest that the requirement for T cells in the
Fc-induced polyclonal response can be replaced with interleukin
(IL-2). B cells obtained either by treatment of conventional
spleen cells with anti-thymus serum plus complement or from
athymic mice do not show a polyclonal response to either Fc
fragments or IL-2 (Table 5). On the other hand, addition of

Table 4. The Requirement for Macrophages
in the Fc Fragment-Induced Polyclonal Antibody Response

Cell Treatment	Stimulator*	cpm ± SE	Anti-TNP PFC/10^6 Cultured Cells ± SE†
None	Fc fragments	31,982 ± 491	176 ± 12
Sephadex G-10 filtered	Fc fragments	3,561 ± 181	30 ± 14
None	LPS	60,590 ± 3,226	388 ± 118
Sephadex G-10 filtered	LPS	81,266 ± 10,790	335 ± 55

*100 μg of Fc fragment and 20 μg LPS/culture.
†Direct PFC response. Background subtracted from experimental response.
(Reprinted in part from Morgan and Weigle [30], © 1980 Williams & Wilkens Co., Balti-
more.)

Table 5. Restoration of Polyclonal Response in T-Depleted Cultures
by Addition of TRF

Cells	Fc*	TRF†	PFC/10^6‡
6×10^5 B cells§	+	+	447 ± 39
	+	−	26 ± 3
	−	+	33 ± 4
6×10^5 Nude spleen cells	+	+	248 ± 26
	+	−	6 ± 3
	−	+	2 ± 1

*50 μg per culture well.
†10 μg per culture well.
‡Direct anti-TNP PFC/10^6 cultured cells ± SE. Background was subtracted.
§Rabbit anti-thymocyte sera and C treated.
(Reprinted from Thoman et al [31], © 1980 Williams & Wilkins Co., Baltimore.)

both Fc fragments and IL-2 to these cells results in a good polyclonal response [31]. Furthermore, polyclonal activation can be obtained in B cell preparations by the addition of both IL-2 and the 14,000-MW Fc subfragment.

It has recently been shown that the addition of Fc fragments to either intact spleen cells or enriched preparations of T cells results in the generation of a thymus-replacing factor (Fc-TRF) that can replace T cells in the polyclonal response induced by the Fc fragment [32]. The addition of Fc fragments, Fc subfragments or Fc-TRF to athymic spleen cells does not cause a polyclonal response. On the other hand, the addition of both Fc fragments and Fc-TRF does result in a polyclonal response (Table 6). This polyclonal response apparently requires macrophages since the removal of macrophages from the athymic spleen cells abolishes the ability of these cells to respond to Fc fragments and Fc-TRF. However, the Fc subfragment combined with Fc-TRF is sufficient to trigger the B cell to a polyclonal response. The addition of Fc fragment or subfragments to the B cell cultures 48 hours prior to the addition of Fc-TRF still results in a good polyclonal response. On the other hand, if the Fc fragments are added after the addition of Fc-TRF, no polyclonal activation occurs. Thus, as others have shown with antigen-specific responses [33, 34], the signal resulting in the proliferative response apparently can

Table 6. Requirement for Macrophages in the Fc-TRF Polyclonal Response

Cells	Culture Additions*			PFC/10⁶†
	Fc	Subfrag.	TRF	
6 × 10^5 Nude spleen cells	+	−	−	25 ± 11
	−	+	−	21 ± 16
	−	−	+	24 ± 15
	+	−	+	147 ± 20
6 × 10^5 G-10-passed nude spleen cells	+	−	−	<10
	−	+	−	<10
	−	−	+	11 ± 13
	+	−	+	<10
	−	+	+	225 ± 9

*Additions were made at culture initiation in the following amounts: Fc, 50 μg/well; subfragment, 50 μg/well; and TRF, 10 μg/well.
†Direct anti-TNP PFC/10⁶ cultured cells + SE.
(Reprinted from Thoman et al [31], © 1980 Williams & Wilkins Co., Baltimore.)

precede the differentiation signal by as much as 48 hours. The generation of Fc-TRF also requires macrophages and the role of the macrophages appears to be that of enzymatic cleavage of the Fc fragment into the active 14,000-MW subfragment [32].

Modulation by Aggregated Immunoglobulin

A similar series of cellular and subcellular events occurs in the activation of B lymphocytes by aggregated immunoglobulin. Aggregated preparations of HGG prepared by heating at 63°C for 25 minutes are effective in activation of B cells, similar to that described above with Fc fragments [35]. Although the intact aggregated material has some activity, the most stimulating material is the soluble aggregates precipitated by 0.62 M sodium sulfate. Soluble aggregated HGG causes both proliferative and polyclonal responses comparable to those observed with Fc fragments (Table 7). As with the Fc fragments, the proliferative response induced in B cells with aggregated preparations of HGG requires macrophages. Sephadex G-10-filtered spleen cells fail to develop either a proliferative or

Table 7. The Ability of AHGG to Induce Proliferation and
Polyclonal Antibody Production

Stimulator	cpm ± SE*	Direct Anti-TNP PFC/10⁶ Cultured Cells ± SE*
	2,792 ± 385	6 ± 2
AHGG†	31,002 ± 1,939	116 ± 8
Fc fragments‡	45,555 ± 1,401	143 ± 6

*Proliferation and polyclonal antibody production were measured on day 3 of culture.
†100 μg/culture heat AHGG.
‡100 μg/culture Fc fragments from HGG.
(Reprinted from Morgan and Weigle [35], © 1980 Williams & Wilkins Co., Baltimore.)

polyclonal response in the presence of aggregated HGG (Table 8). On the other hand, incubation of soluble aggregated HGG with macrophages results in a 14,000-MW subfragment that is capable of stimulating B cells depleted of macrophages to proliferation. The active subfragment prepared by incubation of aggregated HGG with macrophages can be removed by passage over an anti-Fc column. Material subsequently eluted from such columns, however, is very active in both the proliferative and

Table 8. The Requirement for Macrophages in the AHGG-Induced
Proliferative and Polyclonal Antibody Responses

Spleen Cell Treatment	AHGG*	cpm ± SE†	Direct Anti-TNP PFC/10⁶ Cultured Cells ± SE†
None	–	3,314 ± 1,110	3 ± 2
None	+	55,713 ± 2,273	104 ± 4
Sephadex G-10 filtered	–	2,476 ± 1,041	25 ± 5
Sephadex G-10 filtered	+	5,873 ± 752	34 ± 12

*100 μg heat AHGG/culture.
†Proliferation and polyclonal antibody production were measured on day 3 of culture.
(Reprinted from Morgan and Weigle [35], © 1980 Williams & Wilkins Co., Baltimore.)

Table 9. The Ability of the Stimulatory Material from the Macrophage
Supernatant to Bind to an Anti-Fc Affinity Column*

Treatment of Stimulatory Material†	cpm ± SE	Direct Anti-TNP PFC/10⁶ Cultured Cells ± SE
	1,597 ± 241	5 ± 2
None	26,270 ± 1,913	109 ± 3
Anti-Fc column effluent	6,338 ± 62	27 ± 11
Anti-Fc column eluate	27,477 ± 102	105 ± 4

*Sephadex G-10-filtered spleen cells were incubated with 50 μl of the stimulatory material and assayed for proliferation and polyclonal antibody production on day 3 of culture.

†The 14,000-MW pool from the Sephadex G-50 chromatographic separation of AHGG macrophage supernatant.

(Reprinted from Morgan and Weigle, [35], © 1980 Williams & Wilkins Co., Baltimore.)

polyclonal response (Table 9). As evidenced by the failure to obtain polyclonal responses in either spleen cells from athymic mice (Table 10) or B cells (depleted of T cells) from conventional mice, T cells are also required for this response.

Modulation by Antigen-Antibody Complexes

In view of the above observations with aggregated HGG, it is not surprising that B cells can be activated with soluble

Table 10. The Differential Requirement for T Cells in
the AHGG-Induced Proliferative and Polyclonal Antibody Responses

Source of Cells	AHGG*	cpm ± SE†	Direct Anti-TNP PFC/10⁶ ± SE†
nu/nu	−	4,065 ± 598	33 ± 6
nu/+	−	5,538 ± 445	8 ± 2
nu/nu	+	38,331 ± 354	36 ± 3
nu/+	+	37,058 ± 3,007	120 ± 6

*100 μg/culture.

†Culture was assayed for proliferation and polyclonal antibody on day 3 of culture. The lack of T cells in nu/nu mice was monitored with Con A.

(Reprinted from Morgan and Weigle [35], © 1980 Williams & Wilkins Co., Baltimore.)

antibody-antigen complexes [29]. Such complexes prepared between human Fab fragments and antibody to these fragments can generate a proliferative response in murine spleen cells (Fig. 7). This proliferative response appears to depend on the antibody-antigen ratio of the complexes. Complexes in antibody excess are not as effective as complexes prepared from

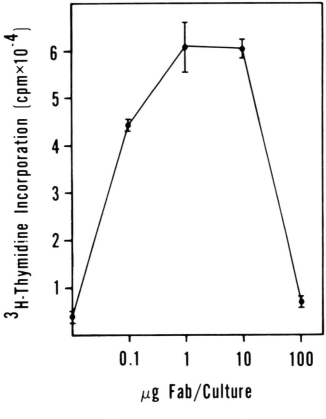

0.5% of Mouse Anti-human Fab
in All Cultures

FIG. 7. Stimulation of DNA synthesis in mouse spleen cells by antigen-antibody complexes. Increasing amounts of Fab fragments were added to a constant amount (0.5%) of mouse anti-Fab fragment.

slight to moderate antigen excess, and complexes prepared from
large antigen excess appear to be ineffective. In addition to the
proliferative response, soluble antibody-antigen complexes can
also induce polyclonal antibody responses in murine splenic
cells. Complexes of mouse anti-ovalbumin and ovalbumin have
been shown to cause polyclonal antibody responses (Fig. 8).
Again, the ratio between the antibody and antigen in such
complexes is critical. It remains to be determined whether

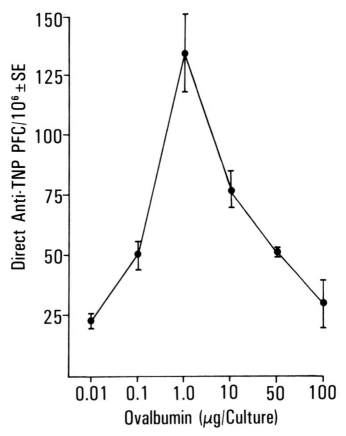

FIG. 8. Antigen-antibody complex-induced polyclonal antibody response.
Varying concentrations of ovalbumin added to constant amount of a
mouse anti-ovalbumin serum (0.5%). The polyclonal response was measured against TNP-SRBC on day 3 of culture.

cellular and subcellular events responsible for proliferative and polyclonal responses induced by antigen-antibody complexes are the same as those responsible for B cell activation by either Fc fragments or aggregated HGG.

Adjuvant Properties of Fc Fragments

In addition to the ability of Fc fragments to activate T and B cells in the proliferative and polyclonal response of B lymphocytes, Fc fragments can regulate humoral and cell-mediated immune responses. Fc fragments derived from human and murine Ig act as potent adjuvants when given with antigen in both the in vitro and in vivo responses to sheep red blood cells (SRBC) [37]. The adjuvant effect is dependent on the dose of antigen used, with the greatest enhancement occurring at suboptimal doses of antigen. In the in vitro response to SRBC, addition of Fc fragments results in a marked enhancement of both the IgM and IgG antibody responses when suboptimal concentrations of sheep red blood cells are used (Table 11). The adjuvant effect is specific for the Fc fragment since Fab fragments or intact IgG did not cause enhancement. Fc fragments also enhance the in vivo immune responses to SRBC [36]. It appears that in this adjuvant effect, the splenic cell population affected by the Fc fragments is the T cell [37]. That Fc fragments do not act directly on the B cell is, in part, evidenced by the failure of Fc fragments to enhance the

Table 11. Enhancement of the In Vitro Secondary IgM and IgG Responses to SRBC with Fc Fragments

| | | Anti-SRBC | |
Fc*	SRBC†	IgM	IgG
		PFC/10^6 ± SE	
−	−	10 ± 2	60 ± 19
−	+	102 ± 19	331 ± 28
+	−	81 ± 16	90 ± 27
+	+	670 ± 37	1,272 ± 73

*100 μg Fc/culture.
†1 × 10^4 SRBC/culture.
(Reprinted from Morgan et al [36].)

response to a thymus-independent antigen (Fig. 9). Thus, the response to the thymus-independent antigen TNP-LPS is not enhanced by addition of Fc fragments. Furthermore, when T cells are replaced with IL-2 in the in vitro antibody response to SRBC, the addition of Fc fragments does not result in enhancement (Fig. 10). It appears that only the antibody responses which involve T cells are enhanced by Fc fragments. Consistent with the adjuvant properties of Fc being at the T cell level is the finding that the mixed lymphocyte reaction (MLR) can be markedly enhanced by Fc fragments [38]. This enhancement is restricted to an MLR resulting from allogeneic differences in the *Ir* gene regions regulating the I-A or I-B gene products. The MLR resulting from allogeneic differences in these regions is due to Lyt $1^+2,3^-$ T cells [39-41]. On the other hand, the MLR generated by a difference in the *K* or *D* regions is not enhanced by Fc fragments [38] and the reactivity resulting from these differences is due to Lyt 2^+ cells [40].

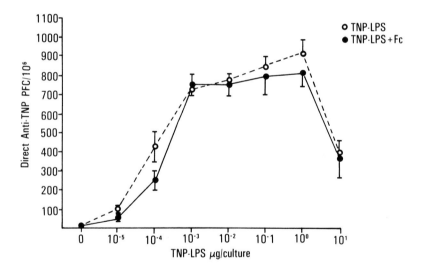

FIG. 9. The primary in vitro response to TNP-SRBC + 100 μg Fc fragment (•———•) or TNP-SRBC alone (o————o). (Reprinted from Morgan et al [37], © 1980 Williams & Wilkins Co., Baltimore.)

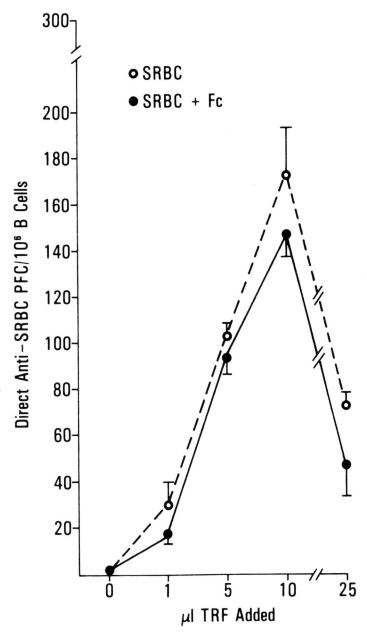

FIG. 10. Restoration of the in vitro anti-SRBC response by T cell-replacing factor (TRF). A constant number of SRBC (1×10^4) (o— — -o) or SRBC + 100 μg Fc (•———•) was added with increasing amounts of TRF. (Reprinted from Morgan et al [31], © 1980 Williams & Wilkins Co., Baltimore.)

Mechanism of Lymphocyte Activation
via Fc Receptors

Subcellular and cellular events involved in the activation of
T and B lymphocytes by Fc fragments and the adjuvant effect
of these fragments on immune responses are summarized in
Figure 11. The first step involves the reaction of antigen with
the antibody, possibly altering a site on the Fc portion of the
antibody that permits it to react more avidly with the
appropriate Fc receptor on macrophages. In step 2a, an enzyme
of the macrophage cleaves the Fc fragment between the second
and third domain, resulting in a Fc subfragment with a site that
is reactive with the Fc receptors on T cells and B cells. In step
3a, reaction of the subfragment (14,000 MW) with B cells
causes the B cells to proliferate. In step 3b, the action of the
subfragment with T cells releases a Fc-TRF to act upon the B
cells, causing the B cells to differentiate. This series of cellular
and subcellular events may be responsible for some of the
enhancement seen by memory B cells where the antibody being
released from B cells reacts with the antigen carried by
macrophages. Cleavage of the antibody in these complexes at

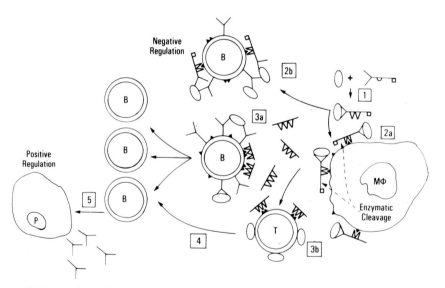

FIG. 11. Possible pathway of antibody-mediated regulation of an immune
response.

the surface of the macrophage may result in further activation of nearby B cells and T cells. The specificity of this enhancement may lie in the effect of dilution of the subfragments as they diffuse away from the specific B and T cells. When the ratio of antigen to antibody is such that the Fc receptors on macrophages are saturated, the complexes may attach to B cells through both their Fc receptors and the antigen (2b), resulting in suppression.

Regulation by Mechanisms of Self-Nonself Discrimination

Immunological Tolerance

Another avenue of regulation of the immune response is through the induction of a specific unresponsive state. In all likelihood it is this type of immune regulation that is responsible for self-nonself discrimination [42] and in many cases the control of the development of autoimmune phenomena. Immunological tolerance can be defined as a refractory state to antigenic stimulation. This type of tolerance is antigen-directed in that the antigen must come into contact with the antigen-reactive cells before the tolerant state is induced. Although there are a variety of conditions that lead to specific unresponsive states, the various types of tolerance can be divided into two categories, i.e. peripheral inhibition and central unresponsiveness [43]. In peripheral inhibition immunologically competent cells are present, but are blocked by some peripheral mechanism. This type of tolerance usually cannot be transferred to irradiated recipients and quite often is accompanied by the transient production of antibody or suppressor cells. Examples of peripheral inhibition are the unresponsive states caused by antibody feedback, antigen blockade and the regulatory T cell circuit which generates suppressor T cells. Peripheral inhibition is not a true tolerant state but most likely represents the negative pole of the normal regulatory mechanisms controlling the immune system. On the other hand, central unresponsiveness results from the functional deletion of specific competent cells. This type of tolerance can be transferred to irradiated recipients, is not accompanied by either the transient production of antibody or antigen blockade, and suppressor T cells are not responsible. It is this type of unresponsiveness that most likely mimics the tolerant state that we enjoy to our own body constituents.

Cellular Mechanism. The classical example of central unresponsiveness is the unresponsive state induced in adult animals injected with deaggregated preparations of heterologous IgG preparations. Commercial preparations of mammalian γ-globulins owe their antigenicity to the presence of a small amount of aggregated material [44]. When this aggregated material is removed by ultracentrifugation, biological filtration or chemical precipitation, the resulting monomeric form is not antigenic. On the other hand, preparations of mammalian γ-globulin aggregated by heating (63°C for 25 minutes) are relatively good antigens. However, if the deaggregated preparations are injected first, there is no immune response to a subsequent injection of aggregated preparations. As can be seen in Table 12, the injection of aggregated HGG into adult A/J mice results in a good antibody response. However, if an injection of deaggregated HGG precedes the injection of aggregated HGG, the animals are tolerant in that they fail to respond [45]. A single injection of 2.5 mg of deaggregated HGG (DHGG) readily induces a complete and lasting unresponsive state in adult A/J mice, as evidenced by their failure to respond to a subsequent injection of aggregated HGG (AHGG). Antigen-binding cells disappear from the spleen shortly after the injection of DHGG [46]. During the period of tolerance induction and the subsequent time that tolerance is maintained, no antibody-producing cells (IgM or IgG) are detectable [47]. In this system, tolerance is maintained neither by suppressor cells [48, 49] nor by antigen blockade [50], and tolerance is not lost when cells

Table 12. Antibody Response to Aggregated (A) Preparations of Human Gamma Globulin (HGG) and Turkey Gamma Globulin (TGG) in A/J Mice Previously Injected with 2.5 mg Deaggregated HGG (DHGG)

Antigen Injected		Indirect PFC Response to HGG or TGG	
Day 0	Days 15 and 25	Day 30	
		HGG	TGG
None	AHGG	+	0
DHGG	AHGG	0	0
DHGG	ATGG	0	+

are transferred to irradiated syngeneic hosts. Both the T and B cells become tolerant [51], although the duration of tolerance differs in the two cell types (Table 13) [52]. Induction of tolerance in either thymus cells or peripheral T cells is rapid and parallels the kinetics of induction observed in intact mice; peripheral B cells are only slightly slower to assume the tolerant state. Conversely, there is a latent period of 8 to 9 days after injection of DHGG before tolerance is detectable in bone marrow cells, and the tolerant state is not complete until day 21. Of more importance to self tolerance is the marked difference in the kinetics of the spontaneous termination of the tolerant state in peripheral B and T cells. Peripheral T cells, like the intact mouse, remain tolerant for 120 to 150 days after injection of DHGG, although peripheral B cells return to complete competency between 50 and 60 days. Another situation in which tolerant T cells coexist with competent B cells is established with low doses of DHGG. The dose of DHGG required to induce tolerance in adult thymus cells is 100 to 1000 times less than that required to induce tolerance in adult bone marrow cells. Similarly, doses required to induce tolerance to bovine serum albumin (BSA) are considerably less in thymus cells compared to bone marrow cells [53] and in peripheral T cells compared to peripheral B cells [54]. Thus, when central unresponsiveness is induced with small doses of antigen, B cells remain competent, while T cells become tolerant. Similar dose-response effects most likely apply to self antigens; antigens present in low concentration in the body fluid would be expected to induce tolerance in only T cells and antigens present in high concentrations should induce tolerance in both

Table 13. Temporal Patterns of Immunologic Unresponsiveness to HGG in A/J Mice*

| Site | Days of | |
	Induction	Maintenance
Thymus	1	120-135
Bone marrow	8-15	40- 50
Spleen: T cells	1	100-150
B cells	2- 4	50- 60
Whole animal	1	130-150

*Injected with 2.5 mg DHGG on day 0.

T and B cells. When T cells are tolerant and B cells are competent, termination of the tolerant state can result by bypassing either the need for, or specificity of, T cells, and the B cells activated by self determinants can produce autoantibody, possibly accompanied by disease. It has been well documented that acquired tolerance induced in experimental animals can be readily terminated when tolerance is only at the T cell level by immunizing with cross-reacting antigen or by injection of B cell activators [reviewed in 55].

A Model of Self-Nonself Discrimination. Since many of the experimental models of central unresponsiveness appear to be the same as tolerance to self antigens, these models have both practical and theoretical implications for the mechanisms involved in self tolerance and autoimmunity. Although autoimmune disease may involve abnormalities in any phase of the complex regulatory system controlling the immune response, events instrumental in initiating autoimmunity are probably dictated by both the manner in which self antigen is presented to the immune system and the immune status of T and B cells in regard to that self antigen. A cellular model of self tolerance can be developed if one accepts the assumption, first, that self tolerance results from a central unresponsive state rather than from peripheral inhibition; second, that self tolerance is dependent on the concentration of the self antigen in the microenvironment of potential self-reactive cells; and third, that the concentration of self antigens required to induce tolerance in T and B cells differs markedly. Thus, the immune status of T and B cells to the self antigen in question may dictate the immunological pathway of a particular autoimmune response. A high degree of tolerance to self antigens such as serum albumin may be present in both T and B cells, although with other antigens (certain classes of Ig, growth hormone and thyroglobulin) a high level of tolerance may exist in T cells while B cells are competent. With still other antigens (cytochrome C, basic protein of myelin, acetylcholine receptor and idiotypic immunoglobulin determinants), both T and B cells may be competent (Fig. 12). In cases of tolerant T cells and competent B cells, the B cells may be triggered by procedures which bypass either the need for, or specificity of, T cells. When neither cell type is tolerant, both can be activated specifically when self antigen is presented in an effective manner. Competent B cells,

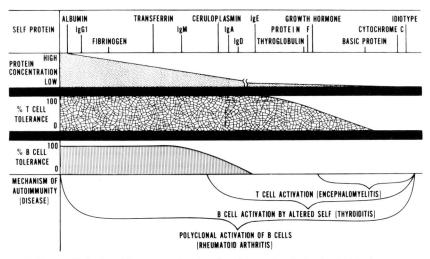

FIG. 12. Relationship among levels of self proteins in body fluids, immune status of T cells and B cells to self proteins and autoimmunity. (Reprinted from Weigle [73].)

of course, are always susceptible to activation by polyclonal B cell activators.

When a self antigen is present in low concentrations, B cells with reactivities ranging from low to high affinity escape tolerance induction and are competent for autologous antigen. Some self antigens present in high concentrations may be able to maintain a tolerant state in both T and B cells with receptors of high to moderate affinity for the antigen; however, even with these antigens the concentration may still be too low to maintain tolerance in those B cells with antigen-reactive receptors of low affinity, since tolerance preferentially affects B cells with a higher affinity for antigen [56]. On the other hand, the affinity of these B cell receptors for self antigen is often inadequate to trigger differentiation and antibody synthesis. However, polyclonal (B cell) activators could trigger such B cells to produce low-affinity antibody. The ability of isolated microbial products as well as microbial, parasitic and viral infections to cause polyclonal activation in vivo is well documented, and often autoantibody has been detected as well [reviewed in 43].

All the incidents of polyclonal activation in vitro are explainable in terms of competent B cells possessing low-affinity receptors to self antigens. How often, or whether, such polyclonal activation occurs in vivo is unclear, but it may be in part responsible for low levels of autoreactive antibody found in the serum of normal individuals. Even if this is antibody to antigens responsible for vital biologic functions and the antibody is plentiful, it would rarely have significant effect because of its negligible affinity and generally low levels of reactivity. A possible exception may be rheumatoid factor in patients with rheumatoid arthritis. The Epstein-Barr (EB) virus has been associated with rheumatoid arthritis in that it is instrumental in producing nuclear antigen reactive with anti-nuclear antibody [57]. It was suggested that EB virus may be an etiologic agent of this disease. EB virus is a potent polyclonal activator of human B cells in vitro, resulting in the production of IgM antibody to HGG [58-60]. Although the avidity of antibody is low, once the HGG-anti-HGG (IgM) complexes are formed, they are relatively stable and biologically active and are capable of activating the complement pathway. In all likelihood, low-avidity antibody is produced by many other self antigens as a result of polyclonal activation, but autoimmune disease does not ensue because of the low affinity of the antibody, or the target antigen is either sequestered or does not play a critical function which is readily interfered with by antibody. Furthermore, most polyclonal activation in vivo may be transient and disappear with elimination of the polyclonal activator, before clinically detectable tissue damage occurs.

Autoimmunity

Experimental Autoimmune Thyroiditis

The classical example of the bypass of tolerant T cells by cross-reacting antigens or altered self antigens is seen with models of experimental autoimmune thyroiditis (EAT) induced with soluble thyroglobulin (Tg). It appears that animals enjoy a high degree of tolerance to syngeneic Tg in their T cells but not in their B cells (Fig. 12). Although EAT has been more commonly produced by immunizing animals with homologous Tg in complete Freund's adjuvant (CFA) [61], it is readily induced by immunization with aqueous preparations of either chemically altered homologous Tg [62] or heterologous

Tg [63]. In rabbits, this model appears to be mediated by antibody and the thyroid lesions are associated with antibody-producing cells to rabbit Tg in the thyroid gland [64]. EAT can also be produced in mice by immunizing with acqueous preparations of heterologous Tg [65, 66]. When thymectomized, irradiated A/J mice are reconstituted with syngeneic spleen cells or a combination of T cells and B cells, but not B cells alone, and immunized with aqueous preparations of heterologous Tg, they produce antibody to both heterologous and mouse Tg and develop lesions [66]. Deleting specific B cells but not specific T cells before reconstituting thymectomized, lethally irradiated mice interferes with the induction of EAT and demonstrates that B cells or a B cell product (antibody) is involved in the induction of this murine model of EAT. In both mice and rabbits, immunization with heterologous Tg apparently bypasses T cell specificity, and the T cells activated by determinants specific for the heterologous Tg supply a second signal for the differentiation of competent B cells that have reacted with self-reactive determinants on the heterologous Tg (Fig. 13). In this model, the rabbit, for example, has both T and B cells that are capable of reacting with nonself (heterologous thyroglobulin) but has only B cells that are capable of reacting

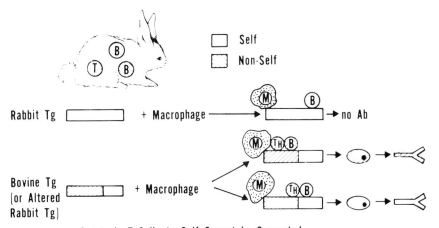

FIG. 13. Cellular events following injection of rabbits with altered homologous and heterologous thyroglobulin (Tg). (Reprinted from Weigle [73].)

with self (syngeneic thyroglobulin). When the rabbit is injected with rabbit thryoglobulin, the macrophage is capable of presenting this self component to competent B cells. However, since self-reactive T cells are not present, the B cells cannot be activated and no antibody is produced. On the other hand, when the rabbit is injected with either a heterologous thyroglobulin or an altered preparation of rabbit thyroglobulin, macrophages present this heterologous antigen to the T cell, which recognizes the nonrelated portion of the molecule, and to the B cell, which recognizes the self portion of the molecule. The B cells are thus turned on to make antibody that is reactive with self and antibody-mediated disease ensues. In this model cytotoxic T cells to self cannot be generated.

In other models in which mice are injected with Tg in CFA, T cells which have a "leaky" tolerance to Tg may become reactive to self-Tg and become a component in the disease process [67].

Experimental Allergic Encephalomyelitis

When the concentration of self antigen is extremely low, complete tolerance is not present in either the T or B cells. In such incidences, an effective exposure to a self antigen may activate both T cells and B cells, resulting in a typical thymus-dependent antibody response. In addition to helper T cells, cytotoxic and possibly suppressor T cells can be activated. However, autoimmunity to these antigens does not usually develop because their concentration is too low. Even if sequestered self antigens are released in high concentrations into the microenvironment of self-reactive lymphocytes as a result of infection or other trauma, the response is transient and probably disappears before clinical symptoms are generated. It is only when antigen is presented so as to persist in an immunogenic form, e.g. when incorporated in CFA, that a progressive autoimmune response accompanied by disease is observed experimentally. The classic example of disease along this pathway is experimental allergic encephalomyelitis (EAE). In contrast to EAT, EAE has been considered to be the result of cell-mediated immunity. EAE is a disease of the central nervous system (CNS) induced by immunization with CNS tissue, basic protein (BP) of myelin or either natural or synthetic polypeptides of BP [reviewed in 68]. In contrast to EAT, binding cells to the responsible antigen (BP) in EAE are present in both the T and B compartments, suggesting that both competent B and competent T cells exist for BP [69]. As an approach to evaluating effector and helper T cells in the initiation of EAE, the EAE-inducing activity of sensitized lymphocytes was assessed after removal of T cells. Lymphocytes were removed from BP-sensitized Lewis rats nine days after injection of BP in CFA, when T cells were no longer required to sustain antibody production, and then used to reconstitute syngeneic, irradiated rats [70]. Without any further stimulation with BP, recipient rats developed antibody, clinical symptoms and histological lesions of EAE. However, prior treatment of the transferred cells with anti-thymus serum plus complement completely circumvented all symptoms and lesions in the recipient, but had no effect on antibody production. Thus, although these recipients had levels of antibody to BP equivalent to those of recipients which received untreated lymphocytes, EAE was not induced. As in the experiments with murine thyroiditis, the selective elimination of BP-specific T and B cells further defined the role of these cells in EAE. Thymectomized, irradiated rats were readily reconstituted with a mixture of purified thymus and bone marrow cells from normal rats in that the recipients, when injected with BP in CFA, developed circulating auto-antibody, clinical symptoms and histological lesions of EAE. On the other hand, neither symptoms, lesions nor antibody to BP resulted when the reconstituting T cells were specifically depleted of BP-reactive cells prior to transfer. However, the specific elimination of BP-reactive cells from B cell preparations prior to transfer along with normal T cells to irradiated recipients did not interfere with either clinical symptoms of EAE or the development of histological lesions following challenge with BP in CFA, although antibody formation was inhibited. The cellular events involved in EAE are depicted in Figure 14. The Lewis rat contains both T and B cells that are capable of reacting with nonself antigens, as well as T and B cells that are capable of reacting with syngeneic basic protein. In this situation when rat basic protein is injected, the macrophage presents this self antigen to cytotoxic T cells (including amplifying T cells), which are the effector cells that cause lesions accompanied by clinical symptoms of EAE.

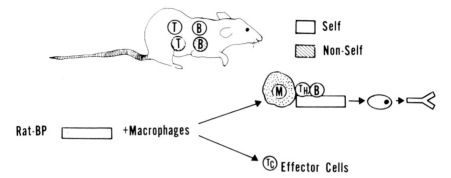

**Effector T Cells Causes Lesions Accompanied by
Clinically Symptoms of EAE**

FIG. 14. Cellular events following immunization of Lewis rats with CFA containing basic protein (BP) of myelin.

Another example of an autoimmune disease in which both competent T cells and competent B cells are present to the self antigen is myasthenia gravis [reviewed in 71]. The antigen involved in this disease is the acetylcholine receptor, which is present in the animals in very small amounts. Tolerance to this self antigen exists in neither the T nor the B cell. Although both T and B cells are activated in the experimental model of myasthenia gravis [72], it is the antibody that is responsible for the disease.

References

1. Janeway, C.A., Jr.: Idiotype, T-cell receptors, and T-B cooperation. Contemp Top. Immunobiol. 9:171-203, 1980.
2. Vadas, M.A., Miller, J.F.A.P., McKenzie, I.F.A. et al: Ly and Ia antigen phenotypes of T cells involved in delayed-type hypersensitivity and in suppression. J. Exp. Med. 144:10-31, 1976.
3. Moorhead, J.W.: Tolerance and contact sensitivity to DNFB in mice. VIII. Identification of distinct T cell subpopulations that mediate *in vivo* and *in vitro* manifestations of delayed hypersensitivity. J. Immunol. 120:137-144, 1978.
4. Faith, R., Luster, M.I. and Moore, J.A.: Chemical separation of helper cell function and delayed hypersensitivity responses. Cell. Immunol. 40:275-284, 1978.
5. Simon, M.M. and Eichmann, K.: T cell subsets participating in the generation of cytotoxic T cells. Springer Semin. Immunopath. 3:39-62, 1980.

6. Cantor, H. and Gershon, R.K.: Immunological circuits: Cellular composition. Symposium. Fed. Proc. 38:2058-2064, 1979.
7. Eardley, D.D.: Feedback suppression: An immunoregulatory circuit. Symposium. Fed. Proc. 39:3114-3116, 1980.
8. Durum, S.K., Eardley, D.D., Green, D.R. et al: Contrasuppression, a newly characterized immunoregulatory circuit: The inducer and acceptor. Fed. Proc. 39:353, 1980.
9. Uhr, J.W. and Möller, G.: Regulatory effect of antibody on the immune response. Adv. Immunol. 8:81-127, 1968.
10. Walker, J.G. and Siskind, G.W.: Studies on the control of antibody synthesis: Effect of antibody affinity upon its ability to suppress antibody formation. Immunology 14:21-28, 1968.
11. Weigle, W.O. and Berman, M.A.: Role of the Fc portion of antibody in immune regulation. In Pernis, B. and Vogel, H. (eds.): Cells of Immunoglobulin Synthesis. New York:Academic Press, Inc., 1979, pp. 223-251.
12. Cerottini, J.-C., McConahey, P.J. and Dixon, F.J.: Specificity of the immunosuppression caused by passive administration of antibody. J. Immunol. 103:268-275, 1969.
13. Feldmann, M. and Diener, E.: Antibody-mediated suppression of the immune response in vitro. IV. The effect of antibody fragments. J. Immunol. 108:93-101, 1972.
14. Sinclair, N.R.St.C., Lees, R.K., Abrahams, S. et al: Regulation of the immune response. X. Antigen-antibody complex inactivation of cells involved in adoptive transfer. J. Immunol. 113:1493-1500, 1974.
15. Kappler, J.W., van der Hoven, A., Dharmarajan, U. and Hoffmann, M.: Regulation of the immune response. IV. Antibody-mediated suppression of the immune response to haptens and heterologous erythrocyte antigens in vitro. J. Immunol. 111:1228-1235, 1973.
16. Hoffmann, M., Kappler, J.W., Herst, J.A. and Oettgen, H.F.: Regulation of the immune response. V. Antibody-mediated inhibition of T and B cell cooperation in the in vitro response to red cell antigen. Eur. J. Immunol. 4:282-286, 1974.
17. Mason, W.M. and Fitch, F.W.: Suppression of the antibody response to SRBC with F(ab')₂ and IgG in vitro. J. Immunol. 110:1427-1429, 1973.
18. Taylor, R.B., Tite, J.P. and Manzo, C.: Immunoregulatory effects of a covalent antigen-antibody complex. Nature 281:488-490, 1979.
19. Rowley, D.A., Fitch, F.W., Axelrod, M.A. and Pierce, C.W.: The immune response suppressed by specific antibody. Immunology 16:549-559, 1969.
20. Morrison, S.L. and Terres, G.: Enhanced immunologic sensitization of mice by the simultaneous injection of antigen and specific antiserum. II. Effect of varying the antigen-antibody ratio and the amount of immune complex injected. J. Immunol. 96:901-905, 1966.
21. Weigle, W.O.: The effect of x-radiation and passive antibody on immunologic tolerance in the rabbit to bovine serum albumin. J. Immunol. 92:113-117, 1964.
22. Berman, M.A. and Weigle, W.O.: B-lymphocyte activation by the Fc region of IgG. J. Exp. Med. 146:241-256, 1977.

23. Morgan, E.L. and Weigle, W.O.: The requirement for adherent cells in the Fc fragment-induced proliferative response of murine spleen cells. J. Exp. Med. 150:256-266, 1979.

24. Higuchi, Y., Ishida, M. and Hayashi, H.: A lymphocyte chemotactic peptide released from immunoglobulin G by neutrophil neutral thiol protease. Cell. Immunol. 46:297-308, 1979.

25. Passwell, J.H., Dayer, J.-M., Gass, K. and Edelson, P.J.: Regulation by Fc fragments of the secretion of collagenase, PGE_2, and lysozyme by mouse peritoneal macrophages. J. Immunol. 125:910-913, 1980.

26. Berman, M.A., Spiegelberg, H.L. and Weigle, W.O.: Lymphocyte stimulation with Fc fragments. I. Class, subclass, and domain of active fragments. J. Immunol. 122:89-96, 1979.

27. Berman, M.A., Morgan, E.L. and Weigle, W.O.: Lymphocyte stimulation with Fc fragments. II. Requirements for mature B lymphocytes. Cell. Immunol. 52:341-349, 1980.

28. Morgan, E.L. and Weigle, W.O.: Regulation of Fc fragment-induced murine spleen cell proliferation. J. Exp. Med. 151:1-11, 1980.

29. Morgan, E.L. and Weigle, W.O.: Regulation of lymphocyte activation by the Fc portion of immunoglobulin. J. Supramol. Struct. (In press.)

30. Morgan, E.L. and Weigle, W.O.: Polyclonal activation of murine B lymphocytes by Fc fragments. I. The requirement for two signals in the generation of the polyclonal antibody response induced by Fc fragments. J. Immunol. 124:1330-1335, 1980.

31. Thoman, M.L., Morgan, E.L. and Weigle, W.O.: Polyclonal activation of murine B lymphocytes by Fc fragments. II. Replacement of T cells by a soluble helper T cell replacing factor (TRF). J. Immunol. 125:1630-1633, 1980.

32. Thoman, M.L., Morgan, E.L. and Weigle, W.O.: Fc fragment activation of T lymphocytes. I. Fc fragments trigger Lyt 1^+23^- T lymphocytes to release a helper T cell replacing activity. J. Immunol. (In press.)

33. Dutton, R.: Separate signals for the initiation of proliferation and differentiation in the B cell response to antigens. Transplant. Rev. 23:66-77, 1975.

34. Schimpl, A. and Wecker, E.: A third signal in B cell activation given by TRF. Transplant. Rev. 23:176-188, 1975.

35. Morgan, E.L. and Weigle, W.O.: Aggregated human γ-globulin-induced proliferation and polyclonal activation of murine B lymphocytes. J. Immunol. 125:226-231, 1980.

36. Morgan, E.L., Walker, S.M., Thoman, M.L. and Weigle, W.O.: Regulation of the immune response. I. The potentiation of in vivo and in vitro immune responses by Fc fragments. J. Exp. Med. 152:113-123, 1980.

37. Morgan, E.L., Thoman, M.L.. Walker, S.M. and Weigle, W.O.: Regulation of the immune response. II. Characterization of the cell population(s) involved in the Fc fragment-induced adjuvant effect. J. Immunol. 125:1275-1279, 1980.

38. Morgan, E.L., Thoman, M.L. and Weigle, W.O.: Enhancement of T-lymphocyte functions by Fc fragments of immunoglobulins. I. Augmentation of allogeneic mixed lymphocyte culture reactions

requires I-A or I-B subregion differences between effector and stimulator. J. Exp. Med. (In press.)

39. Wettstein, P.J., Bailey, D.W., Mobraaten, L.E. et al: T-lymphocytes response to H-2 mutants. I. Proliferation is dependent on Ly 1^+2^+ cells. J. Exp. Med. 147:1395-1404, 1978.

40. Okada, M. and Henney, C.S.: The differentiation of cytotoxic T cells *in vitro*. II. Amplifying factor(s) produced in primary mixed lymphocyte cultures against K/D stimuli require the presence of Lyt 2^+ cells but not Lyt 1^+ cells. J. Immunol. 125:300-307, 1980.

41. Bach, F.H. and Alter, B.J.: Alternative pathways of T lymphocyte activation. J. Exp. Med. 148:829-934, 1978.

42. Weigle, W.O.: Analysis of autoimmunity through experimental models of thyroiditis and experimental allergic encephalomyelitis. Adv. Immunol. 30:159-273, 1980.

43. Weigle, W.O.: Central *versus* peripheral mechanisms in the control of antiself reactions. *In* Sercarz, E. and Cunningham, A.J. (eds.): Strategies of Immune Regulation. New York:Academic Press, Inc., 1980, pp. 121-122.

44. Dresser, D.W.: Specific inhibition of antibody production. II. Paralysis induced in adult mice by small quantities of protein antigen. Immunology 5:378-388, 1962.

45. Habicht, G.S., Chiller, J.M. and Weigle, W.O.: Methods for the study of the cellular basis of immunological tolerance. *In* Zacharia, T.P. (ed.): Methods in Molecular Biology. Immune Response at the Cellular Level. New York:Marcel Dekker, Inc., 1973, pp. 141-160.

46. Louis, J., Chiller, J.M. and Weigle, W.O.: Fate of antigen-binding cells in unresponsive and immune mice. J. Exp. Med. 137:461-469, 1973.

47. Chiller, J.M. and Weigle, W.O.: Cellular events during induction of immunologic unresponsiveness in adult mice. J. Immunol. 106:1647-1653, 1971.

48. Parks, D.E., Doyle, M.V. and Weigle, W.O.: Induction and mode of action of suppressor cells to human gamma globulin. I. An immunologic unresponsive state devoid of suppressor cells. J. Exp. Med. 148:625-638, 1978.

49. Parks, D.E., Shaller, D.A. and Weigle, W.O.: Induction and mode of action of suppressor cells generated against human gamma globulin. J. Exp. Med. 149:1168-1182, 1979.

50. Parks, D.E. and Weigle, W.O.: Maintenance of immunologic unresponsiveness to human γ-globulin. Evidence for irreversible inactivation of B lymphocytes. J. Immunol. 124:1230-1236, 1980.

51. Chiller, J.M., Habicht, G.S. and Weigle, W.O.: Cellular sites of immunologic unresponsiveness. Proc. Natl. Acad. Sci. U.S.A. 65:551-556, 1970.

52. Chiller, J.M., Habicht, G.S. and Weigle, W.O.: Kinetic differences in unresponsiveness of thymus and bone marrow cells. Science 171:813-815, 1971.

53. Katsura, Y., Kawaguchi, S. and Muramatsu, S.: Difference in the target cells for tolerance induction in relation to the dose of tolerogen. Immunology 23:537-544, 1972.

54. Rajewsky, K. and Brenig, C.: Paralysis to serum albumins in T and B lymphocytes in mice. Dose dependence, specificity and kinetics of escape. Eur. J. Immunol. 4:120-125, 1974.

55. Weigle, W.O.: Immunological unresponsiveness. Adv. Immunol. 16:61-122, 1973.

56. Theis, G.A. and Siskind, G.W.: Selection of cell populations in induction of tolerance: Affinity of antibody formed in partially tolerant rabbits. J. Immunol. 100:138-141, 1968.

57. Alspaugh, M.A., Jensen, F.C., Rabin, H. and Tan, E.M.: Lymphocytes transformed by Epstein-Barr virus: Induction of nuclear antigen reactive with antibody in rheumatoid arthritis. J. Exp. Med. 147:1018-1027, 1978.

58. Rosen, A., Gergely, P., Jandel, M., Klein, G. and Britton, S.: Polyclonal Ig production after Epstein-Barr virus infection of human lymphocytes in vitro. Nature 267:52-54, 1977.

59. Luzzati, A.L., Hengartner, H. and Schreier, M.H.: Induction of plaque-forming cells in cultured human lymphocytes by combined action of antigen and EB virus. Nature 269:419-420, 1977.

60. Slaughter, L., Carson, D.A., Jensen, F.C. et al: In vitro effects of Epstein-Barr virus on peripheral blood mononuclear cells from patients with rheumatoid arthritis and normal subjects. J. Exp. Med. 148:1429-1434, 1978.

61. Rose, N.R. and Witebsky, E.: Studies on organ specificity. V. Changes in the thyroid glands of rabbits following active immunization with rabbit-thyroid extracts. J. Immunol. 76:417-427, 1956.

62. Weigle, W.O.: The production of thyroiditis and antibody following injection of unaltered thyroglobulin without adjuvant into rabbits previously stimulated with altered thyroglobulin. J. Exp. Med. 122:1049-1062, 1965.

63. Weigle, W.O. and Nakamura, R.M.: The development of autoimmune thyroiditis in rabbits following injection of aqueous preparations of heterologous thyroglobulins. J. Immunol. 99:223-231, 1967.

64. Clinton, B.A. and Weigle, W.O.: Cellular events during the induction of experimental thyroiditis in the rabbit. J. Exp. Med. 136:1605-1615, 1972.

65. Nakamura, R.M. and Weigle, W.O.: Experimental thyroiditis in complement intact and deficient mice following injections of heterologous thyroglobulins without adjuvant. Proc. Soc. Exp. Biol. Med. 129:412-416, 1968.

66. Clagett, J.A. and Weigle, W.O.: Roles of T and B lymphocytes in the termination of unresponsiveness to autologous thyroglobulin in mice. J. Exp. Med. 139:643-660, 1974.

67. Kong, Y.M., David, C.S., Giraldo, A.A. et al: Regulation of autoimmune response to mouse thyroglobulin: Influence of H-2 D-end genes. J. Immunol. 123:15-18, 1979.

68. Paterson, P.Y.: The demyelinating diseases: Clinical and experimental studies in animals and man. In Samter, M., Talmage, D.W., Rose, B. et al (eds.): Immunological Diseases. New York:Little, Brown and Co., Inc., 1978, pp. 1400-1435.

69. Ortiz-Ortiz, L. and Weigle, W.O.: Cellular events in the induction of experimental allergic encephalomyelitis. J. Exp. Med. 144:604-616, 1976.

70. Ortiz-Oritz, L., Nakamura, R.M. and Weigle, W.O.: T cell requirement for experimental allergic encephalomyelitis induction in the rat. J. Immunol. 117:576-579, 1976.

71. Lindstrom, J.: Autoimmune response to acetylcholine receptors in myasthenia gravis and its animal model. Adv. Immunol. 27:1-50, 1979.

72. De Baets, M.H., Einarson, B., Lindstrom, J.M. and Weigle, W.O.: Cellular and humoral mechanisms in experimental autoimmune myasthenia gravis. Fed. Proc. (In press.)

73. Weigle, W.O.: The discrimination between self and nonself. In Gale, R.P. and Fox, C.P. (eds.): Biology of Bone Marrow Transplantation. New York:Academic Press, Inc., 1980, p. 341.

Antigen-Specific T Lymphocytes: Propagation, Activation and Function

Elaine DeFreitas, Ph.D., Barry Skidmore, Ph.D.,
Scott Young, B.S., Janice White, M.S.
and Jacques M. Chiller, Ph.D.

Introduction

In recent years, studies dissecting the cellular basis of immunity have led to the concept that the immune system is a web of interacting cells and molecules responsive, on one hand, to external stimuli and controlled, on the other hand, by internal regulatory signals and pathways. The most striking example of the progress which has been made in this regard is the analysis of T lymphocyte activation. Thus, it is now generally accepted that specific activation of the T cells by antigen requires the participation of accessory cells, most likely macrophages; that the interactions between T cells and macrophages are restricted by products of the major histocompatibility complex (MHC); that such restriction is a behavior learned or selected for within a particular genetic environment; and that cytokines of either macrophage or lymphocyte origin may provide the intermediatory molecules required for the completion of cellular commitment and expansion.

Antigen- or mitogen-induced T cell proliferation has provided the best experimental system by which to study macro-

Elaine DeFreitas, Ph.D., Barry Skidmore, Ph.D., Scott Young, B.S., Janice White, M.S. and Jacques M. Chiller, Ph.D., Department of Medicine, National Jewish Hospital and Research Center, Denver, Colo.

This work was supported by USPHS grants #AI-13131 and CA-21825, Training Grant AI-00048 (E.D.), NIH Young Investigator Research Award NIH AI-16573 (B.S.) and NIH RCDA AI-00133 (J.C.).

phage-lymphocyte interactions. Although initial studies to that aim used human cells [1, 2], the most salient observations have been made more recently with cells from guinea pigs and mice. Murine cells are particularly useful since they are amenable to purification schemes and can be obtained from recombinant strains, permitting genetic mapping of the elements necessary for interactions. A set of general conclusions emanating from a large number of studies of antigen-induced T cell proliferation can be summarized as follows: Antigen-dependent T cell activation requires accessory cells (Ia$^+$ macrophages) whose function is essential as antigen-presenting cells [3-10]. Furthermore, there is a requirement for compatibility at the I region of the MHC between the interacting sets of cells [3-10], a conclusion which is also applicable to other interactions involving lymphocytes, for example T-B collaboration [11, 12], cytotoxic T cell-target interactions [13] and T cell activity leading to delayed-type hypersensitivity (DTH) [14]. In essence, it appears that most T lymphocytes must recognize specific antigen in the context of self molecules coded by regions of the MHC, either I in the case of T cell proliferation, T-B collaboration and DTH, or K or D in the case of cytotoxic T cells. Suppressor cells may be an example of one T cell subpopulation that may be an exception to this rule [15-17], although it is still not well established whether it is the activation of these cells or their mode of action which reflects lack of restriction.

Recent experiments have provided further understanding of the mechanisms by which accessory cell-dependent T cell activation occurs. Although the process of T cell proliferation per se requires a cell growth factor, recently termed interleukin-2 (IL-2) [18, 19], such factors do not induce growth in resting T cells [20]. However, the latter can be rendered sensitive to IL-2 by a short pulse of specific ligands in the form of either mitogens [21] or antigen [22], a process which apparently leads to T cell activation and the expression of putative receptors for IL-2 [23]. Our own efforts have focused on defining those elements which are necessary to render T cells sensitive to IL-2 [24]. The conclusions from studies to be detailed in this communication are that the process requires macrophage-T cell H-2-restricted cooperation which can be divided into two signals, namely the recognition by T cells of antigen/Ia presented by accessory cells (signal 1) and the action on T cells of a macrophage product in the form of lymphocyte-activating factor (signal 2), more recently termed interleukin-1 (IL-1). IL-1 was described some years ago as a monokine which augments proliferative response to lectins [25, 26], promotes T cell-dependent in vitro antibody responses [27] and enhances the development of cytotoxic T cells [28]. It is of specific interest that IL-1 acts on stimulated T cells (late G_1), causing a calcium-dependent use in cyclic GMP which appears closely linked to the later initiation of DNA synthesis and mitogens [29-31]. The observation that IL-1 is effective if added to stimulated cells only after 14 hours following triggering with mitogen is compatible with other data showing that triggering of DNA synthesis by mitogen [33, 34] or antigen [35] requires two successive stimulatory signals and that the second of these, starting at 15 to 18 hours, may require or be mimicked by the action of macrophage products [35, 36].

A major factor which has hampered the progress and interpretation of studies relating to lymphocyte activation and regulation has been the fact that the cellular components of the immune system are extremely heterogenous, not only from the standpoint of distinct populations of functional cells but also from the perspective of the clonal spectrum within each subpopulation. Recent developments in a number of laboratories have provided the potential means by which to overcome this problem in the capacity to obtain lines of enriched or clonally derived specific T cells [37-46]. Derivation of T cell hybridoma lines whose induction is antigen-specific and MHC-restricted [47] provides an additional experimental tour de force in that specific activation can be quickly and readily monitored. Coupled to the availability of lines of cells which produce quantities of cytokines such as IL-1 [48] or IL-2 [49], conditions now exist which permit a more precise analysis of specific T lymphocyte activation/recognition.

Propagation of Antigen-Specific T Lymphocytes

We have previously described methodologies by which to enrich and propagate antigen-specific murine T lymphocytes which possess specific function. A brief description of such procedures is as follows: Mice are primed subcutaneously at the base of the tail with 50 to 100 μg of antigen emulsified in CFA, and seven days later the para-aortic and inguinal lymph nodes are harvested [50]. These lymph node cells are cultured at 4 × 10^6/ml in Click's medium containing 0.5% to 1.0% fresh syngeneic normal mouse serum and 10 to 100 μg/ml of antigen [22]. After four days of culture, the live cells are recovered on Ficoll-Hypaque gradients and cultured for an additional three to four days in RPMI medium supplemented with 5% FCS and IL-2 obtained either from a Con A-induced T cell hybridoma [49] or as the supernatant fluid (SUP) from normal mouse spleen cells incubated with a mitogenic concentration of Con A for 24 hours, then supplemented with α-methyl mannoside to neutralize residual Con A. This procedure yields a population of cells with the following physical and functional characteristics:

1. The cells are >99% Thy 1^+, Ly 1^+, Ly $2,3^-$.
2. They proliferate in vitro in response to challenge with specific antigen in the presence of I region-compatible macrophages (Table 1).
3. They function as specific helper cells for hapten-primed histocompatible B cells in a modified in vitro Mishell-Dutton system (Table 2).
4. Such proliferative and helper activities are profoundly (>100-fold) enriched as a consequence of in vitro propagation when compared to cells tested directly from primed animals.

Using this methodology, cells specific for the following antigens have been cultured: OVA, HGG, KLH, beef apo-cytochrome c, (T,G)-A--L and Sendai virus.

The methods can be applied to obtain not only short-term propagated T lymphocytes, but, in addition, T cells which can be maintained for prolonged periods (up to 12 months). Further, the technology can be extended to obtain clonally derived lines of antigen-specific, functional T cells in the following fashion. Propagated lines, which after five to eight weeks in culture show proper specificity and restriction, are utilized for cloning by seeding into wells of microtiter plates 100 μl of a suspension containing 5 × 10^5 accessory cells and an appropriate concentration of IL-2. Each well is then supplemented with 100 μl of a suspension containing IL-2 and propagated T cells (averaging less than one cell/well). Plates are

Table 1. Genetic Restriction in Cooperative Interactions Between
OVA-Specific Propagated T Cells and Accessory Cells

T-Cells*	Strain	K	I-A	I-B	I-J	I-E	I-C	D	Response‡ cpm ± (SE) × 10^{-3}
B10.A	B10.A	k̲	k̲	k̲	k̲	k̲	d̲	d̲	63.3 (0.8)
B10.A	B10.TL	s	k̲	k̲	k̲	k̲	k	d̲	72.1 (2.4)
B10.A	B10.S(7R)	s	s	s	s	s	s	d̲	1.7 (0.9)
B10.A	B10.A(4R)	k̲	k̲	b	b	b	b	b	82.9 (0.2)
B10.A	B10.A(5R)	b	b	b	k̲	k̲	d̲	d̲	9.3 (0.8)
B10.A	B10.D2	d	d	d	d	d	d̲	d̲	1.6 (0.5)
B10.A	B10	b	b	b	b	b	b	b	3.3 (0.7)
B10.A	none								0.3 (0.1)

*Lymph node cells obtained from mice immunized IT seven days previously with
100 μg of OVA in CFA were cultured at 4×10^6 cells/ml in Click's medium supplemented
with 1% syngeneic NMS and 100 μg/ml OVA. After four days of culture the viable cells
were isolated on Ficoll-Hypaque gradients and cultured for an additional four days in IL-2-
containing medium (24-hour-culture supernatants from Con A-stimulated mouse spleen
cells). Such IL-2-propagated T cell blasts were cultured at 10^4 cells per microtiter well for
assay of antigen-induced proliferative response.

†Accessory cells were spleen cells obtained from normal donors, exposed in vitro to
3,000 rads of irradiation, and cultured at 5×10^5 cells per microtiter well.

‡The responses shown represent the net incorporation of ^{3}H-TdR obtained in cultures
stimulated with 100 μg/ml OVA after subtraction of incorporation into saline-treated controls, the latter usually ranging between 500 and 2000 cpm. Cultures were harvested at the
peak of the proliferative response (day 3) after a 24-hour pulse with ^{3}H-TdR.

incubated for one week at 37°C, 2% CO_2, after which time 100
μl of the supernatant fluid is removed and replaced with 100 μl
of fresh medium/IL-2 solution. Positive growth usually becomes
evident by 10 to 14 days. Next 100 to 150 μl of the content of
the positive wells is transferred to larger vessels (Costar plates)
with a 1-ml suspension containing fresh IL-2, antigen and
accessory cells (5×10^6). Growth is then followed and cultures
are further expanded to flasks under the same conditions.

The results of a representative experiment are shown in
Table 3. In this case, cells from several clones displayed the
capacity, on one hand, to proliferate in the response to specific
antigen (human γ-globulin) in the presence of restricted
accessory cells and, on the other hand, provided specific help to
a source of hapten-primed B cells/accessory cells in the response

Table 2. Comparative Helper Capacity of Lymph Node Cells, Ag-Induced Blasts and SUP-Propagated Blasts*

Helper Cells No. × 10⁻⁴	Response (PFC/10⁶)†								
	LNC			Ag Blasts			SUP Blasts		
	Med	DNP-O	DNP-K	Med	DNP-O	DNP-K	Med	DNP-O	DNP-K
25	4	3,300	275	—	—	—	—	—	—
5	4	400	60	49	3,100	10	0	1,467	4
1	12	113	56	40	2,000	25	15	4,000	3
0.2	4	20	8	7	380	51	0	1,157	1
0.1	3	0	4	1	0	15	0	219	0
0.1 (NMS + C)‡							—	1,067	—
0.2 (NMS + C)							—	1,328	—
0.1 (Thy 1.2 + C)‡							—	19	—
0.2 (Thy 1.2 + C)							—	3	—

*Comparative helper activity of BDF_1-primed lymph node cells, antigen-activated blast cells and SUP-propagated blast cells as a function of decreasing number of helper cells/well. DNP-KLH-primed BDF_1 spleen cells treated with anti-Thy 1.2 + C were used as a source of B cells (5×10^5 cells/well).

†Indirect plaque-forming cells (PFC) from triplicate cultures expressed as PFC/10^6 spleen cells. The data presented are day 6 responses; similar trends were obtained on days 5 and 3. DNP-OVA (DNP-O), DNP-KLH (DNP-K) or medium (Med.) was added to each source of helper cells evaluated. The anti-Thy 1 + C treatment of the B cell source allowed DNP-KLH was 3,933 before and 87 after removal of Thy 1^+ cells. Nonconjugated SRBC were tested in each group and few, if any, plaques to SRBC were observed. Lymph node cells, antigen-induced or supernatant-grown blast cells cultured without hapten-primed spleen cells did not produce PFC even in the presence of specific antigen.

‡SUP-propagated blast cells were treated with either normal mouse serum (NMS) + C or anti-Thy 1.2 + C before assessment for helper function.

Table 3. Functional Analysis of Clonally Derived T Cells*

| | *Response* | |
Clone No.	PFC/10^6	CPM $\times$ 10^{-3}
72, 71, 57	25,000 → 14,500 (IgM, IgG)	12 → 9
52, 36, 46, 25	7,000 → 4,000 (IgM, IgG)	14 → 8
10, 1, 31, 37	1,500 → 800 (IgM)	12 → 10
75, 48, 45	<100	12 → 9
54, 63, 61	<100	0.2

*BDF_1 cells were derived using a protocol described in the text. Various clones were tested for two functions, namely help and antigen-induced proliferation. The former involved admixing T cells with 1.25×10^5 anti-Thy 1.2 + C-treated spleen cells from BDF_1 mice previously immunized with DNP-KLH. After four or seven days in modified Mishell-Dutton conditions, hapten-specific direct (IgM) and indirect (IgG) PFC were quantitated. Various numbers of T cells were titrated, but data presented represent those obtained with 6×10^3 cells from each clone. No responses were obtained with DNP-KLH as antigen. Numbers represent DNP-lysine-inhibitable PFC. Proliferation (uptake of ^{3}HTdR) involved testing the capacity of 10^4 T cells to respond to specific (HGG) or non-cross-reactive (OVA) antigen in the presence of a source of irradiated accessory cells (2.5×10^5 syngeneic spleen cells). In all cases, only responses to HGG were seen. Data present the range of responses obtained with the various clones tested.

to DNP-HGG. Although the extent of the proliferative response was relatively invariant from one positive line to another, helper function revealed far more heterogeneity. In addition, some lines proliferated in response to specific antigen but did not display help. A number of clones showed neither reactivity; presumably, such lines were selected for their capacity to grow in IL-2.

Activation of Propagated T Lymphocytes

Thus T cells from lymph nodes of immunized animals, after activation in vitro with antigen, can be propagated in the following conditions: (1) with specific antigen and a source of irradiated syngeneic accessory cells, (2) in the absence of antigen and accessory cells but in the presence of a source of IL-2, or (3) using the combination of both approaches. Such cells can be maintained in culture for prolonged periods and show enriched function, defined either by the capacity to proliferate specifically to antigen in the context of H-2 (Ia)-restricted accessory cells or by the ability to provide carrier-specific T help in the response of hapten-primed B cells to haptenated carrier proteins. Those T lymphocytes propagated in a source of IL-2 without either antigen or accessory cells provide an exquisite means by which to study accessory cell-dependent antigen stimulation since, when such cells are removed from the IL-2 source, they will continue to proliferate only when supplemented with specific antigen and syngeneic spleen or LN accessory cells which can be defined as plastic-adherent, Ig^-, Thy 1^-, esterase-staining and 50% to 60% Ia^+. Thus, the technique of in vitro enrichment and propagation of such T lymphocytes provides not only a source of cells whose activation obeys requirements similar to those previously described by others using cells from immune tissues but, in addition, populations which can be markedly enriched for specific activity, even cloned (*vide supra*) so as to permit analysis of the activation of small numbers of cells.

In experiments aimed at delineating the requirement for the specific activation of propagated T lymphocytes, it was observed that whereas antigen and either nontreated or γ-irradiated accessory cells supported T cell proliferation, antigen and UV-irradiated cells did not. Further, the same relationship held when accessory cells were pulsed with antigen prior to treatment with either γ or UV irradiation. However, antigen-pulsed, UV-irradiated accessory cells were capable of stimulating T cells when supplemented with a source of IL-1, usually obtained as the supernatant fluid from a murine macrophage line, P388 D1 (Table 4). It should be stressed that the T cells used in these experiments were those which were propagated in IL-2 to a point when further growth on IL-2 alone did not occur. Such cells could only be restimulated with antigen-pulsed accessory cells. Additional relevant observations in this system were that (1) IL-1 alone failed to stimulate, (2) stimulation was dependent on specific antigen, and (3) the source of antigen-pulsed UV accessory cells needed to be homologous with the T lymphocytes, restriction mapping to the *Ia* region of the MHC, more specifically I-A and I-E/C (Table 5). Further, fractionation

Table 4. Activation of Propagated T Cells*

Accessory Cell Treatment	Response – cpm (SEM) × 10^{-3}
None	0.2 (0.1)
OVA	26.3 (3.4)
OVA-pulsed, γ-irrad. (4000 rads)	36.2 (6.4)
OVA-pulsed, UV-irrad.	2.6 (0.8)
OVA-pulsed, UV-irrad. + Con A SUP	21.7 (3.3)
Con A SUP alone	4.1 (3.1)
OVA-pulsed, UV-irrad. + IL-1	26.9 (2.8)
HGG-pulsed, UV-irrad. + IL-1	1.6 (0.8)
IL-1 alone	1.1 (0.2)

*Lymph node cells obtained from BDF_1 mice, primed at the base of tail seven days previously with OVA in CFA, were cultured with OVA for four days. Following Ficoll separation, viable cells were reseeded with antigen and syngenic irradiated (4000 rads) cells for another four days, at which time Ficoll-separated cells were cultured in the *absence* of antigen and accessory cells, but in the presence of a source of IL-2 (designated as Con A SUP and representing supernatant fluids obtained following a 24-hour incubation of BDF_1 spleen cells and Con A, then supplemented with α-methyl mannoside). Such cells were propagated for 7 to 11 days to a stage where they no longer grew in IL-2 alone. Then 10^4 cells were seeded in microtiter wells with accessory cells (splenic adherent cells) treated in the conditions described in the Table. The source of IL-1 was treated supernatant fluid from the murine macrophage line P388 D1, utilized at a final concentration of 20%. Irradiation consisted of exposure to 4000 rads (γ) or for 5 minutes, 20 cm from a 30-W germicidal lamp (UV). Cells were incubated for three days, pulsed 24 hours with ^{3}HTdR, harvested and uptake of label quantified by scintillation counting.

of the IL-1 source revealed that the activity resided primarily within a peak having a molecular weight of 14,000 to 16,000 daltons, a size compatible with that previously described for murine IL-1.

The following hypothetical scheme thus emerges as a basis underlying the process of antigen-triggered T cell activation. T lymphocytes, more specifically T cells functionally tested for help or for proliferation, require two obligatory signals for activation: the recognition on macrophages of antigen presented in the context of self Ia (signal 1) and the binding of IL-1 (signal 2), itself produced by macrophages as a consequence of back stimulation by T cells. Signal 1 also leads to the expression of IL-1 acceptor sites on T cells. Unless signal 2 (IL-1) is available to signal 1-induced T cells (expressing IL-1 acceptor sites), such

Table 5. Restriction of Stimulation of B10.A T Cells with OVA-Pulsed,
UV-Treated Filler Cells and IL-1*

| UV-Treated Accessory Cells | H-2 Homology | Response ± SE × 10⁻³ | |
		−IL	+IL−1
B10.A	K-D	1.2 (0.6)	12.3 (0.1)
B10	none	0.5 (0.1)	0.2 (0.1)
B10.A(4R)	K, IA	1.8 (1.0)	19.3 (1.6)
B10.A(5R)	IE → D	1.0 (0.3)	5.4 (0.7)
B10.TL	IA, B, K, E, D	2.6 (1.0)	22.2 (2.4)
B10.S(7R)	D	0.1 (0.1)	0.3 (0.1)
None	−	0.1 (0.1)	0.2 (0.1)

*The methods are similar to those described in Table 4, with the exception that
T cells specific to OVA were obtained from B10.A-primed mice. The data shown
represent those derived when 10^4 propagated B10.A T cells were incubated with
IL-1 (P388D-derived; 25% final concentration) and accessory cells (normal spleen
cells) from the sources listed. Such cells were pulsed with OVA (1 mg/ml) for three
hours, then washed and irradiated with UV light.

cells will not become activated but may become specifically
anergic. The sum total of signal 1/signal 2 results in T cell
activation, i.e. differentiation to a stage where IL-2 acceptor
sites are expressed. In the presence of IL-2, T cell proliferation
and amplification proceed. In the absence of IL-2, activated
cells revert to a "resting" stage and subsequent triggering once
again requires the same sequence of signals. Thus three stages
can be envisioned in the process of T cell proliferation, namely
induction, requiring the interaction with antigen-self and
leading, on one hand, to the expression of IL-1 acceptor sites on
T cells and, on the other hand, to back stimulation of the
interacting macrophages; activation, requiring the interaction
with IL-1 and leading to the expression of IL-2 acceptor sites;
and proliferation, requiring the interaction with IL-2 and
leading to cell replication. A diagrammatic representation of the
scheme is presented in Figure 1.
    Although the conceptual genesis postulating that lympho-
cyte triggering requires separate signals has had a long history
[51], perhaps the most thorough treatise of the hypothesis was
elaborated over a decade ago [52] and revised and refined since
then [53-56]. Notwithstanding the controversy which exists for
B cell triggering [43], there is a body of evidence which in

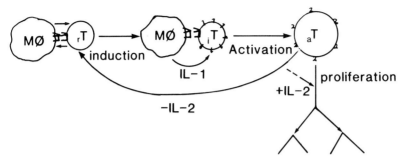

FIG. 1. Hypothetical scheme for T lymphocyte induction, activation and proliferation. Key: $_rT$ = resting T cell; $_iT$ = induced T cell; $_aT$ = activated T cell; 1 = acceptor sites on $_iT$ for IL-1; 2 = acceptor sites on $_aT$ for IL-2.

effect supports the notion that T cell activation may be governed by such a general scheme [24, 58, 59]. An important prediction from this concept is that whereas two signals are necessary for lymphocyte induction, a single signal — more specifically, antigen — in the absence of the second signal may lead to specific lymphocyte anergy or tolerance. Although formal proof for such a pathway has not been presented, data which we have recently obtained are certainly compatible with that possibility. Thus exposure of T cells to antigen/Ia in the absence of IL-1 leads to specific anergy in such lymphocytes [60].

T Lymphocyte Function

While the foregoing experiments add to and extend the notion that T cell induction requires, in part, recognition of antigen presented by macrophages in a self-restricted context, they do not address the question of whether similar restrictions govern interaction with specific B lymphocytes, enabling the latter to produce immunoglobulin. To delve into that issue the following approach was utilized. The in vitro response to DNP was evaluated by using combinations of cells and antigens in the form of (a) propagated T cells with specificity to OVA, (b) B cells/macrophages obtained after anti-Thy 1.2 and complement treatment of spleens from animals originally primed with DNP-KLH, and (c) the antigen DNP-OVA or DNP-KLH. The T lymphocytes used in the experiments to be described were F_1 cells propagated in such a way as to select for populations which were restricted in their response to OVA on one *or* the other parental haplotype. Thus, OVA-primed lymph node T cells from BDF_1 mice (H-$2^{b/d}$) were propagated with antigen and either BDF_1-, B10 (H-2^d)- or B10.D2 (H-2^d)-irradiated accessory cells. Following several alternative cycles of propagation on antigen/accessory cells and in IL-2 alone, cells were obtained with the characteristics seen in Table 6. T cells propagated on F_1 accessory cells were capable of responding to OVA in the presence of irradiated accessory cells possessing either H-2^b (B10), H-2^b (B10.D2) or both (BDF_1) haplotypes. T cells obtained under conditions of propagation with B10 accessory cells responded to antigen in the presence of either B10 or BDF_1 but not in the presence of B10.D2 accessory cells. Reciprocally, cells propagated on B10.D2 cells were capable of responding to OVA in the presence of B10.D2 or BDF_1 but not in the presence of B10 accessory cells. Thus, under the appropriate selective conditions, it is possible to propagate T lymphocytes from F_1 animals which can recognize specific antigen in the context of either one or the other parental

Table 6. Proliferative Response of BDF_1 T Cells Specific to OVA and Selected on F_1 or Parental Haplotypes

T Cells* Selected on	OVA	Accessory Cells:	BDF_1	B10	B10.D2
			\multicolumn{3}{c}{Response† – cpm + SE × 10^{-3}}		
BDF_1	–		1.3 (0.6)	0.6 (0.4)	0.6 (0.3)
BDF_1	+		19.8 (1.3)	16.1 (1.0)	10.2 (1.1)
B10	–		0.4 (0.1)	0.3 (0.2)	0.3 (0.1)
B10	+		26.1 (2.4)	28.9 (3.1)	1.1 (0.6)
B10.D2	–		0.4 (0.1)	0.5 (0.1)	0.7 (0.4)
B10.D2	+		19.6 (1.8)	3.1 (1.9)	20.1 (2.4)

*Lymph node T cells from BDF_1 mice primed with 100 μg OVA in CFA were propagated by three cycles alternating between OVA and irradiated (4000 rads) normal spleen cells + OVA or IL-2. Selection was performed by using irradiated accessory cells from either BDF_1, B10 or B10.D2 animals. In the proliferative assay, 10^4 T cells/well were used.

†Responses represent those obtained by admixing 10^4 T cells, 4×10^5 accessory cells (4000 rad spleen cells) ± OVA (100 μg/ml). Peak ^{3}HTdR incorporation was measured by pulsing cultures (triplicate wells) for 24 hours on day 2 of incubation.

haplotype. Restricted functional activity not only can be obtained in the context of proliferation but also can be observed with specific helper function. The data presented in Table 7 demonstrate that helper activity of B10-selected T cells was evident in the presence of a source of B cells/macrophages from BDF_1 or B10 mice but not from B10.D2 animals. Conversely, the helper activity of B10.D2-selected T cells was restricted to a B cell source with the H-2^d haplotype (F_1, B10.D2) but not with the H-2^b haplotype (B10).

In view of the fact that the process leading to antibody formation involves the interaction between accessory cells (macrophages), T and B lymphocytes, the restriction seen for helper function could reflect that occurring between macrophages and T cells or between T and B lymphocytes, or both. In order to gain insight into the cellular levels of restriction inherent in this system, experiments were performed in which T cells selected to interact with only one parental strain were admixed with antigen and *both* parental types of hapten-primed B cells and macrophages. The haplotype of the responding B cells was determined at the time of assay by typing the

Table 7. Helper Capacity of BDF_1 T Cells Specific to OVA and Selected on F_1 Parental Haplotypes

T Cells*		Response†	PFC/10^6 B Cells		
Selected on	Antigen	B cells/MØ:	BDF_1	B10	B10.D2
BDF_1	DNP-KLH		20	40	20
BDF_1	DNP-OVA		1,890	610	1,040
B10	DNP-KLH		40	20	20
B10	DNP-OVA		1,030	430	20
B10.D2	DNP-KLH		40	40	20
B10.D2	DNP-OVA		1,060	30	1,010

*T cells were selected and propagated as described in Table 6 and used at 10^4 cells/well.

†Responses were evaluated either to specific hapten carrier (DNP-OVA) or non-cross-reactive hapten carrier (DNP-KLH). B cells/macrophages (MØ) were obtained after treating spleens from DNP-KLH-primed mice (BDF_1, B10, B10.D2) with anti-Thy 1.2 and complement; 5×10^5 cells/well were used. Responses represent those specific to TNP by measuring indirect plaque-forming cells (PFC) on day 7 of culture.

antibody-forming cells (PFC) with specific anti-*H-2* sera and complement. If T cell help were restricted only in the step involving macrophage interaction, then both B cell populations would be expected to be stimulated. However, if restriction were to extend to T-B collaboration, only B cells histocompatible with the T cell source should be stimulated to antibody formation.

The data presented in Table 8 illustrate the results of such an approach. The combination of F_1-selected T cells with B cells/macrophages derived from B10 and B10.D2 mice yielded a response in which PFC were derived equally from both strains since either anti-$H-2^d$ or $H-2^b$ sera and complement eliminated approximately the same proportion of PFC. However, where B10-selected T cells were utilized, the vast majority of PFC typed as $H-2^b$; whereas when B10.D2-selected T cells were utilized, most of the PFC typed as $H-2^d$ B cells. Thus, it appears that the selected populations of propagated T cells show restriction not only with respect to T-macrophage interaction but also with respect to T-B collaboration.

The data presented above thus support the concept that T-B interactions, much like T-MØ interactions, are H-2 (Ia)-restricted, an observation initially made some years ago by Katz et al [12] and confirmed since by others [61-63]. Perhaps

Table 8. Selected T Cells Do Not Activate B Cells of the
Inappropriate Haplotype When in the Presence of B Cell/Macrophages
of the Appropriate Haplotype

		Responses:		
		Indirect Anti-TNP PFC/10^6 B Cells‡		
Carrier-Primed T	*Hapten-Primed*		*Contribution by*	
Cells Selected with *	*B cells/macrophages†*	*Whole Culture*	*B10*	*B10.D2*
F_1	B10 + B10.D2	1,090	405	490
B10	B10 + B10.D2	950	1,075	125
B10.D2	B10 + B10.D2	1,285	100	1,260

*BDF$_1$ T cells were selected as described in Table 6. They were used at 10^4 cells/well.

†Cells were obtained after treating with anti-Thy 1.2 and C, spleen populations from either B10 or B10.D2 mice primed with DNP-KLH. They were used at 5×10^5 cells/well.

‡Response to DNP-OVA (5 ng/well) was monitored seven days after initiation of culture.

unique to the experimental conditions presently described is the fact that the use of F_1 T cells selected for interaction with a given parental haplotype and of B cells/M$\emptyset$ populations treated so as to delete T cells obviates the complication that usually results from mixing histocompatible cells, namely enhancing or suppressive effects of allogeneic responses [64].

It should be pointed out that there exist a number of reports which demonstrate that H-2-restricted T-B interaction is not an obligate requirement for specific antibody formation [65-67]. Although the bases for this discrepancy are not known, it is possible that differing requirements reflect differing stages of B lymphocyte activation. For example, while continued growth of B cells triggered with lipopolysaccharide can be supported by an activated T helper cell clone in a non-H-2-restricted fashion [68], activation and growth of small resting B cells appear to require syngeneic, i.e. H-2-restricted, T cells [63]. In this respect, triggering of resting B cells, like the activation of resting specific T cells, may require a dual set of signals, one provided by the specific ligand interaction occurring between T and B lymphocytes and the second in the form of an interleukin. Activated B cells, on the other hand, may be capable of cycling and differentiating by simply binding appropriate factors (?IL-2, IL-3) because they express acceptor sites for such activities. In that light, it may be that B cell triggering can be divided into stages similar to those contemplated for T cell activation, namely (1) induction of resting B cells, requiring both recognition by T cells of antigen in an H-2-restricted fashion and the action of interleukin; (2) proliferation mediated by an interleukin (?IL-2); and (3) differentiation into terminal antibody-forming plasma cells, mediated by another T cell-derived, hormone-like substance (?IL-3). Derivative from such a hypothetical scheme is the possibility that T cells recognize the identical antigenic moieties on macrophages and B cells, namely processed antigen in the context of self Ia, a possibility supported by recently obtained evidence [69].

Acknowledgments

We would like to thank a number of our past and present colleagues who have contributed both physically and intellectually to our efforts: Drs. Giampietro Corradin, Robert Chesnut, Howard Grey, Michael Julius, John Kappler, James Kurnick, Philippa Marrack and Rachel Schrier and Ms. Renee Durant. In addition, we are indebted to Ms. Edna Squillante for the preparation of the manuscript.

One of us (J.C.) is particularly thankful to Basel Institute for Immunology for providing an outstanding setting in which to spend a sabbatical year culturing and nurturing T lymphocytes, among other things. Finally, to Frank Dixon, to whom this symposium is dedicated, my constant gratitude for building the cradle of my scientific birth — Immunology at Scripps Clinic and Research Foundation.

References

1. Hersch, E.M. and Harris, J.E.: J. Immunol. 100:1184, 1968.
2. Cline, M.J. and Sweet, V.C.: J. Exp. Med. 128:1309, 1968.
3. Seeger, R.C. and Oppenheim, J.J.: J. Exp. Med. 132:44, 1970.
4. Rosenthal, A. and Shevach, E.: J. Exp. Med. 138:1194, 1973.
5. Thomas, D.W. and Shevach, E.M.: Proc. Natl. Acad. Sci. U.S.A. 74:2104, 1977.
6. Yano, A., Schwartz, R.H. and Paul, W.E.: Eur. J. Immunol. 8:344, 1978.
7. Schwartz, R.H., Yano, A. and Paul, W.E.: Immunol. Rev. 40:153, 1978.
8. Cowings, C., Pincus, S.H., Sachs, D.H. and Dickler, H.B.: J. Immunol. 121:1680, 1978.
9. Farr, A.G., Kiely, J.M. and Unanue, E.R.: J. Immunol. 122:2413, 1979.
10. Kammer, G.M. and Unanue, E.R.: Clin. Immunol. Immunopathol. 15:434, 1980.
11. Kindred, B. and Shreffler, D.C.: J. Immunol. 109:940, 1972.
12. Katz, D.H. Hamaoka, T., Dorf, M.E. et al: Proc. Natl. Acad. Sci. U.S.A. 70:2624, 1973.
13. Zinkernagel, R.M. and Doherty, P.C.: Nature 251:547, 1974.
14. Vadas, M.A., Miller, J.F.A.P., Whitelaw, A. and Gamble, J.: Immunogenetics 4:137, 1977.
15. Ishizaka, K. and Adachi, T.: J. Immunol. 117:40, 1976.
16. Feldmann, M. and Kontiainen, S. Eur. J. Immunol. 6:302, 1976.
17. Pierres, M. and Germain, R.N.: J. Immunol. 121:1306, 1978.
18. Morgan, D.A., Ruscetti, F.W. and Gallo, G.: Science 193:1007, 1976.
19. Gillis, S. and Smith, K.A.: Nature 268:154, 1977.
20. Coutinho, A., Larsson, E.L., Gronvik, K.O. and Andersson, J.: Eur. J. Immunol. 9:587, 1979.
21. Larsson, E.L. and Coutinho, A.: Nature 280:239, 1979.
22. Schrier, R.A., Skidmore, B.J., Kurnick, J.T. et al: J. Immunol. 119:1048, 1979.

23. Larsson, E.L., Iscove, N.N. and Coutinho, A.: Immunol. Rev. 51:61, 1980.
24. DeFreitas, E.C., Chesnut, R.W., Grey, H.M. and Chiller, J.M.: (Submitted for publication.)
25. Gery, I., Gershon, R.K. and Waksman, B.H.: J. Exp. Med. 136:128, 1972.
26. Lachmann, L.B., Hacker, M.P. and Handschumaker, R.E.: J. Immunol. 119:2019, 1977.
27. Koopman, W.J., Farrar, J.J., Oppenheim, J.J. et al: J. Immunol. 119:55, 1977.
28. Farrar, W.L., Mizel, S.B. and Farrar, J.J.: J. Immunol. 124:1371, 1980.
29. Kierszenbaum, F. and Waksman, B.H.: Immunology 33:663, 1977.
30. Katz, S.P., Kierszenbaum, F. and Waksman, B.H.: J. Immunol. 121:2386, 1978.
31. Rosenstreich, D.L. and Mizel, S.B.: Immunol. Rev. 40:102, 1978.
32. Katz, S.P., Shimamura, T., Dessaint, J.P. et al: Cell. Immunol. 56:68, 1980.
33. Toyoshima, S., Iwata, M. and Osawa, T.: Nature 264:447, 1976.
34. McClain, D.A. and Edelman, G.M.: J. Exp. Med. 144:1494, 1976.
35. Greenberg, P.D. and Bluestein, H.G.: J. Immunol. 121:239, 1978.
36. Tormey, D.C. and Mueller, G.C.: Exp. Cell Res. 74:220, 1972.
37. Nabholz, M., Engers, H.D., Collaro, D. and North, M.: Curr. Top. Microbiol. Immunol. 81:1876, 1978.
38. Fathman, C.G. and Hengartner, H.: Nature 272:617, 1978.
39. Baker, P.E., Gillis, S. and Smith, K.: J. Exp. Med. 149:273, 1979.
40. Bach, F.H., Inouye, H., Hank, J.A. and Alter, B.J.: Nature 281:307, 1979.
41. Von Boehmer, H., Hengartner, H., Nabholz, M. et al: Eur. J. Immunol. 9:592, 1979.
42. Schreier, M.H. and Tees, R.: Int. Arch. Allergy Immunol. 61:227, 1980.
43. Hengartner, H. and Fathman, C.G.: Immunogenetics 10:175, 1980.
44. Lotze, M.T., Strausser, J.L. and Rosenberg, S.A.: J. Immunol. 124:2972, 1980.
45. Sredni, B., Tse, H.Y., Chen, C. and Schwartz, R.H.: J. Immunol. 126:341, 1981.
46. Chiller, J.M. and Julius, M.H.: (Manuscript in preparation.)
47. Kappler, J.W., Skidmore, B.J., White, J. and Marrack, P.: J. Exp. Med. (In press.)
48. Mizel, S.B., Oppenheim, J.J. and Rosenstreich, D.L.: J. Immunol. 120:1497, 1978.
49. Harwell, L., Skidmore, B., Marrack, P. and Kappler, J.: J. Exp. Med. 152:893, 1980.
50. Corradin, G., Etlinger, H.M. and Chiller, J.M.: J. Immunol. 119:1948, 1977.
51. Dresser, D.W.: Immunology 5:378, 1962.
52. Bretcher, P.A. and Cohn, M.: Science 169:1042, 1970.
53. Cohn, M. and Blomberg, B.: Scand. J. Immunol. 4:1, 1975.

54. Lafferty, K.J. and Woolnough, J.A.: Immunol. Rev. 35:231, 1977.
55. Cohn, M. and Epstein, R.: Cell. Immunol. 39:125, 1978.
56. Claman, H.N.: Cell. Immunol. 48:201, 1979.
57. Immunol. Rev. vol. 43, 1979.
58. Talmage, D.W., Woolnough, J.A., Hemmingsen, H. et al: Proc. Natl. Acad. Sci. U.S.A. 74:4610, 1977.
59. Cleveland, R.P. and Claman, H.N.: J. Immunol. 124:474, 1980.
60. Skidmore, B.J., White, J., DeFreitas, E.C. et al: Fed. Proc. (In press.)
61. Marrack, P., Harwell, L., Kappler, J. et al: *In* Barum, P., Battisto, J. and Pierce, C. (eds.): Immunologic Tolerance and Macrophage Function. New York:Elsevier/North-Holland, 1979, p. 31.
62. Hunig, T. and Schimpl, A.: Eur. J. Immunol. 9:730, 1979.
63. Andersson, J., Schreier, M.H. and Melchers, F.: Proc. Natl. Acad. Sci. U.S.A. 77:1612, 1980.
64. Katz, D.H.: Transplant. Rev. 12:141, 1972.
65. McDougal, J.S. and Cort, S.P.: J. Immunol. 120:445, 1978.
66. Singer, A., Hatcock, K.S. and Hodes, R.S.: J. Exp. Med. 149:1208, 1979.
67. Erb, P., Meier, B., Matsunaga, T. and Feldmann, M.: J. Exp. Med. 149:686, 1979.
68. Schreier, M.H., Andersson, J., Lernhardt, W. and Melchers, F.: J. Exp. Med. 151:194, 1980.
69. Chesnut, R.W. and Grey, H.M.: J. Immunol. 126:1075, 1981.

Quantitation and Cloning of Cytolytic T Lymphocytes and Their Precursors

Jean-Charles Cerottini, M.D.

Introduction

Cell-mediated immunity has long been recognized as being instrumental in the elimination of intracellular bacteria and some viruses, the rejection of allografts and destruction of certain types of cancer cells. Since it is well established that thymus-derived (T) lymphocytes are involved in cell-mediated immunity, considerable effort has recently been devoted to the analysis of effector T cells using different in vitro model systems. Thus, it has been shown that effector T cells can exert a variety of functions in vitro, including direct lysis of antigen-bearing target cells, release of soluble factors, collaboration with B cells and suppression of the humoral response. While it is generally accepted that a single effector T cell cannot perform all these functions, there is still much uncertainty as to the actual number of functionally distinct effector cells. For example, are T cells exhibiting helper function in the humoral response also capable of participating in the activation of macrophages? Or, what is the relationship between T cells that proliferate in vitro in response to antigenic stimulation and those that mediate delayed-type hypersensitivity in vivo? Progress along this line has been hampered mostly by the lack of single-cell assays for functional T cells. This problem has been compounded by the fact that most of the assay systems used to assess T cell activities are not quantitative, and therefore

Jean-Charles Cerottini, M.D., Director and Member, Ludwig Institute for Cancer Research, Lausanne Branch, Epalinges, Switzerland.

103

provide little information on the frequency of T cells with a defined function in a given population.

In view of these limitations, a major effort has recently been directed to the development of techniques that allow for (a) the isolation of cloned functional T cell lines, and (b) the enumeration of functionally active T lymphocytes and their precursors.

Among effector T cells, cytolytic T cells (CTL) are the only ones whose specific function can be measured directly in a short-term (three-hour) quantitative in vitro assay using target cells labeled with radioactive chromium (^{51}Cr). Furthermore, it has been well documented that CTL are generated in vivo after injection of allogeneic cells or in vitro in allogeneic mixed leukocyte culture (MLC) systems. Moreover, the formation of CTL is now considered to be a normal component of a host's immune response to cell-associated antigens resulting from viral infection or malignant transformation. Last, but not least, evidence has been provided that CTL, although they are defined by in vitro assay systems, are involved in allograft rejection and may participate in the process of recovery or of tissue injury in many viral infections. It is therefore understandable that initial attempts to isolate functional T cell clones have concentrated on the establishment of cloned CTL lines. Similarly, much work has been directed to the enumeration of CTL precursors (CTL-P) in normal or immune lymphoid cell populations by limiting-dilution analysis.

In the first part of this chapter, I will briefly review the various approaches used to derive murine CTL clones. The basic feature of newly developed limiting-dilution microculture systems that allow quantitation of CTL-P in lymphoid cell populations will be discussed in the second part. Finally, the application of such microculture systems to the determination of CTL-P frequencies in murine model systems of immune responses against alloantigens or virus-associated antigens will be presented.

Establishment of Continuous Cloned CTL Lines

A list of the various experimental approaches used toward the production of "immortalized," cloned CTL lines is given in

Table 1. Early attempts involved repeated stimulation in vitro of allospecific CTL populations generated in MLC using appropriate stimulator cells. Except for one case, these studies showed that the MLC populations, in spite of a persisting proliferative response, lost their lytic activity after several cycles of stimulation. In contrast, CTL populations cultured in medium supplemented with culture supernatant of concanavalin A-stimulated spleen cells were reported to undergo continuous proliferation without losing lytic activity [1]. Subsequent studies indicated that the ability of such supernatant to stimulate continuous growth of CTL populations was mediated by a factor designated T cell growth factor (TCGF) or interleukin 2. Further analysis has established that murine TCGF is a protein of approximately 30,000 molecular weight which is produced by T cells stimulated with mitogen or alloantigen [2]. It should be pointed out that the growth-promoting activity of this factor is not restricted to CTL but appears to affect most, if not all, antigen- or mitogen-activated T cells.

Based on these findings, a general procedure has been developed to derive allospecific CTL clones. Lymphocyte populations are first enriched for CTL by repeated stimulation in MLC, then maintained in continuous proliferation in culture medium supplemented with an appropriate source of TCGF, and finally cloned, usually by limiting dilution, in the presence of TCGF. By this approach, clonal CTL lines with different allospecificities have been isolated and characterized (for further details, see Nabholz et al [3]). A similar approach has been used to derive monoclonal CTL directed against hapten-modified or virus-associated antigens. Some of these cloned

Table 1. Methods Used for the Production of Homogeneous CTL Lines

Method	Success
Repeated antigenic stimulation	No
Transformation by oncogenic viruses	No
Transfer of chromosomes from transformed cells	No
Long-term culture using TCGF	Yes
Short-term culture under limiting-dilution conditions	Yes
Hybridization with thymoma cells	Yes

CTL lines have been maintained in continuous proliferation for several years and therefore appear to have an unlimited life span. It is evident that such cloned lines are useful tools for further analysis of CTL function at the cellular and molecular levels. However, recent evidence suggests that such clones are derived from very few CTL which are selected for during culture in TCGF-supplemented medium. Therefore, these clones do not necessarily represent the whole repertoire of CTL present in the initial cell populations.

In view of this limitation, another procedure has been developed which allows the production of CTL clones with high efficiency [4]. This protocol simply involves culturing very small numbers of cells (one to five cells per microwell) from populations enriched for CTL by a single stimulation in vitro with appropriate antigen-bearing cells. Optimal cloning efficiency is obtained by adding TCGF, irradiated feeder cells and (in some instances) antigen-bearing cells. Clones obtained under these conditions are then expanded using the same culture supplements. By using this approach, we have been able to isolate large numbers of CTL clones which maintained a high degree of stability and specificity over a four-month period of observation [5].

Following the demonstration that hybrids between B cells for immune mice and selected murine myeloma cell lines continue to secrete antibodies with the same specificity as those produced by the parental B cells, several laboratories have tried to produce CTL lines by fusing nonfunctional thymoma lines with CTL populations. While many attempts along this line have been unsuccessful, recent work by Nabholz et al [6] and by Berke (personal communication) indicates that hybrids with cytolytic activity can be produced under special conditions.

Measurement of CTL-P Frequencies

It is generally accepted that CTL are derived from immediate, small-sized precursors which are devoid of lytic activity. Upon appropriate antigenic stimulation, these precursors undergo clonal expansion and differentiation into medium- to large-sized effector cells. It has been well established that CTL are not necessarily end cells, inasmuch as they may further differentiate into small-sized lymphocytes with low cytolytic activity. Although this concept is based primarily on studies concerning the generation of allospecific CTL in MLC, current evidence indicates that similar cellular events take place during the formation in vitro of CTL directed against conventional antigens, including virus-associated antigens.

The induction phase of the CTL response has been the subject of considerable study in recent years. In analogy with the concept of collaboration between macrophages, helper T cells and B cells in antibody responses, it has been suggested that the triggering of CTL-P requires the participation of macrophages and helper T cells in addition to antigen. According to a recently proposed model, CTL-P are first activated as the result of antigen recognition, and then undergo clonal expansion under the influence of TCGF-produced helper T cells.

Whatever the actual mechanism might be, it is evident that a CTL-P, although it is devoid of lytic activity, can be detected through the ability of its clonal progeny to lyse appropriate target cells. On this basis, the following approach has been used to determine the frequency of CTL-P in a given lymphocyte population. Large numbers of microcultures are set up containing decreasing numbers of lymphocytes and a fixed number of antigen-bearing stimulator cells. After an appropriate incubation period (usually seven days), the lytic activity of individual microcultures is assessed using a ^{51}Cr release assay. In theory, detection of CTL activity after antigenic stimulation indicates that the microwell tested contained at least one (or several) CTL-P reactive to the antigen used. When the number of CTL-P per culture becomes limiting, some cultures contain no CTL-P, and thus are negative when assayed for lytic activity after appropriate antigenic stimulation. Since a positive response can result indistinguishably from the presence of any number of precursor cells, whereas a negative response can result only from the absence of precursor cells, the zero-order term of the Poisson equation is used to describe the relation between the number of cells tested per culture and the percentage of nonresponding cultures per group (for discussion of this concept, see Miller et al [7]).

An obvious condition to the use of limiting-dilution assays for the determination of CTL-P frequencies is that no other cell type should be limiting under the culture conditions used.

Recent work has established that, indeed, CTL-P are the only limiting cell type, provided optimal concentrations of stimulating cells, accessory cells and serum are used in conjunction with an appropriate source of TCGF. However, it should be noted that the efficiency of detection of CTL-P cannot be assessed with certainty. Therefore, the frequency estimates obtained with a given assay should be considered as minimal estimates.

An example of the use of such limiting-dilution assays for determining CTL-P frequencies in lymphoid tissues is shown in Table 2 [8]. In this experiment, the frequency of CTL-P directed against DBA/2 (H-2^d) alloantigens was measured in spleen and thymus of adult C57BL/6 (*H-2^b*) mice. It can be seen that the percentage of cytolytically positive microcultures increased with increasing number of lymphocytes per culture. Moreover, the dose of thymus cells required to obtain a given percentage of positive cultures was much higher than that of spleen cells. As calculated by Poisson statistics, the anti-DBA/2 CTL-P frequency in thymus was approximately fivefold lower than that in spleen in this experiment.

Frequencies of Alloreactive CTL Precursors

By using the aforementioned limiting-dilution assay method, it has been possible to obtain minimal estimates of the

Table 2. Cytolytic Response by Limiting Number of
Allostimulated Spleen or Thymus Cells

Source of Lymphoid Cells	Number of Cells per Well	Number of Positive Wells	Reciprocal of CTL-P Frequency
Spleen	250	7/24	
	500	12/24	480
	750	18/24	
Thymus	1000	9/33	
	1500	12/33	2440
	2000	19/33	

Groups of 24 to 33 microcultures containing the indicated number of C57BL/6 lymphoid cells were incubated with 10^6 irradiated DBA/2 spleen cells in medium supplemented with secondary MLC supernatant as a source of TCGF. After seven days, each microwell was assayed for cytotoxicity against ^{51}Cr-labeled P815 (DBA/2) tumor target cells. The CTL-P frequencies were determined according to the Poisson distribution. (For further details, see reference 8.)

frequency of CTL-P reactive against alloantigens in various lymphoid populations [4]. Thus, the mean frequency of CTL-P in C57BL/6 spleen reactive against DBA/2 alloantigens was found to be 1 in 400. The frequency of such CTL-P was even higher in lymph node and in peripheral blood lymphocytes (1/70 and 1/180, respectively). Thus, these results confirmed and extended previous observations indicating a high frequency of alloreactive lymphocytes as judged by the percentage of cells proliferating in MLC. This high frequency could possibly be explained by the large number of antigenic determinants involved since C57BL/6 and DBA/2 strains differ at the whole major histocompatibility complex as well as at multiple minor histocompatibility loci. However, further studies showed that the mean frequency measured in a congenic H-2^b/anti-H-2^d combination was not very different (Table 3). Moreover, the frequencies of CTL-P reactive with K^d and D^d determinants were similar and approximately equal to 50% of the frequency of CTL-P reactive against the whole haplotype. Unexpectedly, the mean frequency of CTL-P in C57BL/6 spleen which were reactive against three independently derived K^b mutants was found to be within the range of frequencies observed in entirely H-2-incompatible combinations [9]. Since there is biochemical evidence that the glycoproteins encoded by these mutated loci

Table 3. A Summary of CTL-P Frequency Determinations
in Normal Female C57BL/6 (H-2^b) Spleen

Antigenic Stimulus	Antigen(s) Involved	Reciprocal of CTL-P Frequency
DBA/2	H-2^d and non-H-2	400
B10.D2	H-2^d	737
B10.HTG	H-2K^d	1,438
B10.A (5R)	H-2D^{dd}	1,216
B6-H-2^d	Mutant H-2K^b	772
C57BL/6 ♂	H-Y	100,000

Groups of microcultures containing limiting numbers of C57BL/6 spleen cells were incubated with 10^6 irradiated spleen cells (as indicated) in medium supplemented with secondary MLC supernatant as a source of TCGF. After 7 days, each microculture was assayed for cytotoxicity against ^{51}Cr-labeled blast cells of the appropriate genotype. CTL-P frequencies were determined according to the Poisson distribution. (For further details, see reference 4.)

differ from the native H-2K^b molecules by very few amino acids, these results thus indicate that limited genetic alterations of H-2 molecules can result in complex antigenic changes, at least at the level of CTL-P recognition.

From these few examples, it is evident that the availability of limiting-dilution assays for alloreactive CTL-P frequency provides a novel approach to the quantitation of such cells in various experimental conditions. Thus, it is now feasible to study in quantitative terms changes in frequency resulting from specific immunization [10] or induction of tolerance, to follow the development of CTL-P during ontogeny [11], or to test the in vivo effect of drugs [8], to name but a few of the applications that have been carried out recently.

The search for qualitative and quantitative effects of specific immunization on allospecific CTL responses has been the subject of several investigations. The concept that memory existed at the level of CTL responses was first suggested by the observation that mice preimmunized with allogeneic tumor cells developed, after challenge with the same tumor cells, an anamnestic CTL response in vivo, with accelerated kinetics and higher peak levels of activity. Subsequent studies showed that the expression of memory after in vitro secondary antigenic stimulation was even greater than after in vivo challenge [12]. However, the cellular basis for anamnestic CTL responses remains to be defined. In particular, whether memory reflects (a) quantitative changes, e.g. an increase in the number of CTL-P; (b) qualitative changes, e.g. selection of precursor cells with high-avidity receptors; or (c) persistence of effector cells generated during primary immunization, is unclear.

Recently, direct evidence has been provided that immunization in vivo may be accompanied by a selective increase in CTL-P directed against the immunizing alloantigens. Thus, spleens of C57BL/6 mice injected IP one month earlier with DBA/2 tumor cells were found to contain up to three times as many anti-DBA/2 CTL-P as compared to unprimed spleens [10]. Further studies showed that the frequency of anti-DBA/2 CTL-P was strikingly increased in the peritoneal lymphocyte population collected from these mice at the peak of the primary response (Table 4). Similarly, the frequency of anti-DBA/2 CTL-P was very much increased after in vitro stimulation of

Table 4. Effect of Immunization on the Frequency of C57BL/6
CTL-P Directed Against DBA/2 Alloantigens

Immunization	Lymphoid Cell Population	Reciprocal of CTL-P Frequency
None	Spleen	399
	Peritoneal exudate	1,224
In vivo*	Spleen (day 60)	154
	Peritoneal exudate (day 12)	15
In vitro†	MLC (day 5)	5
	MLC (day 14)	9

*C57BL/6 mice were injected IP with 3×10^7 P815 (DBA/2) tumor cells.
†Spleen cells from normal C57BL/6 mice were stimulated with irradiated DBA/2 spleen cells in MLC.

C57BL/6 spleen cells in MLC [13]. Since both peritoneal lymphocyte and MLC populations contained relatively large numbers of mature, active CTL, the question arose whether these effector cells behaved operationally as CTL-P. Suggestive evidence that this was indeed the case was obtained by comparing CTL activity and CTL-P frequency in MLC populations separated according to size by velocity sedimentation [13]. More recently, this question was directly resolved by demonstrating that up to 50% of individual peritoneal lymphocytes which could be identified as CTL, using the single-cell assay described by Zagury et al [14], behaved as CTL-P, e.g. gave rise to a cytolytic progeny, upon stimulation in microcultures. Since other studies showed that high CTL-P frequencies were observed in long-term MLC populations, i.e. at a time when CTL had reverted to small lymphocytes devoid of lytic activity [10], it is evident that limiting-dilution microculture systems can detect cells of the CTL lineage irrespective of whether or not they express cytolytic function; i.e., they detect the original CTL-P, CTL and memory CTL-P derived from CTL.

Frequencies of CTL-P Against
Retrovirus-Associated Antigens

Recently, the CTL-P assay has been adapted to a syngeneic CTL model system. It is well documented that inoculation of

Moloney sarcoma leukemia virus (MoSV-MoLV) complex into adult mice results in the development of a sarcoma at the site of injection which spontaneously regresses. Previous studies established that CTL specific for MoLV-associated cell surface antigens could be detected in spleen and in tumor at the onset of tumor regression. Moreover, MoLV-specific CTL activity could be generated in vitro by stimulating spleen cells from normal or immune mice with irradiated MoLV-induced lymphomas in mixed leukocyte-tumor cell cultures (MLTC). Studies of the specificity of CTL activity indicated H-2 restriction of recognition of MoLV-associated antigens [15, 16].

Based on the work in allogeneic systems, we have developed a MLTC microculture system which allows the determination of the frequency of CTL-P directed against MoLV-associated antigens [17]. Optimal culture conditions for stimulating limiting numbers of CTL-P involved the addition of irradiated syngeneic spleen cells, TCGF and irradiated MoLV-induced lymphoma cells as a source of antigen. Under these conditions, anti-MoLV CTL-P frequencies could be determined in the same manner as anti-allogeneic frequencies. Thus, it was found that the frequency of CTL-P against MoLV was 10- to 20-fold lower than that of anti-DBA/2 CTL-P in normal C57BL/6 spleen [4]. However, anti-MoLV CTL-P frequencies were dramatically increased in spleens of C57BL/6 mice which had rejected a MoSV-MoLV-induced tumor, reaching values comparable to anti-DBA/2 CTL-P frequencies. Thus, these results provide direct evidence that immunization in vivo is not only characterized by the generation of specific CTL, but also results in quantitative changes in the number of CTL-P directed against the immunizing antigens.

It is of interest that operationally defined CTL-P were also found among the leukocytes infiltrating the tumor [4]. As compared with that of blood lymphocytes from the same animals, the anti-MoLV CTL-P frequency in leukocyte populations recovered from disaggregated tumors was significantly enriched, thus indicating a selective accumulation of specific effector cells within the tumor.

All together, these results indicate that quantitation of CTL-P directed against conventional (non-H-2) antigens is now feasible. Such CTL-P assays should facilitate further study of the specificity repertoire of CTL-P in mice of different genetic background. In addition, they should be useful for a detailed analysis of the specificity and function of cells which accumulate at the site of viral infections or tumors.

Conclusion

Until recently, studies of CTL generated either in vivo or in vitro have been limited to qualitative analysis of heterogeneous populations. The recent identification of soluble growth-promoting factors active on T cells has led to the development of methods that allow the generation and propagation of homogeneous, antigen-specific CTL. It is clear that the availability of large amounts of cloned CTL will facilitate further detailed analysis of the surface characteristics and biochemical properties of these effector cells. In addition, such factors have been utilized successfully in limiting-dilution microculture systems to determine the frequency of CTL-P directed against foreign H-2 antigens and conventional antigens associated with self H-2 products in lymphoid tissues. Using this novel approach, it has been demonstrated that the frequency of CTL-P reactive against individual alloantigens coded for by the *K* or *D* regions of the major histocompatibility complex is relatively high (1 in 1000 lymphocytes), whereas the frequency of CTL-P against conventional antigens is 10- to 100-fold lower. However, after immunization in vivo, the frequency of such CTL-P can reach values comparable to that against foreign H-2 antigens. It appears that such assays should be very useful for further analysis of the acquisition and the maintenance of the CTL repertoire as well as the functional activity of lymphocytes accumulating at the site of immunopathological reactions.

References

1. Gillis, S. and Smith, K.A.: Long-term culture of tumour-specific cytotoxic T cells. Nature 268:154-156, 1977.
2. Watson, J. and Mochizuki, D.: Interleukin 2: A class of T cell growth factors. Immunol. Rev. 51:257-278, 1980.
3. Nabholz, M., Conzelmann, A., Acuto, O. et al: Established murine cytolytic T-cell lines as tools for a somatic cell genetic analysis of T-cell functions. Immunol. Rev. 51:125-156, 1980.
4. MacDonald, H.R., Cerottini, J.-C., Ryser, J.-E. et al: Quantitation and cloning of cytolytic T lymphocytes and their precursors. Immunol. Rev. 51:93-123, 1980.

5. Weiss, A., Brunner, K.T., MacDonald, H.R. and Cerottini, J.-C.: Antigenic specificity of the cytolytic T lymphocyte (CTL) response to murine sarcoma virus-induced tumors. III. Characterization of CTL clones specific for Moloney leukemia virus-associated cell surface antigens. J. Exp. Med. 152:1210-1225, 1980.

6. Nabholz, M., Cianfriglia, M., Acuto, O. et al: Cytolytically active murine T-cell hybrids. Nature 287:437-440, 1980.

7. Miller, R.G., Teh, H.-S., Harley, E. and Phillips, R.A.: Quantitative studies of the activation of cytotoxic lymphocyte precursor cells. Immunol. Rev. 35:38-58, 1977.

8. Taswell, C., MacDonald, H.R. and Cerottini, J.-C.: Limiting dilution analysis of alloantigen-reactive T lymphocytes. II. Effect of cortisone and cyclophosphamide on cytolytic T lymphocyte precursor frequencies in the thymus. Thymus 1:119-131, 1979.

9. Widmer, M.B. and MacDonald, H.R.: Cytolytic T lymphocyte precursors reactive against mutant K^b alloantigens are as frequent as those reactive against a whole foreign haplotype. J. Immunol. 124:48-51, 1980.

10. Ryser, J.-E.,and MacDonald, H.R.: Limiting dilution analysis of alloantigen-reactive lymphocytes. III. Effect of priming on precursor frequencies. J. Immunol. 123:128-132, 1979.

11. Ceredig, R.: Frequency of alloreactive cytotoxic T cell precursors in the mouse and spleen during ontogeny. Transplantation 28:377-381, 1979.

12. Cerottini, J.-C., Engers, H.D., MacDonald, H.R. and Brunner, K.T.: Generation of cytotoxic T lymphocytes in vitro. I. Response of normal and immune mouse spleen cells in mixed leukocyte cultures. J. Exp. Med. 140:703-717, 1974.

13. Maryanski, J.L., MacDonald, H.R. and Cerottini, J.-C.: Limiting dilution analysis of alloantigen-reactive T lymphocytes. IV. High frequency of cytolytic T lymphocyte precursor cells in MLC blasts separated by velocity sedimentation. J. Immunol. 124:42-47, 1980.

14. Zagury, D., Bernard, J., Thierness, N. et al: Isolation and characterization of individual functionally reactive cytotoxic T lymphocytes: Conjugation, killing and recycling at the single cell level. Eur. J. Immunol. 5:818-822, 1975.

15. Plata, F., Jongeneel, V., Cerottini, J.-C. and Brunner, K.T.: Antigenic specificity of the cytolytic T lymphocyte (CTL) response to murine sarcoma virus (MSV)-induced tumors. I. Preferential reactivity of in vitro generated secondary CTL with syngeneic tumor cells. Eur. J. Immunol. 6:823-829, 1976.

16. Gomard, E., Duprez, V., Reme, T. et al: Exclusive involvement of $H\text{-}2D^b$ or $H\text{-}2K^d$ product in the interaction between T-killer lymphocytes and syngeneic $H\text{-}2^b$ or $H\text{-}2^d$ viral lymphomas. J. Exp. Med. 146:909-922, 1977.

17. Brunner, K.T., MacDonald, H.R. and Cerottini, J.-C.: Antigenic specificity of the cytolytic T lymphocyte (CTL) response to murine sarcoma virus-induced tumors. II. Analysis of the clonal progeny of CTL precursors stimulated in vitro with syngeneic tumor cells. J. Immunol. 124:1627-1634, 1980.

The Role of Major Histocompatibility Gene Complex in T Cell Restriction, Effector Function and Responsiveness

Rolf M. Zinkernagel, M.D., Ph.D.

Introduction

Relationships between cell-mediated immune responses and major transplantation antigens were first noticed in the early 1960s; e.g., the susceptibility of inbred strains of mice to certain tumors or to tumor induction was in some way related to the major histocompatibility gene complex (MHC). Then, in the mid and to late 1960s it became clear that infections with viruses and rejection of foreign grafts had many mechanisms in common. The classical experiments of Svet-Moldavsky showed that skin from mice neonatally injected with murine sarcoma virus (MSV), when transplanted on syngeneic but noninjected normal control mice, was rejected as quickly as skin originating from a completely foreign strain of mice. Soon thereafter, McDevitt showed in mice, as Benacerraf had observed a few years earlier in two guinea pig strains (2 and 13), that the response to antigen was in some way related to the MHC. That observation led ultimately to experiments that demonstrated the phenomenon (MHC) restriction.

This paper illustrates, using examples of cell-mediated immunity against intracellular parasites (e.g. viruses), how MHC products function in the interactions between thymus-derived lymphocytes and other cells. The major points of this paper on T cell interactions are the following: First, MHC products

Rolf M. Zinkernagel, M.D., Ph.D., Institute of Pathology, University of Zurich Medical School, Zurich, Switzerland.

determine the T cell effector function. Second, because of this functional correlation, immune response phenomena arise. Third, T cell differentiation is open-ended; there is some evidence that the thymus and the antigen-presenting cells have a role in the differentiation of the T cell repertoire within the individual, and that during this T cell differentiation a selection in favor of structures for self-MHC recognition is made. These findings may probably explain the phenomenon of MHC polymorphism, the fact that we have so many transplantation antigens.

Let us look at a classical infectious disease in which T cell-mediated immunity plays a major role, both in recovery and protection: the smallpox infection. As studied by Fenner in the late 1940s, and later by Blanden in Australia, it is thought that viral infection occurs in the skin first; then after migration to the lymph node, further spreading through the lymphatics and blood vessels into secondary organs occurs. When we look at the viral titers in such an infection model, we find that virus grows rather rapidly and reaches a peak early, at three to four days, and thereafter declines, so that after seven or eight days, one cannot demonstrate free virus any longer in the host. Thereafter, antibody responses usually become demonstrable, but sometimes antibodies may come up earlier, by three to four days of infection. It is important to remember that antibody titers stay high for quite a while. Somewhere between the decline of viral titers and when the antibody comes up, delayed-type hypersensitivity or other T cell responses become detectable. The easiest method for measuring T cell responses is the chromium 51 release assay according to Brunner et al. Six or seven days after virus infection, mice are killed and splenic lymphocytes are exposed to radiolabeled target cells that are infected with either the same virus used to immunize the mouse or an irrelevant virus, or to uninfected target cells. Cytotoxic activity assessed by release of radiolabel is found only against targets of appropriate specificity. Cytotoxic effector T cells are extremely efficient not only in vitro but also in vivo.

Immune Protection vs. Immunopathology

Virus as intracellular parasite can be characterized by two main parameters: First, virus usually undergoes an eclipse phase;

that is, after absorption and integration of the viral genetic material into the host cell, there is a certain lag period before new viral progeny is fully assembled and released. If, during that period of time, the target cell is killed, not only the host cell is eliminated but also the infectious particle. If immune T cells kill the target cell only after viral progeny is assembled, antiviral protection is not achieved during the same growth cycle; but eventually T cells will catch up with virus spread. Second, viruses have the capacity to infect nonphagocytic as well as phagocytic cells; that is, viruses as a class of infectious agents can infect all sorts of somatic cells. Thus, to make the system of T cell-mediated killing of infected target cells efficient, the following conditions must be fulfilled. First, the killing mechanism is to be expressed on all cells, i.e. phagocytic and nonphagocytic cells, and second, the effector mechanism is a lytic mechanism. Both seem to be operating: during virus infections T cells that kill infected target cells are generated; on all cells that can be infected by virus, there is a receptor for lytic signals, i.e. major transplantation antigens.

What about intracellular bacteria and fungi? They differ from viruses in that they do not undergo an eclipse phase; secondly, they must be phagocytized before they become associated with cells. In order to take care of these types of intracellular parasites, T cells must concentrate on phagocytic types of cells. Lysis of such a target cell would not help much because the bacterium or the fungus would be released because neither of them undergoes an eclipse phase. Therefore, there must be some sort of intracellular digestion going on. It looks as if the I region product within the major histocompatibility gene complex codes exactly for such receptors for signals that induce macrophages, for example, to increase their digestive potential.

Antiviral immune protection against certain viruses is thus mediated essentially by T cell-mediated host cell destruction, and immune T cells have been created to take care of these intracellular parasites. Obviously, the evolutionary pressure to control such viruses would not have evolved if viruses were not cytopathic; that is, if pathogenic viruses would not destroy the cells in which they grow. What happens to poorly or noncytopathic viruses, such as lymphocytic choriomeningitis virus (LCMV), herpes virus, measles virus and cytomegolovirus?

Because the immune system has been trained to take care of acute cytopathic viruses, it reacts similarly against noncytopathic viruses. However, since the latter do not threaten the survival of the cell, nor of the host, no immune protection would be needed against these viruses. The consequence is that immune protection against this latter class of viruses does not decrease or eliminate the nonexisting pathology caused by the virus, but instead the immune response against these viruses manifests itself as cell-mediated immunopathology. Thus, immunoprotection and immunopathology are two sides of the same coin.

MHC Restriction of T Cells

The effector function of T cells is determined by their restriction specificity. This is documented in the following example: virus X generates immune T cells that kill virus-infected cells of type A infected with X, but the same immune T cells cannot kill virus-infected target cells of type B, and vice versa. With the inbred and genetically defined strains of mice, it was easy to map this restriction to the major histocompatibility gene complex on the 17th chromosome: for cytotoxic T cells these restrictions mapped to either K or D.

All T cells seem to be doubly specific for self and for the foreign antigenic determinant. The restricting element within the major histocompatibility gene complex seems to determine the effector function of T cells. Lytic T cells are restricted to K or D. With regard to other T cell functions — be it help, as described by Katz and Benacerraf and by Kindred and Shreffler, or T cell proliferation, as originally worked out by Shevach and Rosenthal, and more recently in the mouse mainly by Schwartz and collaborators; be it delayed-type hypersensitivity, as worked out by Jacques Miller and his collaborators, or the macrophage activation by T cells in the *Listeria* system — all of these T cell effector functions that trigger differentiation processes are restricted to one of the I subregions and are nonlytic.

Thus, all of the classical MHC regions code not only for the misnomer major transplantation antigens, but they code for restricting elements and are all somehow responsible for immune regulation.

How can the dual specificity of T cells be explained? One explanation is that T cells have two receptor sites, one for self and one for the foreign antigenic determinant X (it is unknown whether they are on two molecules or on one molecule close together); i.e., there are two distinguishable receptor sites on each T cell. The single-recognition model proposes that T cells do not see self alone or the foreign antigenic determinant X alone, but rather see a new antigenic determinant formed by the complex of self and the foreign antigenic determinant.

How do T cells or the stem cells learn to recognize the self marker as self? How do they select the restrictive specificity? An experiment that gave some insight used mice that were devoid of T cells and had no thymus. For example, heterozygote mice (H-2^a $\times$ H-2^b)F$_1$ were thymectomized, lethally irradiated on bone marrow reconstituted and grafted with a thymus of H-2^a type. Such F$_1$ stem cells mature in a H-2^a thymus and their restriction specificity is determined by the grafted thymus. These experiments are not yet fully understood. There is, however, no doubt that the thymus has some sort of selective influence on the restriction repertoire; whether this is an artifact caused by the experimental design is an open question. Thymic selection of a restriction specificity seems to be a necessary step, but by itself is not sufficient to promote full maturation of T cells; there is something more to the process of maturation. Probably the important additional step is the amplification of T cells upon exposure to peripheral lymphohemopoietic antigen-presenting cells.

We have stated so far that, at the T cell level, T cell recognition is for self and for foreign antigenic determinant, that the generation of the repertoire for self and for foreign has to undergo certain differentiation processes, with the thymus and the periphery playing some role.

MHC Restriction and Ir Phenomena

The selection of a restriction specificity for self seems in one way or another to limit the potential of the cells to recognize foreign antigenic determinants; that is, each restriction receptor seems to create in the field of vision of a T cell a certain blind spot. Why this blind spot arises, we do not know.

This phenomenon of immune-response-gene regulation is illustrated in the following example. A homozygote inbred mouse is expected to possess cytotoxic T cells restricted to K and other cytotoxic T cells restricted to D. If this mouse is immunized with pox virus, or with lymphocytic chorio-meningitis virus, one would expect about 50% of cytotoxic T cells to be restricted to the K, and another 50% of cytotoxic T cells to be restricted to the D allele of that particular H-2 type. But that is not the case; for example, with pox virus, one finds that all of the response is associated with K and no response whatsoever is associated with the restricting D^k allele. In contrast, the immune response against LCMV is mostly associated with D^k restriction and little with K^k. The effect of the restriction specificity expressed by T cells on this T cell's capacity to recognize foreign antigens indicates why MHC polymorphism may exist within the species, i.e. to minimize the risk of low responsiveness to cytopathic viruses optimally in a population.

Two explanations for these immune response regulations are being entertained; they follow the discussed models of T cell recognition. First, the choice of the restriction receptor for self either precludes or limits the numbers of receptors available to be chosen against X; thus the choice of a receptor for self creates a hole in the receptor repertoire for antigenic determinants X. Alternatively, the defect is not a defect at the level of antigen recognition or at the level of the receptor, but the foreign antigenic determinant X cannot associate or complex properly with the restricting self marker. There is no evidence whatsoever at the moment for one or the other of these possibilities. Restriction specificites and the so-called *Ir* genes, the genes that influence the capacity of T cells to respond to certain foreign antigenic determinants, map to exactly the same subregions or regions within the major histocompatibility gene complex. It would therefore be simplest to argue that because the T cell effector function is determined by the restriction specificity, there is probably, for some evolutionary reason, a linkage between the repertoire of T cells for the restricting elements and the receptor repertoire for foreign antigenic determinants.

MHC Disease Associations

Immune protection and immunopathology induced by intracellular parasites have been major selective forces in driving polymorphism of major transplantation antigens and the diversification of the T cell receptor repertoire. As a consequence of this linkage and the fact that immune protection and immunopathology are two sides of the same mechanism, we see MHC disease associations. MHC disease associations may therefore not necessarily be caused by defects in immunoprotection against acute cytopathic viruses, but rather by immunopathology modulated by *Ir* gene influence. There obviously remains a lot of work to be done in this area to find the linkage between infectious diseases and MHC-dependent T cell responses. One may, however, guess that MHC disease association itself may provide an indication that a particular disease is in fact immunopathologically mediated.

Suggested Reading

Immunol. Rev. vol. 42, 1978.
Katz, D.H.: Lymphocyte Differentiation, Recognition and Regulation. New York:Academic Press, 1977.
Transplant. Rev. vol. 19, 1974.
Transplant. Rev. vol. 29, 1976.
Zinkernagel, R.M. and Doherty, P.C.: Adv. Immunol. 29:52, 1979.

Interaction of Immunoglobulins of Different Classes and Subclasses with Fc Receptors on Leukocytes

Hans L. Spiegelberg, M.D.

Immunoglobulin Classes and Subclasses

It is well established that all antibodies (immunoglobulins, Ig) are composed of two types of polypeptide chains, heavy (H) and light (L), which are linked by disulfide bonds (Fig. 1). The amino acid sequence of the first 110 amino acids of both chains is variable, whereas the remainder of the chain is constant except for minor genetically controlled substitutions [1, 2]. The immunoglobulins can be fragmented by papain into three fragments [3], two Fab fragments consisting of a light chain and the Fd portion of the heavy chain and one Fc fragment representing a dimer of the COOH-terminal halves of the heavy chains. The antibodies can also be cleaved by pepsin, resulting in one fragment made up of two covalently linked Fab fragments called F(ab')$_2$ [4]. The Fc fragment is usually degraded into dialyzable peptides by pepsin. The functions of antibodies can be divided into a primary function which is binding of antigen accomplished by the Fab fragments and secondary or effector functions which are mediated by the Fc fragment [5]. Typical effector functions are activation of complement, binding to Fc receptors on leukocytes, transfer of antibodies through membranes and control of the rate of in vivo

Hans L. Spiegelberg, M.D., Department of Immunopathology, Scripps Clinic and Research Foundation, La Jolla, Calif.

This is publication No. 2323 from the Department of Immunopathology, Scripps Clinic and Research Foundation. The work was supported by USPHS grants AI-10734 and AI-15350 and Biomedical Research Support Program Grant RRO-5514.

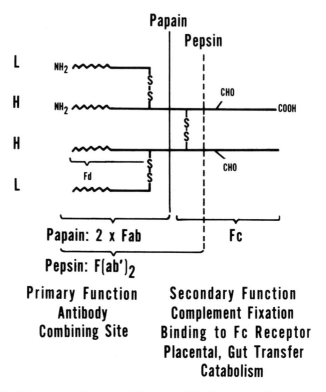

FIG. 1. Schematic diagram of immunoglobulin molecules demonstrating the structures responsible for the primary function and the secondary or effector functions of antibodies. H: Heavy chain; L: Light chain; Fd: Fd fragment representing the NH_2-terminal half of the H chain; CHO: Carbohydrate moiety.

turnover. The Fc fragment also contains the major antigenic determinants on which the division of immunoglobulins into five classes — IgG, IgA, IgM, IgE, IgD — and four IgG and two IgA subclasses is based (Table 1). Antibodies of different classes and subclasses differ in their effector functions: e.g., human IgG1, IgG2, IgG3 and IgM activate the classical complement pathway, whereas IgG4, IgA, IgD and IgE do not. It is difficult to purify normal IgG of different subclasses because they are structurally very similar. It is also difficult to obtain normal IgE and IgD because of their low serum concentration, less than 1

Table 1. Nomenclature of Immunoglobulin Classes and Subclasses
in Three Species

Man	Mouse	Rat
IgG1	IgG2a	IgG2a
IgG2	IgG1	IgG1
IgG3	IgG2b	IgG2b
IgG4	IgG3	IgG2c
IgA1	IgA	IgA
IgA2		
IgM	IgM	IgM
IgD	IgD	IgD
IgE	IgE	IgE

The correspondence between human and rodent IgG subclasses in unknown.

and 30 μg/ml, respectively. Patients with multiple myeloma form large quantities of monoclonal immunoglobulins of one class or subclass and these can be isolated in relatively pure form. Because the Fc fragment that mediates the secondary effector functions is common to all immunoglobulins of one class or subclass, myeloma proteins either in monomeric or chemically aggregated form can be used to study effector functions of antibodies of different classes and subclasses [5]. As mentioned above, white blood cells have receptors reacting specifically with the Fc fragment of antibodies (Fc receptors). In order to determine the interaction of immunoglobulins of different classes and subclasses with Fc receptors, we have studied the interaction of purified myeloma proteins with different white cell types.

Concept of Fc Receptors

The concept of Fc receptors is shown in Figure 2. White blood cells have membrane-bound glycoproteins which specifically bind the Fc fragment of a particular Ig class or subclass. The immunoglobulins bind to the Fc receptors with a certain affinity varying from 10^6 to 10^9 L/M, and there exists an equilibrium between free and bound immunoglobulins [6, 7]. In classical Fc receptor functions, binding of monomeric Ig to Fc receptors does not affect the cell. In contrast, when Ig

Fc RECEPTORS

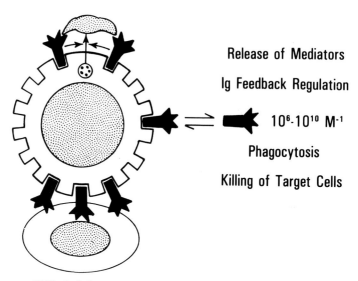

Release of Mediators

Ig Feedback Regulation

10^6-10^{10} M^{-1}

Phagocytosis

Killing of Target Cells

FIG. 2. Schematic diagram of the Fc receptor concept.

bound to Fc receptors reacts with antigen, a signal is given to the cell. The signal can induce the release of mediators from the cell, promote phagocytosis or induce lysis of a target cell. Classical examples of such Fc receptor-mediated activities are the release of histamine by IgE from basophilic granulocytes or mast cells [7, 8], phagocytosis of IgG-coated erythrocytes by monocytes and macrophages [9, 10] and lysis of IgG-coated chicken erythrocytes by K (killer) lymphocytes [11]. The exact mechanism by which the Fc receptors provide a signal to the cell is unknown. Two models of action, called the allosteric model and the associative model, have been proposed (Fig. 3). In the allosteric model, it is assumed that the Fc fragment changes its configuration after reaction with antigen and that this provides the signal to the cell. This model is not generally believed to be correct, because few if any changes in the Fc fragments could be detected after reaction with antigen. Recently, it was shown that anti-IgE Fc receptor antibodies can induce histamine release from basophils in the absence of IgE [12]. At present, it seems more likely that bridging of at

MEDIATION OF BIOLOGICAL ACTIVITIES BY Fc RECEPTORS

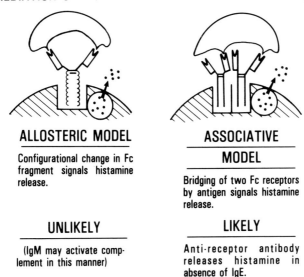

ALLOSTERIC MODEL	ASSOCIATIVE MODEL
Configurational change in Fc fragment signals histamine release.	Bridging of two Fc receptors by antigen signals histamine release.
UNLIKELY	**LIKELY**
(IgM may activate complement in this manner)	Anti-receptor antibody releases histamine in absence of IgE.

FIG. 3. Schematic diagram of the two models which have been proposed for the mechanism of Fc receptor functions.

least two Fc receptors provides the functional signal to the cell [7].

Fc receptors can be detected by several methods. First, binding of radiolabeled immunoglobulins can be quantitated [6]. Second, binding of fluoresceinated, usually aggregated Ig can be detected [13]. Third, binding of Ig-coated red cells to white cells, the so-called rosette assay (Fig. 4), can be used [14] for detection of Fc receptors. Finally, the function of Fc receptors can be analyzed after interaction of the cells with aggregated Ig. In all instances, it should be shown that the interaction is Fc fragment-specific. The binding to Fc receptors should be shown to be specifically inhibitable by Ig of only one particular class of antibodies to avoid interpreting a nonspecific "stickiness" of Ig to surfaces as an indication of the presence of Fc receptors. The membrane proteins representing the Fc receptors will be physicochemically characterized in the near future since many laboratories are working on their isolation and chemical characterization.

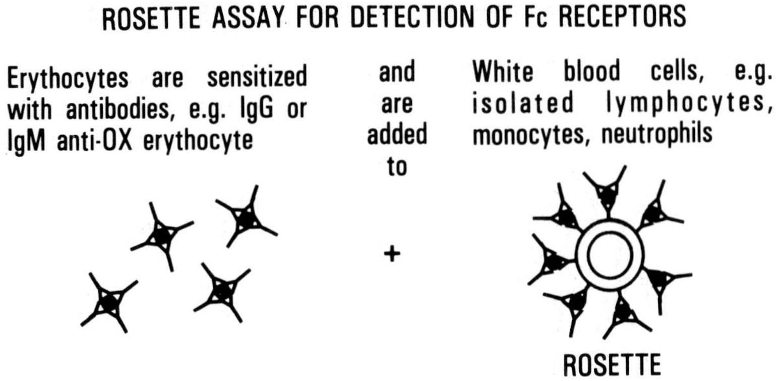

ROSETTE ASSAY FOR DETECTION OF Fc RECEPTORS

Erythocytes are sensitized with antibodies, e.g. IgG or IgM anti-OX erythocyte   and are added to   White blood cells, e.g. isolated lymphocytes, monocytes, neutrophils

+

ROSETTE

FIG. 4. Schematic diagram of the rosette assay.

Fc Receptors on Granulocytes

In order to detect Fc receptors on human neutrophils, we measured the binding of radiolabeled myeloma proteins of different classes and subclasses, either in monomeric form or aggregated with rabbit F(ab)$_2$ anti-human Fab fragments [15]. We found that unaggregated IgG1, IgG3, IgA1 and IgA2 bound to neutrophils. When aggregated, more of these immuno-globulins bound and, in addition, IgG2 and IgG4 also bound. In contrast, neither monomeric nor aggregated IgM, IgD nor IgE bound to neutrophils. These data suggested that neutrophils have Fc receptors only for IgG and IgA. This was confirmed by measuring a functional property of the neutrophil Fc receptors, the release of the granule enzyme β-glucuronidase [16]. As shown in Figure 5, aggregated IgG and IgA of all subclasses but not IgM, IgE or IgD caused significant release of β-glucuronidase from neutrophils.

Basophilic granulocytes have been well documented to have high-affinity Fc receptors for IgE whose function is to release histamine and other vasoactive substances [7, 8, 12]. Basophils also have Fc receptors for IgG; however, it appears that they do not mediate histamine release [17].

Eosinophils have Fc receptors for IgG and most likely for IgE also [18, 19].

Fc Receptors on Platelets

It is difficult to study binding of radiolabeled immuno-globulins to platelets because large quantities of cells are

NEUTROPHILS IN SUSPENSION

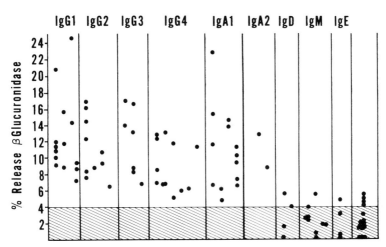

FIG. 5. Percentage of β-glucuronidase released from human neutrophils after incubation with chemically aggregated myeloma proteins of different classes and subclasses.

necessary for such studies. Therefore, in order to determine the class specificity of Fc receptors on platelets, we analyzed a function of Fc receptors, the release of serotonin after addition of aggregated Ig [20]. As can be seen in Figure 6, aggregated IgG of all subclasses caused significant release of serotonin. In contrast, aggregated myeloma proteins of the other classes did not release serotonin. It appears, therefore, that platelets have Fc receptors for IgG but not for other immunoglobulin classes. Whether these Fc_γ receptors are related in structure to Fc_γ receptors on other cell types remains to be elucidated.

Fc Receptors on Monocytes and Macrophages

Historically, "Fc receptors" were first detected on macrophages. Boyden and Sorkin [21] incubated rabbit macrophages with anti-bovine serum albumin antiserum. After washing, the macrophages bound bovine serum albumin, apparently through "cytophilically" bound antibodies. Subsequently, Berken and Benacerraf [9] analyzed this phenomenon further and demonstrated that this binding is related to the Fc fragment of IgG. They also showed the class specificity of Fc receptors by

PLATELETS

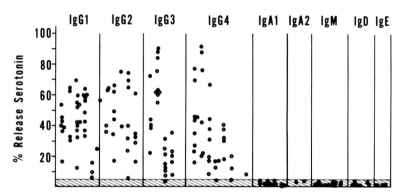

FIG. 6. Percentage of ^{3}H-labeled serotonin released from human platelets after incubation with chemically aggregated myeloma proteins.

demonstrating that guinea pig IgG2 but not IgG1 binds to macrophages. These studies led to the concept of Fc receptors and extensive research on the binding of Ig to cells in many laboratories. The first function of Fc receptors found was promotion of phagocytosis of IgG-coated particles by macrophages. Until recently, macrophages and monocytes were only studied for IgG receptors. One Fc receptor reacting in the order IgG3 > IgG1 > IgG4 > IgG2 was found on human monocytes. In contrast, murine macrophages have been shown to have two IgG receptors, one specific for mouse IgG2a and the other for IgG1 and IgG2b [22, 23]. Studies presently performed in our laboratory indicate that rat macrophages also have more than one IgG Fc receptor (Boltz-Nitulescu and Spiegelberg, in preparation).

Capron and his colleagues [24] first demonstrated that rat macrophages also interact with IgE and kill schistosomules in the presence of IgE-containing immune sera. The presence of Fc receptors for IgE (Fc$_\epsilon$) was shown by Dessaint et al [25] by demonstrating binding of radiolabeled IgE and measuring release of β-glucuronidase from these cells [26]. We have confirmed these observations by demonstrating that over 80% of normal rat alveolar macrophages form specific rosettes with IgE-coated red cells [27]. Furthermore, we showed by a rosette assay that approximately 20% of human peripheral blood monocytes have Fc_ϵ receptors [28]. In contrast to nonallergic donors, up to 80% of monocytes from severely allergic patients had Fc_ϵ receptors and showed significant increased lysis of IgE-coated target cells [29]. No correlation between percentage of Fc_ϵ^+ monocytes and IgE serum level was found in the allergic patients. However, when rats were injected with purified myeloma proteins, rat peritoneal and alveolar macrophages expressed more Fc_ϵ receptors, as shown by rosette assays employing undersensitized cells (Boltz-Nitulescu and Spiegelberg, unpublished observations). These experiments indicate that the IgE serum concentration is at least one factor which governs the expression of Fc_ϵ receptors on macrophages. It has recently been shown that phagocytosis stimulates macrophages to release slow-reacting substance of anaphylaxis (SRS-A) [30, 31]. This suggests that IgE may cause the release of SRS-A from monocytes and macrophages and represents another pathogenic pathway causing allergic diseases.

Whether monocytes and the closely related macrophages have Fc receptors for IgM (Fc_μ) and IgA (Fc_α) is not clearly established. In our laboratory, we could not show Fc_μ and Fc_α receptors by rosette assays. Similarly, Reynolds et al [32] reported that IgG antibodies are far superior in killing *Pseudomonas aeruginosa* than are IgA antibodies, suggesting that Fc_α receptors are low in number or absent on most macrophages. However, the presence of Fc_α receptors on monocytes was recently reported by Fanger et al [33].

Fc Receptors on Lymphocytes

Lymphocytes have been extensively studied for Fc receptors in many laboratories [34]. Fc receptors to all five major Ig classes have been detected on subpopulations of lymphocytes. The majority (40% to 70%) of T cells have Fc receptors for IgM (T_μ) and 10% to 15% have Fc receptors for IgG (T_γ) [35]. Small subpopulations (5% to 15%) of T cells have Fc receptors for IgA [36], IgE [37] and IgD [38]. Most B cells have Fc receptors for IgG [13, 34]. As in T cells, small subpopulations of B cells have Fc receptors for IgM [39], IgA [40], IgE [41] and IgD [38]. K lymphocytes which lyse antibody-coated target cells have Fc receptors for IgG [11]. Whether K cells exist with Fc receptors for IgM is controversial and K cells with

Fc receptors for IgA, IgE and IgD have not been reported. Most normal lymphocytes express only one type of Fc receptors at a time, e.g. T cells are Fc_μ or Fc_γ positive [35] and B cells are Fc_ϵ or Fc_γ positive [41]. In contrast, leukemic B cells can express two or more Fc receptors simultaneously [42, 43]. Lymphocytes can be modulated to change the expression of Fc receptors. A portion of T_γ cells become T_μ cells after interaction with IgG antigen-antibody complexes [44]. Similarly, Fc_γ-positive B cells change to Fc_ϵ-positive cells in the mesenteric lymph nodes of rats infected with parasites [37] or after in vitro incubation with IgE [45].

Relatively little is known about the function of Fc receptors on lymphocytes. The only proven function is that of Fc_γ receptors on K cells, which mediate lysis of IgG-coated target cells [11]. The function of Fc receptors on T and B cells is unknown, but may be regulation of antibody synthesis. Moretta and co-workers [46] showed that T_γ cells suppress and T_μ cells help the in vitro synthesis of Ig induced by pokeweed mitogen. However, the mechanism by which Fc receptors mediate these functions is unknown.

Subpopulations of T and B cells with specific Fc receptors have been studied in patients with different disorders, but no clear correlation between one or another subpopulation and a particular disease was found. The T_γ population is decreased in lupus erythematosus [47], in atopic patients [48] and in the aged population [49]. Drugs can affect the percentages of Fc receptor-bearing lymphocytes. Compounds which increase cAMP, such as theophylline and isoproterenol, cause a decrease of the T_μ cell population [50], and allergic patients treated with corticosteroids have fewer lymphocytes with Fc_ϵ receptors than do normals [51].

Most likely, Fc receptors for a particular Ig class are not restricted to a functional subpopulation of lymphocytes such as helper or suppressor cells. Lymphocytes can probably express more than one type of Fc receptor, depending on their functional state.

Our laboratory first described the B lymphocyte subpopulation which bears Fc receptors for IgE [15, 41, 52]. Since the function of Fc receptors on lymphocytes is unknown, we investigated the Fc_ϵ^+ lymphocyte population in patients and experimental animals having increased IgE levels. Three conditions are known in which IgE serum concentrations are elevated: first, in patients with allergic disorders; second, in patients or experimental animals infected with parasites; and third, in patients or animals bearing IgE-producing myeloma. To determine how these disease states affect the Fc_ϵ^+ lymphocytes, we studied peripheral blood lymphocytes from allergic patients and spleen and mesenteric lymph node lymphocytes from rats infected with *Nippostrongylus brasiliensis* parasites [53] and from rats bearing the IgE-producing tumor IR-162 [54]. Allergic patients who were relatively free of symptoms at the time of testing did not have significantly increased numbers of Fc_ϵ^+ lymphocytes despite elevated serum IgE concentrations [51]. In contrast, severely atopic patients had a fivefold increase of Fc_ϵ^+ B cells as compared to nonallergic or mildly affected patients. Recently, we examined a group of patients known to suffer from seasonal allergic rhinitis resulting from grass pollen allergies [55]. Before and after the grass pollen season, these patients only had slightly more Fc_ϵ^+ cells, on the average 2.1%, as compared to 1.4% for the nonallergic controls. However, during the pollen season all patients showed an increase over the preseason level and had on the average 4.7%, as compared to 1.7% for the controls. All patients had elevated IgE levels and positive RAST scores to three grass pollens. Neither the IgE nor RAST scores were significantly changed during the six-month period of study and, in particular, they were not elevated when the Fc_ϵ^+ cells were significantly increased. These studies provide evidence that the percentage of Fc_ϵ^+ lymphocytes in the peripheral blood is not directly related to IgE level but correlates with the disease state.

Recently, Yodoi and Ishizaka [37] reported that rats infected with the parasite *Nippostrongylus brasiliensis* have significantly increased percentages of Fc_ϵ^+ lymphocytes in their mesenteric lymph nodes 20 days after infection. We repeated these experiments and, as shown in Table 2, we confirmed these observations. Normal rats had 1.9% ± 1.1% Fc_ϵ^+ lymphocytes in the msenteric lymph nodes, whereas the infected rats had 20.3% ± 7.8%. No differences in cells forming rosettes with optimally coated rabbit IgG anti-ox erythrocyte antibodies were found. The spleen lymphocytes of normal rats had 13.9% ±

Table 2. Fc_ϵ- and Fc_γ-Positive Lymphocytes in Rats Infected with
Nippostrongylus brasiliensis Parasites and Rats
Bearing the IgE Myeloma Tumor IR-162

| | % Rosetting Cells | | | |
| | Fc_ϵ (IR-162)* | | Fc_γ (Rabbit IgG) | |
	Spleen	Lymph Node	Spleen	Lymph Node
Normal (12)	13.9 ± 2.4	1.9 ± 1.1	34.3 ± 10.6	22.2 ± 5.9
N. brasiliensis (5) (14-30 days)	21.5 ± 2.9	10.3 ± 7.8	27.8 ± 5.1	21.4 ± 6.6
IR-162 myeloma (5) (12-15 days)	8.7 ± 2.1	10.3 ± 3.7	50.6 ± 7.8	27.4 ± 5.8

*Fixed ox indicator erythrocytes coated with IgE myeloma protein IR-162 [57].

2.4% Fc_ϵ^+ cells and the infected rats 21.5% ± 2.9%. These rats
were tested two to four weeks after infection and had 100 to
200 μg IgE per milliliter. Six rats bearing the rat IgE myeloma
IR-162 and having 3 to 8 mg IgE per milliliter were then tested.
As shown in Table 2, these rats had 10% Fc_ϵ^+ lymphocytes in
their mesenteric lymph nodes and 9% in the spleen. The low
number in the spleen was presumably the result of Fc_ϵ-negative
tumor cells because the spleens were large and infiltrated with
tumor. The lymph nodes, however, were small like those of
normal rats and did not contain many tumor cells. Since the
percentage of Fc_ϵ^+ lymphocytes in mesenteric lymph nodes of
tumor-bearing rats was lower than in infected rats, despite the
fact that they had 10 to 40 times more IgE in their sera, a direct
correlation between IgE serum concentration and percentage of
Fc_ϵ^+ cells may also not exist in rats, suggesting that multiple
factors may be involved in the regulation of the Fc_ϵ^+
lymphocyte population. In contrast, Yodoi et al [45] reported
that in vitro incubation of normal rat lymphocytes with IgE
causes formation of Fc_ϵ^+ cells, suggesting that IgE itself could
induce Fc_ϵ^+ lymphocytes. In order to determine whether an in
vivo elevation of the serum IgE level, in the absence of either
parasitic disease or myeloma, would cause an increase of Fc_ϵ^+
lymphocytes, we injected Lou/M rats IP with 5 mg isolated IgE
myeloma protein IR-162, which resulted in an IgE serum level
of 150 to 250 μg/ml, a concentration similar to that found in *N.
brasiliensis*-infected rats. As shown in Table 3, the percentage of

Table 3. Fc_ϵ- and Fc_γ-Positive Lymphocytes in 150-gm Lou/M Rats
Injected Daily IP with 5 mg IgE Myeloma Protein IR-162

| | % Rosetting Cells | | | |
| | Fc_ϵ (IR-162) | | Fc_γ (Rabbit IgG) | |
	Spleen	Lymph Node	Spleen	Lymph Node
Normal (12)	13.9 ± 1.4	1.9 ± 1.1	34.3 ± 10.6	22.2 ± 5.9
Native IgE				
1 Day (3)	20.2 ± 3.7	11.0 ± 6.0	44.2 ± 12.8	22.0 ± 14.8
2 Days (3)	11.4 ± 2.0	8.7 ± 1.4	38.1 ± 1.2	17.9 ± 1.5
3 Days (2)	18.9 ± 1.6	8.1 ± 4.6	45.3 ± 1.4	28.5 ± 0.4
Reduced and Alkylated IgE				
1 and 2 Days (4)	9.6 ± 4.0	3.0 ± 2.4	49.1 ± 1.8	25.6 ± 2.3

Fc_ϵ^+ mesenteric lymph node lymphocytes of these rats indeed increased from approximately 2% in normal rats to 10%, which is significantly less, however, than the percentage of Fc_ϵ^+ cells in infected rats. The percentage of positive cells in rats injected once was slightly higher than that of rats injected for two and three days, indicating that not more than 24 hours, probably less, was necessary to create or recruit Fc_ϵ^+ lymphocytes into the mesenteric lymph nodes. As a control, four rats were injected with reduced and alkylated IR-162 IgE. No significant increase of Fc_ϵ^+ lymphocytes was observed in these four control rats. These experiments show that an increase of the IgE serum level can cause an increase of Fc_ϵ^+ cells in vivo. However, as mentioned above, there must also be other factors governing the population of Fc_ϵ^+ lymphocytes. In man, culturing lymphocytes with IgE did not result in formation of Fc_ϵ^+ lymphocytes unless the antigen to which the allergic donors were sensitive was added [56]. Monkeys injected with an IgE myeloma protein did not show an increase in Fc_ϵ^+ peripheral lymphocytes [51]. Experiments presently under investigation in our laboratory showed that rats infected with *N. brasiliensis* still had elevated percentages of Fc_ϵ^+ lymphocytes four and six months after infection when the IgE levels had decreased to less than 1.0 and 0.1 $\mu g/ml$, respectively, and the rats were completely cured of disease. Furthermore, normal Lou/M rats which had less than 20 ng IgE per milliliter had 10% to 18% Fc_ϵ^+ lymphocytes in the spleen and 8% in the blood.

Most of the Fc_ϵ^+ lymphocytes in normal rats are B cells [37, 57]. The Fc_ϵ^+ lymphocytes of *N. brasiliensis*-infected rats are also mainly B cells, but up to one third are T cells [37]. We have not yet studied the lymphocytes of rats injected with IgE myeloma protein for B and T cells. Hoover and Lynch [58] showed that mice bearing an IgA myeloma have an increase of Fc_α-bearing lymphocytes and that these cells are mainly T cells. Although more work is necessary to elucidate the role of Fc receptors on T and B cells, the studies demonstrating an increase of Fc receptor-positive lymphocytes under conditions where the Ig level is increased suggest that these cells are involved in the regulation of Ig formation.

Conclusion

Fc receptors for different classes of immunoglobulins are found on all white cell types and mediate many functions (Table 4). A particular cell type can have Fc receptors for more than one Ig class but usually has not more than two. Lymphocytes normally show Fc receptors to only one class, but

Table 4. Function of FcReceptors

1. *Mast cells, basophils granulocytes*
   IgE: Release of vasoactive substances, histamine

2. *Neutrophil granulocytes*
   IgG, IgA: Phagocytosis, release of lysosomal enzymes

3. *Monocytes, macrophages*
   IgG, IgE: Phagocytosis, release of slow-reacting substance of anaphylaxis (SRS-A)

4. *Platelets*
   IgG: Release of serotonin, platelet factors

5. *Lymphocytes*
   IgG: Lysis of IgG-coated targets by K cells
   IgG: ? T_γ supressor cells, ? B_γ cells
   IgM: ? T_μ helper cells, ? B_μ cells
   IgA, IgE: ? T_α, T_ϵ ? B_α, B_ϵ cells

they can change the expression of Fc receptors from one class to another [44, 45]. The role of Fc receptors on phagocytic cells is promotion of phagocytosis. Another function of Fc receptors is induction of the release of intracellular constituents such as vasoactive amines from basophils and mast cells and granule enzymes from neutrophils, monocytes and macrophages. Furthermore, Fc receptors mediate killing of antibody-coated target cells by K lymphocytes and monocytes. The role of Fc receptors on T and B cells is as yet unknown; however, they appear to be involved in regulation of Ig synthesis. The presence of Fc receptors on all white cell types demonstrates their great importance as the link in the cooperation between antibodies and white cells in numerous immune functions.

Acknowledgments

The author thanks Ms. Gloria Portillo for reviewing, and Mrs. Margaret Stone for preparing, the manuscript.

References

1. Edelman, G.M., Cunningham, B.A., Gall, W.E. et al: The covalent structure of an entire γG immunoglobulin molecule. Proc. Natl. Acad Sci. U.S.A. 63:78, 1969.
2. Natvig, J.B. and Kunkel, H.G.: Human immunoglobulins: Classes, subclasses, genetic variants and idiotypes. Adv. Immunol. 16:1, 1973.
3. Porter, R.R.: The hydrolysis of rabbit gamma globulin and antibodies with crystalline papain. Biochem. J. 73:119, 1959.
4. Nisonoff, A., Wissler, F.C., Lipman, L.N. and Woernly, D.L.: Separation of univalent fragments from bivalent rabbit antibody molecule by reduction of disulfide bonds. Arch. Biochem. Biophys. 89:230, 1960.
5. Spiegelberg, H.L.: Biological activities of immunoglobulins of different classes and subclasses. Adv. Immunol. 19:259, 1974.
6. Segal, D.M. and Hurwitz, E.: Binding of affinity cross-linked oligomers of IgG to cells bearing Fc receptors. J. Immunol. 118:1338, 1977.
7. Metzger, H. and Bach, M.: The receptor for IgE on mast cells and basophils: Studies on IgE binding and on the structure of the receptor. *In* Bach, M. (ed.): Immediate Hypersensitivity. New York: Marcel Decker, 1978, p. 561.
8. Ishizaka, K.: Human reaginic antibodies. Ann. Rev. Med. 21:187, 1970.
9. Berken, A. and Benacerraf, B.: Properties of antibodies cytophilic for macrophages. J. Exp. Med. 123:119, 1966.

10. Lobuglio, A.F., Cotran, R.S. and Teudl, J.H.: Red cells coated with immunoglobulin G: Binding and sphering by mononuclear cells in man. Science 158:1582, 1967.

11. Perlmann, H., Perlmann, P., Pape, G.R. and Hallden, G.: Purification, fractionation and assay of antibody dependent lymphocyte effector cells (K cells) in human blood. Scand. J. Immunol. 5 (suppl. 5):57, 1976.

12. Ishizaka, T. and Ishizaka, K.: Triggering of histamine release from rat mast cells by divalent antibodies against IgE-receptors. J. Immunol. 120:800, 1978.

13. Dickler, H.B. and Kunkel, H.G.: Interaction of aggregated γ-globulin with B lymphocytes. J. Exp. Med. 136:191, 1972.

14. Hallberg, T., Gurner, B.W. and Coombs, R.R.A.: Opsonic adherence of sensitized ox red cells to human lymphocytes as measured by rosette formation. Int. Arch. Alllergy Appl. Immunol. 40:500, 1973.

15. Lawrence, D.A., Weigle, W.O. and Spiegelberg, H.L.: Immunoglobulins cytophilic for human lymphocytes, monocytes and neutrophils. J. Clin. Invest. 55:368, 1975.

16. Henson, P.M., Johnson, H.B. and Spiegelberg, H.L.: Release of granule enzymes from human neutrophils stimulated by aggregated immunoglobulins of different classes and subclasses. J. Immunol. 109:1182, 1972.

17. Ishizaka, T., Sterk, A.R. and Ishizaka, K.: Demonstration of Fc_γ receptors on human basophil granulocytes. J. Immunol. 123:578, 1979.

18. Ishikawa, T., Wicher, K. and Arbesman, C.E.: In vitro and in vivo studies of uptake of antigen-antibody complexes by eosinophils. Int. Arch. Allergy Appl. Immunol. 46:230, 1974.

19. Hubscher, T.: Role of the eosinophil in the allergic reactions. I. EDI — An eosinophil-derived inhibitor of histamine release. J. Immunol. 144:1379, 1975.

20. Henson, P.M. and Spiegelberg, H.L.: Release of serotonin from human platelets induced by aggregated immunoglobulins of different classes and subclasses. J. Clin. Invest. 52:1282, 1973.

21. Boyden, S.V. and Sorkin, E.: The adsorption of antigen by spleen cells previously treated with antiserum in vitro. Immunology 3:272, 1960.

22. Unkeless, J.: The presence of two Fc receptors on mouse macrophages: Evidence from a variant cell line and differential trypsin sensitivity. J. Exp. Med. 145:931, 1977.

23. Mellman, I.S. and Unkeless, J.C.: Purification of a functional mouse Fc receptor through the use of a monoclonal antibody. J. Exp. Med. 152:1048, 1980.

24. Capron, A., Dessaint, J.P., Capron, M. and Bazin, H.: Specific IgE antibodies in immune adherence of normal macrophages to Schistosoma mansoni schistosomules. Nature 253:474, 1975.

25. Dessaint, J.P., Torpier, G., Capron, M. et al: Cytophilic binding of IgE for the macrophage. I. Binding characteristics of IgE on the surface of

macrophages in the rat. Cell. Immunol. 46:12, 1979.

26. Dessaint, J.P., Capron, A., Joseph, M. and Bazin, H.: Cytophilic binding of IgE to the macrophage. II. Immunologic release of lysosomal enzyme from macrophages by IgE-anti-IgE in the rat: A new macrophage activation. Cell. Immunol. 46:24, 1979.

27. Boltz-Nitulescu, G. and Spiegelberg, H.L.: Receptors specific for IgE on rat alveolar and peritoneal macrophages. Cell. Immunol. 59:106, 1981.

28. Melewicz, F.M. and Spiegelberg, H.L.: Fc receptors for IgE on a subpopulation of human peripheral blood monocytes. J. Immunol. 125:1026, 1980.

29. Melewicz, F.M., Zeiger, R.S., Mellon, M.H. et al: Increased IgE cytotoxicity by blood mononuclear cells of allergic patients. Clin. Exp. Immunol. 143:526, 1981.

30. Rouzer, A.C., Scott, W.A., Cohn, Z.A. et al: Mouse peritoneal macrophage release leukotriene C in response to a phagocytic stimulus. Proc. Natl. Acad. Sci. U.S.A. 77:4928, 1980.

31. Bretz, U., Dewald, B., Payne, T. and Schnyder, J.: Phagocytosis stimulates the release of a slow reacting substance (SRS) in cultured macrophages. Br. J. Pharmacol. 71:631, 1980.

32. Reynolds, H.Y., Kazmierowski, J.A. and Newball, H.H.: Specificity of opsonic antibodies to enhance phagocytosis of Pseudomonas aeuroginosa by human alveolar macrophages. J. Clin. Invest. 56:376, 1975.

33. Fanger, M.W., Shen, L., Pugh, J. and Bernier, G.M.: Subpopulations of human peripheral granulocytes and monocytes express receptors for IgA. Proc. Natl. Acad. Sci. U.S.A. 77:3640, 1980.

34. Dickler, H.B.: Lymphocyte receptors for immunoglobulin. Adv. Immunol. 24:167, 1976.

35. Moretta, L., Ferrarini, M., Durante, M.L. and Mingari, M.C.: Expression of a receptor for IgM by human T cells in vitro. Eur. J. Immunol. 5:565, 1975.

36. Lum, L.G., Muchmore, A.V., Keren, D. et al: A receptor for IgA on human T lymphocytes. J. Immunol. 122:65, 1979.

37. Yodoi, J. and Ishizaka, K.: Lymphocytes bearing Fc receptors for IgE. I. Presence of human and rat T lymphocytes with Fc$_\epsilon$ receptors. J. Immunol. 122:2577, 1979.

38. Sjöberg, O.: Presence of receptors for IgD on human T and non-T lymphocytes. Scand. J. Immunol. 11:377, 1980.

39. Ferrarini, M., Hoffman, T., Fu, S.H. et al: Receptors for IgM on certain human B lymphocytes. J. Immunol. 119:1525, 1977.

40. Lum, L.G., Muchmore, A.V., O'Connor, N. et al: Fc receptors for IgA on human B and human non-B non-T lymphocytes. J. Immunol. 123:714, 1979.

41. Gonzalez-Molina, A. and Spiegelberg, H.L.: A subpopulation of normal human peripheral B lymphocytes that bind IgE. J. Clin. Invest. 59:616, 1977.

42. Pichler, W.J. and Knapp, W.: Receptors for IgM-coated erythrocytes on chronic lymphatic leukemia cells. J. Immunol. 118:1010, 1977.

43. Spiegelberg, H.L. and Dainer, P.M.: Fc receptors for IgG, IgM and IgE on human leukemic lymphocytes. Clin. Exp. Immunol. 35:286, 1979.

44. Pichler, W.J., Lum, L. and Broder, S.: Fc receptors on human T lymphocytes. I. Transition of T_γ to T_μ cells. J. Immunol. 121:1540, 1978.

45. Yodoi, J., Ishizaka, T. and Ishizaka, K.: Lymphocytes bearing Fc receptors for IgE. II. Induction of Fc_ϵ-receptor bearing rat lymphocytes by IgE. J. Immunol. 123:455, 1979.

46. Moretta, L., Webb, S.R., Gross, C.E. et al: Functional analysis of two human subpopulations: Help and suppression of B cell responses by T cells bearing receptors for IgM (T_M) or IgG (T_G). J. Exp. Med. 146:184, 1977.

47. Moretta, A., Mingari, M.C., Santoli, D. et al: Human T lymphocyte subpopulations: Alterations in systemic erythematosus. Scand. J. Immunol. 10:222, 1979.

48. Canonica, G.W., Mingari, M.C., Melioli, G. et al: Imbalances of T cell subpopulations in patients with atopic diseases and effect of specific immunotherapy. J. Immunol. 123:2669, 1979.

49. Gupta, S. and Good, R.A.: Subpopulations of human T lymphocytes. X. Alterations in T, B, third population cells, and T cells with receptors for immunoglobulin M (T_μ) or G (T_γ) in aging humans. J. Immunol. 122:1214, 1979.

50. Gupta, S.: Subpopulations of human T lymphocytes. XII. *In vitro* effect of agents modifying intracellular levels of cyclic nucleotides on T cells with receptors for IgM (T_μ), IgG (T_γ) or IgA (T_α). J. Immunol. 123:2664, 1979.

51. Spiegelberg, H.L., O'Connor, R.D., Simon, R.A. and Mathison, D.A.: Lymphocytes with immunoglobulin E Fc receptors in patients with atopic disorders. J. Clin. Invest. 64:714, 1979.

52. Gonzalez-Molina, A. and Spiegelberg, H.L.: Binding of IgE myeloma proteins to human cultured lymphoblastoid cells. J. Immunol. 117:1838, 1976.

53. Jarrett, E. and Bazin, H.: Elevation of total serum IgE in rats following helminth parasite infection. Nature 251:613, 1974.

54. Bazin, H. and Becker, A.: IgE myelomas in rats. *In* Johansson, S.G.O., Strandberg, K. and Uvnäs, B. (eds.): Molecular and Biological Aspects of the Acute Allergic Reaction. New York:Plenum Publishers, 1976, pp. 125-152.

55. Spiegelberg, H.L. and Simon, R.A.: Increase of lymphocytes with Fc receptors for IgE during the grass pollen season in patients with allergic rhinitis, abstracted. Allergy Clin. Immunol. (In press.)

56. Yodoi, J. and Ishizaka, K.: Induction of Fc_ϵ-receptor bearing cells *in vitro* in human peripheral lymphocytes. J. Immunol. 124:934, 1980.

57. Fritsche, R. and Spiegelberg, H.L.: Fc receptors for IgE on normal rat lymphocytes. J. Immunol. 121:471, 1978.

58. Hoover, R.G. and Lynch, R.G.: Lymphocyte surface membrane immunoglobulin in myeloma. II. T cells with IgA-Fc receptors are markedly increased in mice with IgA plasmacytomas. J. Immunol. 125:1280, 1980.

The Human Complement Protein C3: Its Unusual Functional and Structural Versatility in Host Defense and Inflammation

Hans J. Müller-Eberhard, M.D.

Introduction

The third component, or C3, is historically the oldest of the 20 complement proteins known to date. It was recognized and described as a distinct protein entity in 1960 [1, 2]. It is related through evolution to two other components, C4 and C5. The three proteins share homology in primary structure [3] and are likely to have arisen by gene duplication. Along with C3, C4 and C5 evolved specific cell surface receptors allowing these proteins to communicate with cells involved in host defense and inflammation. C3 may be phylogenetically the older protein of the three because it is the least specialized, the most versatile and multifunctional. C3 is the precursor of multiple physiological derivatives which display different biological activities.

That complement is essential in host defense against infections has become abundantly clear through the occurrence of life-threatening or lethal infections in individuals with homozygous complement deficiencies [4]. Individuals with C5, C6, C7 or C8 deficiencies often present with meningococcal septicemia and meningitis or disseminated gonococcal infec-

Hans J. Müller-Eberhard, M.D., Chairman, Department of Molecular Immunology; Cecil H. and Ida M. Green Investigator in Medical Research, Research Institute, Scripps Clinic and Research Foundation, La Jolla, Calif.

This is publication No. 2523 from the Research Institute of Scripps Clinic. This work was supported by United States Public Health Service grants AI 17354, CA 27489 and HL 16411.

tions. Clinically the most serious deficiency is that of C3. Recurrent, life-threatening septicemia, pneumonitis, meningitis, otitis media, skin and intestinal infections have been common in the few cases observed to date.

That complement may participate in disease mechanisms has also become clear, largely through the illuminating work done at Scripps Clinic and Research Foundation by Drs. Dixon, Cochrane, Oldstone, Wilson and their associates [5-7]. A complement-dependent pathogenesis has been demonstrated for certain experimental disease models such as nephritis, immune vasculitis, immune arthritis, LCM disease and myasthenia gravis. By analogy and on the basis of clinical investigations, it is probable that the corresponding diseases in man also involve complement in a similar manner.

Complement generates a plethora of biological activities, namely the ability to lyse viral membranes [8], kill gram-negative bacteria [9], kill nucleated cells [10], attract chemotactically inflammatory cells [11], cause the release of their hydrolytic enzymes [12], cause release of SRS-A [13], release histamine from mast cells [14] and opsonize foreign particles so that they may be ingested by phagocytic cells [15, 16]. Generation of these activities is accomplished by highly specific protein-protein interactions, protein-carbohydrate and protein-phospholipid interactions, involving, in part, limited proteolysis and conformational changes. As such, complement has become a model of complex, macromolecular biological systems.

The system is organized in three pathways: the classical [17], the alternative [18] and the common membrane attack pathway [19]. The initial enzyme of the classical pathway, C1, is activated by contact with antigen-antibody complexes. The initial enzyme of the alternative pathway is activated spontaneously, without antibody, by a very simple event, the reaction of native C3 with H_2O. In the course of complement activation, a unique molecular strategy becomes operative that allows transfer of the system from solution to the solid surface of a target particle [20]. The classical pathway establishes firm physical contact with a target particle through C4b; the alternative pathway does so through C3b. The target-bound classical C3 convertase is formed when C2, a proenzyme, binds to C4b and is activated by C1s. The target-bound alternative C3 convertase is formed when factor B, also a proenzyme, binds to

C3b and is activated by factor D. The action of either enzyme on C3 results in the binding to the target of multiple C3b molecules. One such C3b molecule is required for the transient binding and modulation of C5 in such a manner that it can be cleaved by the classical or alternative pathway enzyme. Cleavage of C5 initiates the self-assembly of the membrane attack complex. The three activation peptides C3a, C4a and C5a are released as anaphylatoxins in the process. It is clear from this brief description of the complex reaction sequence that C3 plays a dominant role.

Early History

C3 was first observed in 1958/59 in the Department of Clinical Chemistry at the University of Uppsala, Sweden, and was described in 1960 [1, 2]. The initial observations were simple: A minor β-globulin detectable by immunoelectrophoresis assumed a faster electrophoretic mobility upon incubation of fresh human serum with antigen-antibody complexes or with zymosan. After both proteins were isolated, it was found that the protein isolated from untreated serum was an essential ingredient of hemolytic complement and that the protein isolated from treated serum was hemolytically inactive. Second, C3 was fragmented in the course of complement activation because the reaction product, now called C3c, was found to be antigenically deficient compared to C3, and to have a lower sedimentation coefficient (7S) than C3 (9.5S). Third, prolonged exposure of isolated C3 to aqueous solvents under sterile conditions resulted in the gradual decay of its hemolytic activity and concomitant change in its electrophoretic mobility. The half-life at 37° was 111 hours and the rate of decay 0.45% per hour. A few years later it was observed that chaotropic agents such as KSCN greatly enhanced the spontaneous decay of C3 [21]. Chaotropic agents are known to perturb the tertiary structure of proteins, thus facilitating access of water to their interior. In 1961 it was found that treatment of C3 with low concentrations of simple amines such as hydrazine abolished both its hemolytic activity and its binding ability [22]. Thus, the very initial work on C3 described important properties of the protein such as its fragmentation during complement activation and its sensitivity to water, chaotropes and amines. When, in 1963, hydrazine was shown also to abolish the binding capacity of C4, the possibility was considered that the hydrazine effect might be due to nucleophilic attack on an internal ester [23].

The Internal Thioester of C3

Present evidence indicates that native C3 contains an internal thioester and that the reactions of this thioester are crucial for two basic events: (a) the initiation of the alternative pathway, and (b) the binding of activated C3 to biological particles. The thioester hypothesis was independently advanced in 1980 by Tack et al [24], Law et al [25] and Pangburn and Müller-Eberhard [26]. Treatment of C3 with radiolabeled methylamine instead of hydrazine resulted in inactivation of its hemolytic activity and in incorporation of 1 mole of methylamine into the protein. Concomitant with methylamine incorporation, 1 mole of sulfhydryl was liberated. Both the liberated sulfhydryl and the methylamine binding site were found in the 35,000-dalton d-domain of the α-chain of C3, suggesting a close topological relationship between the two sites. Swenson and Howard [27] had reported that serum α_2-macroglobulin is sensitive to treatment with methylamine and that methylamine was bound within the α_2-macroglobulin molecule to the γ-carboxyl group of a glutamyl residue which was contained in the sequence -Gly-Cys-Gly-Glu-Glu-Asn-. Subsequently, Tack et al [24] showed that C3 contained an identical sequence, that the methylamine binding residue of C3 was glutamic acid in postion 26 of the d-domain of the α-chain, and that the sulfhydryl group that was liberated on methylamine binding belonged to the cysteine residue in position 23 of the d-domain. The occurrence of this sequence in the α-chain of C3 was confirmed by Campbell et al [28]. The finding that the methylamine-reactive glutamyl residue and the iodoacetamide-reactive cysteinyl residue were separated only by two amino acid residues lent much weight to the concept of the existence of an internal thioester.

Molecular models indicated that the thioester bond within the hexapeptide might be relatively strain-free. Therefore, the hexapeptide was synthesized and the crucial thioester linkage was formed by activation of the penultimate glutamyl residue with 1-hydroxybenzotriazol and reaction of the resulting active ester with the cysteinyl thiol group [29]. The cyclized hexapeptide resembled native C3 in that it exhibited spontaneous hydrolysis and bound 1 mole of methylamine, with the concomitant liberation of 1 mole of sulfhydryl. Thus, the 15-membered thiolactone ring may indeed constitute a structural feature of native C3.

The Molecular Architecture of C3

Figure 1 shows schematic representations of the overall architecture of the C3 molecule and its physiological derivatives. C3 has a molecular weight of 185,000 and is composed of two nonidentical polypeptide chains. The molecular weight of the α-chain is 110,000 and that of the β-chain 75,000. The chains are linked by disulfide bonds and non-covalent forces. The internal thioester, which constitutes the precursor of the metastable binding site, is located in the α-chain and separated from the N-terminus by a mass of approximately 46,000 daltons. Its location was deduced from the observation that the α-chain is autocatalytically cleaved when C3 is exposed to sodium dodecyl sulfate and elevated temperatures. The bond cleaved under these conditions has been identified as the -Glu-Glu- bond within the thiolactone ring [30, 31].

C3 is activated by cleavage of peptide bond 77 (-Arg-Ser-) of the α-chain. Removal of the 9000-dalton activation peptide, C3a, leads to the activation of the metastable binding site in the C3b fragment (see below). C3b consists of the α'-chain and the intact β-chain. In its bound or unbound form, C3b is susceptible to attack by the endopeptidase factor I (C3b inactivator) and its cofactor, factor H (β1H). The product, C3bi, consists of two α'-chain fragments (67,000 and 40,000 daltons) which are linked by disulfide bonds to the intact β-chain [32, 33]. The molecular weight of C3bi is identical to that of C3b, but C3bi has none of the functional properties that characterize C3b. A tryptic plasma enzyme then cleaves the 67,000-dalton α'-fragment and thereby severs C3c from C3d. C3c has a molecular weight of 150,000 and consists of two α'-fragments (35,000 and 40,000 daltons) and the β-chain. The 35,000-dalton C3d fragment contains the liberated sulfhydryl group that in native C3 is part of the thiolactone ring. C3d that is derived from

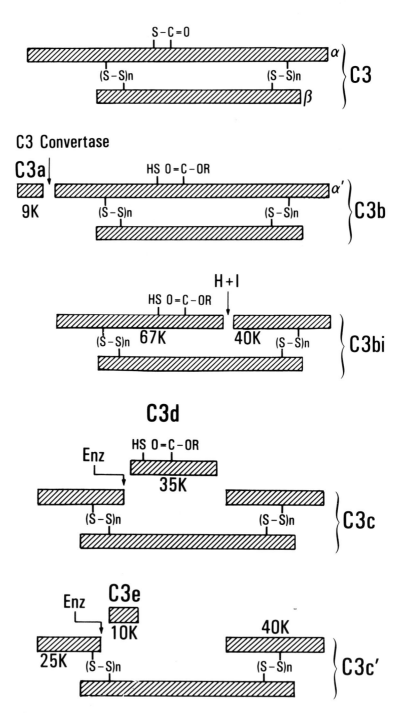

FIG. 1. Chain structure of C3, including approximate topology of the thioester and of the physiological reaction products.

bound C3b remains bound to the target particle. The 10,000-dalton acidic C3e fragment is derived from C3c, probably by tryptic attack on the 35,000-dalton α'-fragment [34].

The biological functions of the various C3 fragments are as follows (for detailed references, see Müller-Eberhard and Schreiber [18]). C3a is one of the three anaphylatoxins; it addresses specific receptors on smooth muscle cells, mast cells and polymorphonuclear leukocytes. In vivo, C3a, like C4a and particularly C5a, exhibits phlogogenic activity. C3b has multiple functions, including the recognition function of the alternative pathway. It constitutes a subunit of the classical C5 convertase and of the alternative C3/C5 convertase. It is the ligand for C3b-specific cell surface receptors which occur on polymorphonuclear leukocytes, monocytes, macrophages and B lymphocytes. C3bi lacks the foregoing activities but is specific for C3bi receptors occurring on the surface of polymorphs, monocytes, mast cells and K lymphocytes that serve as effector cells in antibody-dependent cellular cytotoxicity (ADCC) reactions. C3d also reacts with specific C3d cell surface receptors which occur on K lymphocytes. The interactions of the C3 fragments with cellular receptors enhance phagocytosis, extracellular killing and the K cell-dependent ADCC. Finally, C3e is a leukocytosis-inducing peptide.

Metastable C3b and the Function of Its Thioester Site

The concept of the metastable binding site of activated C3 was proposed in 1966 [35]. It had been known that complement cannot accomplish its opsonic and cytolytic functions unless C3 becomes physically bound to the target particle. The problem was this: Isolated, native C3 was unable to bind to targets of complement attack such as cells. In the classical pathway, which was then studied exclusively, C4 and C2 were required for the mediation of C3 binding. The possibility existed that the C4,2 complex acted as a receptor for native C3 with a binding capacity for one molecule. This hypothesis could be ruled out when differentially radiolabeled C3 and C4 were utilized for quantitative binding studies. It could be established that one C4,2 complex on the surface of a target cell was capable of mediating the binding of a large multiplicity of C3 molecules. In addition, many more C3 molecules accumulated in physically and chemically altered form in the fluid phase. These results not only established the enzymatic nature of the C4,2 complex, but they also led to the realization that the altered C3 molecules in the fluid phase were unable to bind to the target cell, in spite of their having been turned over by the activating enzyme. A labile intermediate form of activated C3 was therefore postulated which was thought to be endowed with a metastable binding site. It was proposed that C3 activated by C3 convertase could bind to targets through this metastable binding site, but failing attachment to the target the metastable C3 would decay and accumulate in inactive form in the fluid phase [35]. A similar mechanism of binding was proposed for activated C4 [36]. This concept was entirely new in protein chemistry and envisaged unique properties for these two proteins that were without precedent. More than ten years later, Law and Levine [37] made the important observation that C3b is bound to zymosan, an insoluble polysaccharide of yeast cell walls, through a hydroxylamine-labile bond. They also found that hydroxamate was associated with the protein that was released from zymosan upon hydroxylamine treatment [38]. The hydroxamate group was located in the d-domain, which, according to the foregoing, also contains the thioester.

In present language, the enzymatically catalyzed binding of C3 to complement targets may be described in the following manner (Fig. 2). When native C3 is attacked by one of its two activating enzymes and the activation peptide, C3a, is removed, the thioester of the d-domain of the α-chain is revealed and comes under stress. The reactive carbonyl in the thioester bond can now transfer to an ester bond formed with a hydroxyl group on the surface of the target [38]. Alternatively, it is conceivable that it may also form an amide bond with an amino group on the receptive surface [39, 40]. C3b becomes thus covalently bound to a target and exhibits a free sulfhydryl group. Metastable C3b that fails to undergo transesterification of its thioester reacts with water and thereby loses its activated binding site. This form of C3b has gained a free sulfhydryl group and an extra carboxyl group and remains henceforth in the fluid phase. However, as will be seen, unbound C3b exhibits most, if not all, functional properties of bound C3b. Thus, binding of C3 to biological particles is covalent in nature and critically involves the internal thioester.

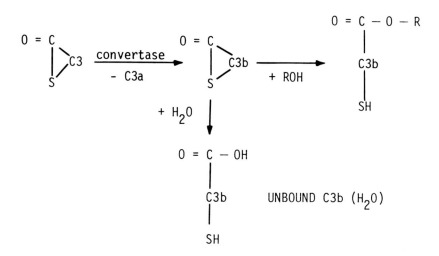

FIG. 2. The binding reaction of C3: Formation of metastable C3b and transesterification of the carbonyl group in the thioester to an ester with a hydroxyl group on the receptive surface.

Multiple Functional Sites of C3b

Perhaps nothing expresses the versatility of C3 more than the occurrence of the multiple functional sites on the C3b fragment. In addition to the metastable binding site, C3b possesses binding sites for (a) factor B, without which the alternative C3 convertase could not be formed; (b) C5, without which C5 could not be properly presented to activated factor B or C2 for cleavage into C5a and C5b; (c) properdin, which allows properdin to stabilize the C3 convertase C3b,Bb; (d) factor H, which allows factor H to exercise control over the C3/5 convertase; and (e) factor I, at which site factor I acts to convert C3b to C3bi. There are also the molecular regions which specifically bind to the C3b receptor of certain cells and, as yet hidden in the C3b molecule, the sites that are specific for the cell surface C3bi and C3d receptors.

Brief mention should be made also of a hypothetical recognition site on the target-bound C3b molecule [18, 41, 42].

Depending on the microenvironment of bound C3b, it either binds preferentially factor B to form the C3 convertase of the alternative pathway, or it binds factor H and is subsequently degraded by factor I. For instance, human C3b on human or on sheep erythrocytes is rapidly degraded, while on rabbit erythrocytes or *E. coli* it is not [42-44]. The diminished binding of factor H to C3b in the latter two situations has been interpreted to suggest that C3b is endowed with a recognition or discriminating site that can engage itself with a select variety of cell surface constituents. Engagement of this site then results in a relative abolition of the factor H binding site of C3b [42].

It is hoped that the various binding sites on C3b may be accessible to mapping and to chemical studies. Certain monoclonal antibodies raised to C3b and to other C3 fragments were capable of inhibiting binding of factor H to C3b, but not that of factor B or properdin. Other monoclonal antibodies inhibited the binding of properdin, but not of factor B or factor H (J.D. Tamerius, M.K. Pangburn and H.J. Müller-Eberhard, unpublished observations). Since C3 and C3b have a characteristic ultrastructure, as electron microscope studies have shown (C. Smith, M.K. Pangburn and H.J. Müller-Eberhard, unpublished observations), it may be possible to correlate functional regions with submolecular topology.

Functionally C3b-Like C3 Generated Nonenzymatically by Nucleophilic Attack or Hydrolysis of the Thioester in Native C3

Native C3 expresses no detectable biological activity. There is no evidence, for instance, that it can bind factor B. Yet, when native C3, factors B, D and Mg^{++} are admixed in physiological concentrations, C3 convertase activity rapidly appears [18, 45]. It was hypothesized, therefore, that a C3 conformer, representing a very small proportion of native C3, might have C3b-like functional properties [18].

Recent evidence strongly suggests that the postulated C3 conformer constitutes C3 that has lost the internal thioester by reacting with water. It was found that C3 with its thioester hydrolyzed ($C3[H_2O]$) exhibits all functional properties of C3b [46]. $C3(H_2O)$ appears to be the first reaction product in the intitiation of the alternative pathway (see below).

When studies of the effect of CH_3NH_2 on C3 made it likely that an internal thioester was opened up without any effect on the primary peptide structure of the protein, $C3(CH_3NH_2)$ was subjected to functional and conformational analyses. It was found that $C3(CH_3NH_2)$ can bind factors B and H, can form a fluid-phase C3 convertase with factors B, D and Mg^{++} and can be cleaved and inactivated by factors H and I [26].

Circular dichroism studies and fluorescence measurements of binding of 1-anilino-8-naphthalene sulfonate (ANS) detected the occurrence of marked spectral changes when C3 was converted to $C3(CH_3NH_2)$ [47]. The spectra of $C3(CH_3NH_2)$ resembled those of C3b [48]. There was, however, a considerable difference in the rate of methylamine uptake by C3 and the rate of conformational rearrangement, which was considerably slower than the former. Further, the appearance of functional properties correlated with the rate of conformational change rather than the rate of chemical modification. And the acquisition of factor H binding capacity by methylamine-modified C3 was slower than the acquisition of factor B binding sites. For instance, at a given methylamine concentration and at $37°$ the methylamine uptake was essentially complete at 5 minutes, whereas 50% factor B and factor H binding activity became expressed at 25 and 35 minutes, respectively [47]. These kinetics suggest that C3, modified at the thioester site, has temporarily a slightly greater chance to form the fluid-phase C3 convertase than to become enzymatically degraded by factors H and I.

The studies of $C3(CH_3NH_2)$ prompted a reinvestigation of the spontaneous decay of C3 in aqueous solution [2] and of the effect of chaotropic agents on C3 [21]. It was found [46] that the rate of spontaneous loss of the C3 binding site in neutral buffer at $37°$ was 0.005% per minute. In the presence of 0.33 M KSCN the rate of inactivation was 1250-fold enhanced, or 6.25% per minute. With progression of inactivation, a free sulfhydryl group appeared which is not present in native C3. The final product has been considered C3 with its thioester hydrolyzed $(C3[H_2O])$. As listed in Table 1, $C3(H_2O)$ exhibits all functional properties of fluid-phase C3b. And, as shown in Figure 3, $C3(H_2O)$ is structurally distinct from C3b in that it contains an intact α-chain rather than the α'-chain, which lacks the C3a domain. Although $C3(H_2O)$ is structurally indis-

Table 1. The C3b-Like Functions of C3(H$_2$O)

Properties	C3	C3b	C3(H$_2$O)
Binding of B	−	+	+
Formation of C3 convertase	−	+	+
Binding of H	−	+	+
Cleavage by I	−	+	+
Binding to cellular C3b receptors	−	+	+
Cleavage by C3 convertase	+	−	±
Metastable binding site	+	−	−

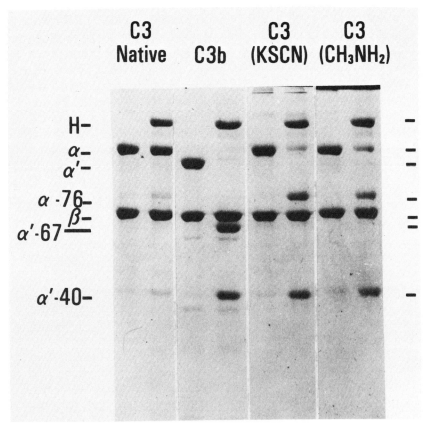

FIG. 3. Susceptibility of C3 modified at the thioester site either by water (C3[KSCN]) or methylamine (C3[CH$_3$NH$_2$]) to cleavage by factors H and I. For comparison, the behavior of native C3 and C3b is shown after treatment with the control proteins (modified from Pangburn et al [46]).

tinguishable from native C3 by its appearance on SDS-poly-acrylamide gel electrophoresis, unlike native C3, its α-chain is susceptible to cleavage by factor I. Factor I cleaves the α-chain of C3(H_2O) (and C3[CH_3NH_2]) into a 76,000- and a 40,000-molecular weight fragment. The 76,000-dalton fragment contains the 67,000-dalton piece of the α′-chain of C3bi, plus the covalently linked 9,000-dalton C3a domain.

The Role of C3(H_2O), Metastable C3b and Target-Bound C3b in the Initiation of the Alternative Pathway

As schematically presented in Figure 4, it is proposed [46] that the initial event in the alternative pathway is the spontaneous generation of C3(H_2O) which is formed continuously at a slow rate. Due to the differential rate of appearance of binding sites during the transition of native C3 to the

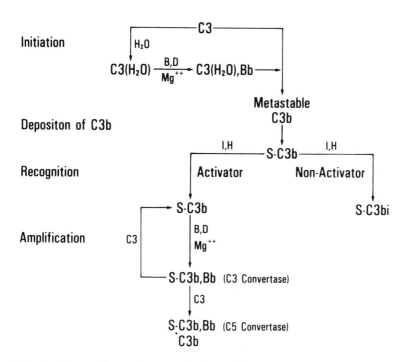

FIG. 4. Proposed reaction mechanism of the alternative pathway of complement activation [46].

C3b-like form of the molecule, the fluid-phase C3 convertase C3(H_2O)Bb may form and generate metastable C3b from native C3 before the enzyme becomes fully susceptible to control by factors H and I. Metastable C3b so generated may randomly attach to surrounding receptive surfaces. Deposited C3b then exercises its discriminatory ability of distinguishing between different cells. On nonactivators of the alternative pathway it is rapidly degraded by factors H and I to C3bi and subsequently by other enzymes to smaller fragments. On activators, the affinity of C3b for factor H is reduced and degradation is sufficiently retarded to allow C3 convertase formation on the target particle, amplification by the C3b-dependent positive feedback and C5 convertase assembly with stabilization of the enzyme by properdin [18, 49].

The recognition of C3(H_2O) [26, 46] as a new functional form of C3 and the observation that C3(H_2O) arises spontaneously may resolve the long-standing question as to the manner in which the alternative pathway is initiated [18, 41, 45, 50, 51].

Evolutionary Relationship Between C3, C4 and C5

The three proteins exhibit many similarities and differences. All three proteins are synthesized as a single polypeptide chain which is processed after translation into the respective chain structures [52]. The α-chain of each protein contributes one of the three anaphylatoxins in the form of the activation peptide. These peptides exhibit similar biological activities, 36% to 38% homology in primary structure and approximately 45% α-helical content [3, 11, 53]. C4 contains the same type of metastable binding site as does C3 [36, 54, 55], but C5 does not. In fact, the sequence around the internal thioester is identical in C3 and C4 [28]. C4 is genetically linked to the MHC; C3 and C5 are not (for references, see Raum et al [4]). C3 binds factor B and C4 binds C2, and these constitute two very similar serine proteases [56] that are genetically linked to the MHC and to each other (for references, see Raum et al [4]).

Membrane Attack: The Dependence of C5
Functions on C3 and C4

C5 is the nucleus in the assembly of the membrane attack complex (MAC), which is formed from five hydrophilic precursor proteins: C5, C6, C7, C8 and C9. C5 has binding sites for C6, C7 and C8. In order to initiate fusion of the five precursor proteins into the amphiphilic and membranolytic MAC, C5 must be cleaved by one of the two C5 convertases into C5a and C5b. Cleavage of C5 is absolutely dependent on C3b, to which it must bind in order to be rendered susceptible to enzymatic attack. In the case of the classical pathway, this enzymatic attack is dependent on C4b, which functions as modulator of the enzyme C2. In the case of the alternative pathway, it is C3b that functions as modulator of the activating enzyme factor B. The point to be emphasized is that the participation of C5 in MAC assembly is entirely dependent on functions of its two homologues, especially on those of C3.

After cleavage of C5, the phlogogenic peptide C5a is removed and C5b, the major reaction product, remains momentarily associated with C3b to await C6 with which it fuses into a bimolecular complex. Upon collision with C7, the resulting trimolecular complex acquires a metastable binding site (which is chemically distinct from that of C3 and C4) through which it can non-covalently bind to phospholipid membranes. C8 then endows the complex with a C9 binding and polymerization site. Two such supramolecular organizations dimerize to a 2 million-dalton tubular structure which is composed of 20 tightly fused molecules and which may be described by the formula $(C5b,C6,C7,C8,C9_6)_2$ [57]. Evidence is accumulating suggesting that the poly-C9 structure within the MAC is primarily responsible for the lipid binding and membranolytic capacity of the MAC [58-61]. The MAC exerts its cell-killing and membrane-disassembling effects by weakening the plasma membrane structure and by formation of transmembrane channels.

Conclusion

Instead of presenting an overview of the present status of complement research covering all areas of chemistry and biology of complement, only one protein was singled out for discussion: C3. It fulfills many functions in host defense and inflammation. While native C3 as such possesses no discernible biological activity, it harbors many distinct structures that constitute the precursors of functional sites. The internal thioester represents not only a novel chemical structure, but it is the strategic center that controls the expression of many functions of the molecule. Upon its spontaneous hydrolysis, native C3, without enzymatic modification, acquires the ability to form a fluid-phase C3 convertase together with factors B, D and Mg^{++}. The reaction of native C3 with one molecule of water may therefore constitute the simple, nonspecific event that initiates perpetually the alternative pathway of complement activation which is regarded as one of the mechanisms of nonspecific resistance to infections. Enzymatic attack of native C3 by the C3 convertase of the classical or the alternative pathway generates metastable C3b. Although enzymatic cleavage occurs near the N-terminus of the α-chain, it is the thioester in the d-domain of the α-chain, which is far removed from the cleavage site, that is affected. Within microseconds the reactive carbonyl group of the thioester in metastable C3b can undergo transesterification and form an ester bond with a hydroxyl group on the surface of biological particles. Thus is effected the transfer of C3 from solution to the solid phase of complement targets. Deposited on a target by the classical pathway, it becomes a subunit of its C5 convertase. Deposited via the alternative pathway, it exercises a low-specificity discriminatory function, furnishes two of the three subunits of the C3/C5 convertase and ignites the unique amplification reaction which is the driving force of the alternative pathway. C3b also functions as an opsonin by serving as a ligand for specific cell surface receptors. Its degradation products, C3bi and C3d, fulfill similar ligand functions. The activation peptide C3a constitutes one of the three anaphylatoxins, which have inflammation-producing activity. The other two anaphylatoxins are derived from C4 and C5. These two proteins are considered evolutionary relatives of C3 because limited sequence analysis has revealed a degree of homology in primary structure.

References

1. Müller-Eberhard, H.J., Nilsson, U. and Aronsson, T.: Isolation and characterization of two β_1-glycoproteins of human serum. J. Exp. Med. 111:201, 1960.
2. Müller-Eberhard, H.J. and Nilsson, U.: Relation of a β_1-glycoprotein of human serum to the complement system. J. Exp. Med. 111:217, 1960.
3. Gorski, J.P., Hugli, T.E. and Müller-Eberhard, H.J.: Characterization of human C4a anaphylatoxin. J. Biol. Chem. 256:2707, 1981.

4. Raum, D., Donaldson, V.H., Alper, C.A. and Rosen, F.S.: Genetics of complement and complement deficiencies. *In* Fougereau, M. and Dausset, J. (eds.): Immunology 80, Progress in Immunology IV. London:Academic Press, 1980, p. 1244.

5. Dixon, F.J. and Wilson, C.B.: Immunological renal injury produced by formation and deposition of immune complexes. *In* Wilson, C.B., Brenner, B.M. and Stein, J.H. (eds.): Immunologic Mechanisms of Renal Disease; Contemporary Issues in Nephrology. New York: Churchill Livingstone, 1979, vol. 3., p.1.

6. Wilson, C.B. and Dixon, F.J.: Renal injury from immune reactions involving antigens in or of the kidney. *In* Wilson, C.B., Brenner, B.M. and Stein, J.H. (eds.): Immunologic Mechanisms of Renal Disease; Contemporary Issues in Nephrology. New York:Churchill Livingstone, 1979, vol. 3, p. 35.

7. Cochrane, C.G.: Mediation systems in neutrophil-independent immunologic injury of the glomerulus. *In* Wilson, C.B., Brenner, B.M. and Stein, J.H. (eds.): Immunologic Mechanisms of Renal Disease; Contemporary Issues in Nephrology. New York:Churchill Livingstone, 1979, vol. 3, p. 106.

8. Esser, A.F., Bartholomew, R.M., Jensen, F.C. and Müller-Eberhard, H.J.: Disassembly of viral membranes by complement independent of channel formation. Proc. Natl. Acad. Sci. U.S.A. 76:5843, 1979.

9. Schreiber, R.D., Morrison, D.C., Podack, E.R. and Müller-Eberhard, H.J.: Bactericidal activity of the alternative complement pathway generated from eleven isolated plasma proteins. J. Exp. Med. 149:870, 1979.

10. Schreiber, R.D., Pangburn, M.K., Medicus, R.G. and Müller-Eberhard, H.J.: Raji cell injury and subsequent lysis by the purified cytolytic alternative pathway of human complement. Clin. Immunol. Immunopathol. 15:384, 1980.

11. Hugli, T.E. and Müller-Eberhard, H.J.: Anaphylatoxins: C3a and C5a. Adv. Immunol. 26:1, 1978.

12. Chenoweth, D.E. and Hugli, T.E.: Human C5a and C5a analogs as probes of the neutrophil C5a receptor. Mol. Immunol. 17:151, 1980.

13. Stimler, N.P., Brocklehurst, W.E., Bloor, C.M. and Hugli, T.E.: Complement anaphylatoxin C5a stimulates release of SRS-A-like activity from guinea-pig lung fragments. J. Pharm. Pharmacol. 32:804, 1980.

14. Johnson, A.R., Hugli, T.E. and Müller-Eberhard, H.J.: Release of histamine from rat mast cells by the complement peptides C3a and C5a. Immunology 28:1067, 1975.

15. Gagli, I. and Nelson, R.A., Jr.: Complement dependent immune phagocytosis. I. Requirements for C'1, C'4, C'2, C'3. Exp. Cell Res. 51:45, 1968.

16. Huber, H., Polley, M.J., Linscott, W.D. et al: Human monocytes: Distinct receptor sites for the third component of complement and for immunoglobulin G. Science 162:1281, 1968.

17. Porter, R.R. and Reid, K.B.: Activation of the complement system by

antibody-antigen complexes: The classical pathway. Adv. Protein Chem. 33:1, 1979.

18. Müller-Eberhard, H.J. and Schreiber, R.D.: Molecular biology and chemistry of the alternative pathway of complement. Adv. Immunol. 29:1, 1980.

19. Podack, E.R., Esser, A.F., Biesecker, G. and Müller-Eberhard, H.J.: Membrane attack complex of complement: A structural analysis of its assembly. J. Exp. Med. 151:301, 1980.

20. Müller-Eberhard, H.J.: Complement. Annu. Rev. Biochem. 44:697, 1975.

21. Dalmasso, A.P. and Müller-Eberhard, H.J.: Hemolytic activity of lipoprotein-depleted serum and effect of certain anions on complement. J. Immunol. 97:680, 1966.

22. Müller-Eberhard, H.J.: Isolation and description of proteins related to the human complement system. Acta Soc. Med. Upsal. 66:152, 1961.

23. Müller-Eberhard, H.J. and Biro, C.E.: Isolation and description of the fourth component of human complement. J. Exp. Med. 118:447, 1963.

24. Tack, B.F., Harrison, R.A., Janatova, J. et al: Evidence for presence of an internal thiolester bond in third component of human complement. Proc. Natl. Acad. Sci. U.S.A. 77:5764, 1980.

25. Law, S.K., Lichtenberg, N.A. and Levine, R.P.: Covalent binding and hemolytic activity of complement proteins (inactivation by amines). Proc. Natl. Acad. Sci. U.S.A. 77:7194, 1980.

26. Pangburn, M.K. and Müller-Eberhard, H.J.: Relation of a putative thioester bond in C3 to activation of the alternative pathway and the binding of C3b to biological targets of complement. J. Exp. Med. 152:1102, 1980.

27. Swenson, R.P. and Howard, J.B.: Characterization of alkylamine-sensitive site in α_2-macroglobulin. Proc. Natl. Acad. Sci. U.S.A. 76:4313, 1979.

28. Campbell, R.D., Gagnon, J. and Porter, R.R.: Amino acid sequence around the proposed thiolester bond of human complement component C4 and comparison with the corresponding sequences from C3 and α_2-macroglobulin. Bioscience Rep. 1:423, 1981.

29. Khan, S.A., Pangburn, M.K., Müller-Eberhard, H.J. and Erickson, B.W.: The cyclic thioester form of a synthetic hexapeptide from human complement protein C3 resembles the C3b metastable binding site. Fed. Proc. 40:1679, 1981.

30. Sim, R.B. and Sim, E.: Autolytic fragmentation of complement components C3 and C4 under denaturing conditions, a property shared with α_2-macroglobulin. Biochem. J. 193:129, 1981.

31. Howard, J.B.: Methylamine reaction and denaturation-dependent fragmentation of complement component 3: Comparison with α_2-macroglobulin. J. Biol. Chem. 255:7082, 1980.

32. Pangburn, M.K., Schreiber, R.D. and Müller-Eberhard, H.J.: Human complement C3b inactivator: Isolation, characterization and demonstration of an absolute requirement for the serum protein $\beta 1H$ for cleavage of C3b and C4b in solution. J. Exp. Med. 146:257, 1977.

33. Lachmann, P.J.: Complement. *In* Sela, M. (ed.): The Antigens. New York:Academic Press, 1979, vol. 5, p. 284.
34. Ghebrehiwet, B. and Müller-Eberhard, H.J.: C3e: An acidic fragment of human C3 with leukocytosis inducing activity. J. Immunol. 123:616, 1979.
35. Müller-Eberhard, H.J., Dalmasso, A.P. and Calcott, M.A.: The reaction mechanism of β_{1C}-globulin (C′3) in immune hemolysis. J. Exp. Med. 123:33, 1966.
36. Müller-Eberhard, H.J. and Lepow, I.H.: C′1 esterase effect on activity and physicochemical properties of the fourth component of complement. J. Exp. Med. 121:819, 1965.
37. Law, S.K. and Levine, R.P.: Interaction between the third complement protein and cell surface. Proc. Natl. Acad. Sci. U.S.A. 74:2701, 1977.
38. Law, S.K., Lichtenberg, N.A. and Levine, R.P.: Evidence for an ester linkage between the labile binding site of C3b and receptive surfaces. J. Immunol. 123:1388, 1979.
39. Campbell, R.D., Dodds, A.W. and Porter, R.R.: The binding of human complement component C4 to antibody-antigen aggregates. Biochem. J. 189:67, 1980.
40. Sim, R.B., Twose, T.M., Paterson, D.S. and Sim, E.: The covalent-binding reaction of complement component C3. Biochem. J. 193:115, 1981.
41. Schreiber, R.D., Pangburn, M.K., Lesavre, P. and Müller-Eberhard, H.J.: Initiation of the alternative pathway of complement: Recognition of activators by bound C3b and assembly of the entire pathway from six isolated proteins. Proc. Natl. Acad. Sci. U.S.A. 75:3948, 1978.
42. Pangburn, M.K., Morrison, D.C., Schreiber, R.D. and Müller-Eberhard, H.J.: Activation of the alternative complement pathway: Recognition of surface structures on activators by bound C3b. J. Immunol. 124:977, 1980.
43. Fearon, D.T. and Austen, K.F.: Activation of the alternative complement pathway due to resistance of zymosan-bound amplification convertase to endogenous regulatory mechanisms. Proc. Natl. Acad. Sci. U.S.A. 74:1683, 1977.
44. Pangburn, M.D. and Müller-Eberhard, H.J.: Complement C3 convertase: Cell surface restriction of β1H control and generation of restriction on neuraminidase treated cells. Proc. Natl. Acad. Sci. U.S.A. 75:2416, 1978.
45. Fearon, D.T. and Austen, K.F.: Initiation of C3 cleavage in the alternative complement pathway. J. Immunol. 115:1357, 1975.
46. Pangburn, M.K., Schreiber, R.D. and Müller-Eberhard, H.J.: Formation of the initial C3 convertase of the alternative complement pathway: Acquisition of C3b-like activities by spontaneous hydrolysis of the putative thioester in native C3. J. Exp. Med., vol. 154, 1981. (In press.)
47. Isenman, D.E., Kells, D.I.C., Cooper, N.R. et al: Nucleophilic modification of human complement protein C3: Correlation of

conformational changes with acquisition of C3b-like functional properties. Biochemistry, 1981. (In press.)

48. Isenman, D.E. and Cooper, N.R.: The structure and function of the third component of human complement. I. The nature and extent of conformational changes accompanying C3 activation. Mol. Immunol. 18:331, 1981.

49. Müller-Eberhard, H.J.: Complement reaction pathways. *In* Fougereau, M. and Dausset, J. (eds.): Immunology 80, Progress in Immunology IV. London:Academic Press, 1980, p. 1001.

50. Müller-Eberhard, H.J. and Götze, O.: C3 proactivator convertase and its mode of action. J. Exp. Med. 135:1003, 1972.

51. Nicol, P.A.E. and Lachmann, P.J.: The alternate pathway of complement activation. The role of C3 and its inactivator (KAF). Immunology 24:259, 1973.

52. Ooi, Y.M. and Colten, H.R.: Genetic deficiency of C5 in mice: A defect in secretion. J. Immunol. 124:1534, 1980.

53. Gorski, J.P., Hugli, T.E. and Müller-Eberhard, H.J.: C4a: The third anaphylatoxin of the human complement system. Proc. Natl. Acad. Sci. U.S.A. 76:5299, 1979.

54. Gorski, J.P. and Howard, J.B.: Effect of methylamine on the structure and function of the fourth component of human complement, C4. J. Biol. Chem. 255:10025, 1980.

55. Janatova, J. and Tack, B.F.: The fourth component of human complement: Studies of an amine-sensitive site comprised of a thiol component. Biochemistry 20:2394, 1981.

56. Medicus, R.G., Götze, O. and Müller-Eberhard, H.J.: The serine protease nature of the C3 and C5 convertases of the classical and alternative complement pathways. Scand. J. Immunol. 5:1049, 1976.

57. Podack, E.R. and Müller-Eberhard, H.J.: Membrane attack complex of complement. Evidence for its dimeric structure based on hybrid formation. J. Biol. Chem. 256:3145, 1981.

58. Podack, E.R., Biesecker, G. and Müller-Eberhard, H.J.: Membrane attack complex of complement: Generation of high affinity phospholipid binding sites by the fusion of five hydrophilic, plasma proteins. Proc. Natl. Acad. Sci. U.S.A. 76:897, 1979.

59. Tschopp, J. and Podack, E.R.: Membranolysis by the ninth component of human complement. Biochem. Biophys. Res. Commun. 100:1409, 1981.

60. Hu, V.W., Esser, A.F., Podack, E.R. and Wisnieski, B.J.: The membrane attack mechanism of complement: Photolabeling reveals insertion of terminal proteins into target membrane. J. Immunol. 127:380, 1981.

61. Podack, E.R., Stoffel, W., Esser, A.F. and Müller-Eberhard, H.J.: Membrane attack complex of complement: Distribution of subunits between the hydrocarbon phase of target membrane and water. Proc. Natl. Acad. Sci. U.S.A., vol. 78, 1981. (In press.)

Application of
Basic Immunobiology to
Immunopathology

The Pathogenesis of Inflammatory Injury Produced by Bacterial Lipopolysaccharides

Charles G. Cochrane, M.D.

Following the injection of bacteria or bacterial lipopoly-saccharide (LPS) intravenously into experimental animals, many of the pathophysiologic changes occur that are observed in bacteremia shock of human beings [1]. Hypotension [2-6], disseminated intravascular coagulation (DIC) [3, 4, 7-11], changes in peripheral leukocytes and platelets [3-5, 12] and death are all observed. The mechanisms responsible for these changes are poorly understood, even though much is known of the biologic activity of LPS. LPS is capable of activating both classical and alternative pathways of complement [13-18], as well as Hageman factor [19]; induces release of vasoactive and coagulation-promoting substances from platelets [12, 20, 21], damages endothelial cells [22-24]; and promotes release of effector substances from neutrophils [25], monocytes [26] and macrophages [17].

The Complement System in LPS-Induced Shock

With the correlation having been drawn between the diminution of complement levels and the severity of shock in bacteremic human beings, we undertook studies of the role of complement in the development of pathophysiologic changes in

Charles G. Cochrane, M.D., Member, Department of Immunopathology, Scripps Clinic and Research Foundation, La Jolla, Calif.

This is publication No. 2326 from the Department of Immunopathology, Scripps Clinic and Research Foundation. This work was supported in part by NIH grants AI-07007 and HL-16411, the Office of Naval Research and the Council for Tobacco Research.

rabbits and rhesus monkeys. Intravenous infusion of highly purified LPS of *E. coli* 0111:B4 and *S. minnesota* R595 were performed in normal and complement-depleted animals and in rabbits genetically deficient in the sixth component of complement. Complement depletion was accomplished using the purified anticomplementary factor in cobra venom [27], which depleted over 95% of C3 and terminal components in both species of animals. Hypotension, prolonged thrombocytopenia, neutropenia, DIC and death occurred to the same extent in all animals whether or not they were deficient in complement components [28]. A similar lack of effect of complement depletion on the prolonged hypotension and shock was noted in dogs [5]. In order to effect a hypotensive response with activated complement, a massive and rapid activation was required, leading to a fall in C3 levels of 30% in the first few minutes. The hypotension and thrombocytopenia were of short (<20 minutes) duration as opposed to that occurring in the shock phase of LPS-induced injury noted above, where thrombocytopenia, hypotension and DIC developed after 90 minutes. The immediate, evanescent hypotension caused by rapid activation of complement in vivo was inhibited with the histamine H_2-receptor antagonist, burimamide [29]. We have concluded that while complement is activated by LPS in vivo, the full spectrum of sustained pathophysiologic changes can be induced in rhesus monkeys and rabbits that have been depleted of C3 and terminal components, frequently beyond detection, and in rabbits genetically deficient in the sixth component of complement. The conclusions are supported by recent data, described below, in which a lipoprotein-complexed LPS fails to activate complement and yet induces hypotensive shock and DIC.

The Hageman Factor System in LPS-Induced Shock

Another system of plasma components that must be considered in the pathogenesis of LPS-induced injury is the Hageman factor (HF) system [30]. As noted above, HF is activated when, in the presence of prekallikrein, it interacts with LPS [19]. In man, during sepsis [31-36] a decrease in prekallikrein has been observed along with a depletion of kallikrein inhibitor [31, 35, 36]. Activation of prekallikrein in the blood stream has been postulated by virtue of a conversion in electrophoretic migration of prekallikrein to correspond to that of a complex with kallikrein inhibitor, C1s inh [33]; and more commonly, by the appearance of arginine esterase activity in the plasma. Concomitantly, Hageman factor [31, 36] and kininogen [34, 36] levels of the plasma are reportedly diminished in patients and free kinin has been detected [34].

In experimental hypotensive shock, a fall in kininogen level and appearance of free kinin activity has been correlated with a fall in peripheral arterial resistance in rhesus monkeys [37], or in monkeys infected with *S. typhimurium* [38]. Similar changes in components of the system have been detected in rabbits [39] and dogs [40, 41].

We have examined directly the effect of LPS shock on the level of circulating human high-molecular weight kininogen in rabbits and rhesus monkeys. In rabbits given lethal doses of LPS, ^{125}I-high-MW kininogen circulated normally and failed to undergo cleavage [42]. The ^{125}I-high-MW kininogen in rabbit plasma was fully reactive when the plasma contacted a negatively charged surface. The data may be explained by an insufficient consumption and removal of the circulating high-MW kininogen for detection during development of shock and probably not to rapid loss of kallikrein-cleaved high-MW kininogen from the circulation, since fully cleaved high-MW kininogen circulated with a half-life of 38 hours, compared to 44 hours of the native molecule. Similarly, in rhesus monkeys, a minimal increased loss of circulating ^{125}I-high-MW kininogen was observed (unpublished data). However, when the labeled protein was infused into the bronchoalveolar space of six rhesus monkeys five hours after infusion of either *E. coli* organisms or LPS of *S. minn.* R595, cleavage of the high-MW kininogen occurred as demonstrated in SDS-acrylamide gel after extraction from the lung. Lavage fluid of the bronchoalveolar tree of LPS-treated monkeys (but not normals) contained enzyme that also cleaved the ^{125}I-high-MW kininogen (unpublished observations).

Thus the Hageman factor system may participate in inflammatory reactions outside of the blood vessels and a reflection of their participation may not be observed intravascularly. Whether the cleavage of components in the tissues or by fluid obtained from the bronchoalveolar space bears on the pathogenesis of the inflammatory disease induced by bacterial LPS will be determined by future studies.

Localization of LPS In Vivo

Another experimental approach to the pathogenesis of LPS-induced injury in the whole animal has been our examination of the tissue distribution and cellular localization of LPS during development of lesions. Studies employing radiolabeled LPS or endotoxins [43-54] or immunofluorescence [55-58] have revealed rapid deposition of the radiolabel in the tissues, predominantly in the liver, after IV injection. Leukocytes and macrophages were found to be the preferred sites. However, the type of chemical bond between LPS and the radiolabel was not known, significant loss of label occurred immediately after injection, and loss of biologic activity in the labeling process has made these data difficult to interpret.

Recently, these problems have been overcome by ^{125}I covalently coupled to purified LPS as performed by Ulevitch [59]. These preparations of ^{125}I-LPS are of high specific activity and the LPS retains full biologic activity. The ^{125}I-LPS recovered from the tissues after IV injection showed no apparent changes in physical characteristics. When infused IV, the ^{125}I-LPS was observed to disappear from the circulation in two phases, one being rapid ($t_{1/2}$ = <30 minutes) and a second having a prolonged circulation time ($t_{1/2}$ = 12 hours). The LPS that was cleaved rapidly (five minutes) was found predominantly in liver (approximately 40%), with lesser amounts in lung, spleen, kidney and adrenal. When expressed as ^{125}I-LPS/gm of tissue, the ^{125}I-LPS was found predominantly in liver and spleen at five minutes [60]. Greater than 80% of the infused ^{125}I-LPS was recovered. Autoradiography of 6 μm and electron microscopic sections taken five minutes after injection showed ^{125}I-LPS in phagocytic vacuoles of macrophages in the liver and spleen and in leukocytes. After 180 minutes, the tissue distribution remained the same, with the notable exception of three- to four-fold increase in the adrenal. The deposition of LPS in tissues over a prolonged period will be discussed below.

After 30 minutes in the blood stream, the ^{125}I-LPS was found to be converted to a low-density form [61], having a $t_{1/2}$

of about 12 to 16 hours. Recent studies of the conversion of LPS from high density (ρ = 1.38 − 1.44 gm/cm^3) to low density (ρ <1.2 gm/cm^3) in plasma or serum by Ulevitch et al have provided significant information for our understanding of the biologic effects of LPS. In agreement with previous data of Skarnes [62], radiolabeled LPS extracted from both *S. minn.* R595 and *E. coli* 0111:B4, when added to serum of rabbits, was found to undergo a marked decrease in buoyant density as determined in isopycnic density gradient centrifugation in CsCl [61]. The shift in density was time-dependent, with the density changing from >1.38 gm/cm^3 of the parent molecule to an intermediate position of 1.3 to 1.4 and a low density of <1.2 gm/cm^3 as noted above. The shift was readily observed after one minute of incubation and was complete in 30 to 60 minutes with LPS of *E. coli* 0111:B4, and in about one minute using *S. minn.* R595 in the presence of EDTA. One milliliter of NRS converted at least 100 μg R595 LPS to a density of <1.2 gm/cm^3 in the presence of EDTA.

A similar shift in density was noted when the ^{125}I-LPS preparations were injected intravenously in rabbits, with complete conversion of the LPS to low density being observed in the rabbit plasma by between 5 and 15 minutes.

Serum-treated, low-density LPS was isolated by ultracentrifugation and the biologic activity assessed. The anticomplementary, pyrogenic and early neutropenia-producing capacities of the LPS were lost. However, the capacity of the low-density LPS to induce hypotension, DIC and lethal effects was retained [61, 63]. The finding that despite the loss of anticomplementary activity, the low-density LPS still produced hypotension, DIC and death supports the conclusions of previous studies in this laboratory that complement does not play a significant role in the pathologic effect of LPS.

The alteration in buoyant density was found to be dependent upon the presence of high-density lipoprotein (HDL) [64]. Delipidated plasma or serum by itself was found not to support the conversion of the ^{125}I-LPS to low density. However, addition of HDL but not other classes of lipoproteins to the delipidated plasma or serum reconstituted the LPS-converting ability. Further studies [65] have shown that a complex of HDL and LPS can be removed from rabbit plasma by affinity chromatography using antibody specific to LPS. The

HDL was characterized and found to have as its major protein a single polypeptide of M_r 26,000. Its size and amino acid composition were identical to those of rabbit apoprotein AI, the major protein of rabbit HDL.

Two important specificites are apparent in these studies. The first involves the reaction between the LPS and HDL of plasma, and the second, the reaction between the complex and certain cells in vivo. The explanations of these two specificities are unclear. An association between molecules bearing amphipathic helices, such as occur with the apolipoproteins and lipid, is known to require opposing polar and nonpolar faces of the proteins. Quite possibly the LPS, also an amphipath, could have polar and nonpolar faces which would allow binding to the apoprotein or the lipids of the HDL. An explanation of its specificity for HDL remains unclear at present. That this complex is important in determining the cellular target in vivo seems clear, and this specificity may well reside in the apoprotein of the HDL. Thus the long (approximately 14 hours) circulation time of the LPS-HDL complex could allow the complex to react with the target tissues, namely, those whose cells normally recognize the apoprotein of the HDL, i.e. the macrophage and the adrenal cells.

The recognition of these reactions and their specificites has provided new insight into the pathogenesis of LPS-induced diseases.

References

1. McCabe, W.R.: Gram negative bacteremia. Adv. Intern. Med. 19:135, 1974.
2. Gilbert, R.P.: Mechanisms of the hemodynamic effects of endotoxin. Physiol. Rev. 40:245, 1960.
3. Garner, R., Chater, B.V. and Brown, D.L.: The role of complement in endotoxin shock and disseminated intravascular coagulation: Experimental observations in the dog. Br. J. Haematol. 28:393, 1974.
4. Kitzmiller, J.L., Lucas, W.E. and Yelenosky, P.F.: The role of complement in feline endotoxin shock. Am. J. Obstet. Gynecol. 112:414, 1972.
5. From, A.H.L., Gewurz, H., Gruninger, R.P. et al: Complement in endotoxin shock: Effect of complement depletion on the early hypotensive phase. Infect. Immun. 2:38, 1970.

6. Guenter, C.A., Fiorica, V. and Hinshaw, L.B.: Cardiorespiratory and metabolic responses to live *E. coli* and endotoxin in the monkey. J. Appl. Physiol. 26:780, 1969.
7. Beller, F.K.: The role of endotoxin in disseminated intravascular coagulation. Thromb. Diath. Haemorrh. 36 (suppl.):125, 1969.
8. McKay, D.G.: Vessel wall and thrombogenesis-endotoxin. Thromb. Diath. Haemorrh. 29:11, 1973.
9. Brown, D.L.: Complement and coagulation. *In* Brent, L. and Holbrow, J. (eds.): Progress in Immunology II. Amsterdam:North-Holland Publishing Company, 1974, vol. 1, p. 191.
10. Muller-Berghaus, G. and Lohmann, E.: The role of complement in endotoxin induced disseminated intravascular coagulation. Studies in congenitally C6-deficient rabbits. Br. J. Haematol. 28:403, 1974.
11. Corrigan, J.J. and Jordan, C.M.: Heparin therapy in septicemia with disseminated intravascular coagulation. N. Engl. J. Med. 283:778, 1970.
12. Brown, D.L. and Lachmann, P.J.: The behavior of complement and platelets in lethal endotoxin shock in rabbits. Int. Arch. Allergy Appl. Immunol. 75:193, 1972.
13. Gilbert, V.E. and Braude, A.I.: Reduction in serum complement in rabbits after injection of endotxin. J. Exp. Med. 116:477, 1962.
14. Phillips, J.K., Snyderman, R. and Mergenhagen, S.E.: Activation of complement by endotoxin: A role for γ^2 globulin, C1, C4, and C2 in the consumption of terminal complement components by endotoxin coated erythrocytes. J. Immunol. 109:334, 1972.
15. Snyderman, R. and Pike, M.C.: Interactions of complex polysaccharides with the complement system: Effect of calcium depletion on terminal component consumption. Infect. Immun. 11:273, 1975.
16. Mergenhagen, S.E., Snyderman, R., Gewurz, H. and Shin, H.S.: Significance of complement to the mechanism of action of endotoxin. Curr. Top. Microbiol. Immunol. 50:37, 1969.
17. McCabe, W.R.: Serum complement levels in bacteremia due to gram-negative organisms. N. Engl. J. Med. 288:21, 1973.
18. Fearon, D.T., Ruddy, S., Schur, P.H. and McCabe, W.R.: Activation of the properdin pathway of complement in patients with gram-negative bacteremia. N. Engl. J. Med. 292:937, 1975.
19. Morrison, D.C. and Cochrane, C.G.: Direct evidence for Hageman factor (factor XII) activation by bacterial lipopolysaccharides endotoxins. J. Exp. Med. 140:797, 1974.
20. Henson, P.M. and Cochrane, C.G.: Immunological induction of increased vascular permeability. II. Two mechanisms of release from rabbit platelets involving complement. J. Exp. Med. 129:167, 1969.
21. Zimmerman, T.S., Arroyave, C.M. and Müller-Eberhard, H.J.: A blood coagulation abnormality in rabbits deficient in the sixth component of complement (C6) and its correction by purified C6. J. Exp. Med. 134:1591, 1971.
22. Stewart, G.J. and Anderson, M.J.: An ultrastructural study of endotoxin induced damage in rabbit mesenteric arteries. Br. J. Exp. Pathol. 52:75, 1971.

23. Evensen, S.A. and Shepro, D.: DNA synthesis in rat aortic endothelium: Effect of bacterial endotoxin and trauma. Microvasc. Res. 8:90, 1974.
24. McGarth, J.M. and Stewart, G.J.: The effect of endotoxin on vascular endothelium. J. Exp. Med. 129:833, 1969.
25. Melmon, K.C. and Cline, M.J.: The interactions of leucocytes and the kinin system. Biochem. Pharmacol. 17 (suppl.):271, 1968.
26. Rivers, R.P.A., Hathaway, W.E. and Weston, W.L.: The endotoxin-induced coagulant activity of human monocytes. Br. J. Haematol. 30:311, 1975.
27. Cochrane, C.G., Aikin, B.S. and Müller-Eberhard, H.J.: Depletion of plasma complement in vivo by a protein of cobra venom: Its effect on various immunologic reactions. J. Immunol. 105:55, 1970.
28. Ulevitch, R.J., Cochrane, C.G., Henson, P.M. et al: Mediation systems in bacterial lipopolysaccharide-induced hypotension and disseminated intravascular coagulation. I. The role of complement. J. Exp. Med. 142:1570, 1975.
29. Ulevitch, R.J. and Cochrane, C.G.: Complement-dependent hemodynamic changes in the rabbit. Inflammation 2:199, 1977.
30. Cochrane, C.G.: Biochemistry and pathophysiologic effects of the Hageman factor system. In Miescher, P.A. (ed.): Immunopathology VIII. Basel:Schwabe and Co., 1981. (In press.)
31. Mason, J.M., Kleeberg, V., Dolan, P. and Colman, R.W.: Plasma kallikrein and Hageman factor in gram-negative bacteremia. Ann. Intern. Med. 73:545, 1970.
32. Robinson, J.A., Kloduycky, M.L., Lock, H.H. et al: Endotoxin, prekallikrein, complement and systemic vascular resistance. Am. J. Med. 59:61, 1975.
33. Colman, R.W., Edelman, R. and Scott, C.F.: Plasma kallikrein activation and inhibition during typhoid fever. J. Clin. Invest. 61:287, 1978.
34. Hirsch, E.F., Nakayima, T., Oshima, G. et al: Kinin system responses in sepsis after trauma in man. J. Surg. Res. 17:147, 1974.
35. O'Donnell, T.F., Clowes, G.H., Jr. and Talamo, R.C.: Kinin activation in the blood of patients with sepsis. Surg. Gynecol. Obstet. 143:539, 1976.
36. Aasen, A.O., Gallimore, M.J., Lyngass, K. et al: Studies on components of the plasma kallikrein-kinin system in normal subjects and patients with septicemia. In Proceedings of the VIIIth International Congress on Thrombosis and Haemostasis, 1979, p. 235.
37. Nies, A.S., Forsyth, R.P., Williams, H.E. and Melmon, K.L.: Contributions of kinins to endotoxin shock in unanesthetized rhesus monkeys. Circ. Res. 22:155, 1968.
38. Wing, D.A., Yamada, T., Hayley, H.B. and Pettit, G.W.: Model for disseminated intravascular coagulation: Bacterial sepsis for rhesus monkeys. J. Lab. Clin. Med. 92:239, 1978.
39. Erdos, E.G. and Miwa, I.: Effect of endotoxin shock on the plasma kallikrein-kinin system of the rabbit. Fed. Proc. 27:92, 1968.

40. Gallimore, M.J., Aason, A.O., Lyngaas, K.H.N. et al: Falls in plasma levels of prekallikrein, high molecular weight kininogen, and kallikrein inhibitors during lethal endotoxin shock in dogs. Thromb. Res. 12:307, 1978.

41. Aasen, A.O., Frolish, W., Saugstad, O.D. and Amundsen, E.: Plasma kallikrein activity and prekallikrein levels during endotoxin shock in dogs. Eur. Surg. Res. 10:50, 1978.

42. Cochrane, C.G. and Revak, S.D.: The participation of high molecular weight kininogen in hypotensive shock and intravascular coagulation. Clin. Immunol. Immunopathol. 15:367, 1980.

43. Braude, A.I., Carey, F.J. and Zalesky, M.: Studies with radioactive endotoxin. II. Correlation of physiologic effects with distribution of radioactivity in rabbits injected with lethal doses of E. coli endotoxin labelled with radioactive sodium chromate. J. Clin. Invest. 34:858, 1955.

44. Howard, J.G., Rowley, D. and Wardlaw, A.C.: Investigations on the mechanism of stimulation of non-specific immunity by bacterial lipopolysaccharides. Immunology 1:181, 1958.

45. Carey, F.J., Braude, A.I. and Zalesky, M.: Studies with radioactive endotoxin. III. The effect of tolerance on the distribution of radioactivity after intravenous injection of Escherichia coli endotoxin labeled with [51]Cr. J. Clin. Invest. 37:441, 1958.

46. Noyes, H.E., McInturf, C.R. and Blahuta, G.J.: Studies on distribution of Escherichia coli endotoxin in mice. Proc. Soc. Exp. Biol. Med. 100:65, 1959.

47. Smith, R.T., Braude, A.I. and Carey, F.J.: The distribution of ^{51}Cr labeled E. coli endotoxin in the generalized Schwartzman reaction. J. Clin. Invest. 36:695, 1957.

48. Herring, W.B., Herion, J.C., Walker, R.I. and Palmer, J.G.: Distribution and clearance of circulating endotoxin. J. Clin. Invest. 42:79, 1963.

49. Brunning, R.D., Woolfrey, B.F. and Schrader, W.H.: Studies with tritiated endotoxin. II. Endotoxin localization in the formed elements of the blood. Am. J. Pathol. 44:401, 1964.

50. Schrader, W.H., Woolfrey, B.F. and Brunning, R.D.: Studies with tritiated endotoxin. III. The local Schwartzman reaction. Am. J. Pathol. 44:597, 1964.

51. Chedid, L., Parant, F., Parant, M. and Boyer, F.: Localization and fate of ^{51}Cr-labeled somatic antigens of smooth and rough Salmonellae. Ann. N.Y. Acad. Sci. 133:712, 1966.

52. DiLuzio, N.R. and Crafton, C.G.: Influence of altered reticulo-endothelial function of vascular clearance and tissue distribution of S. enteritidis endotoxin. Proc. Soc. Exp. Biol. Med. 132:686, 1969.

53. Greisman, S.E., Hornick, R.B., Wagner, H.N., Jr. et al: The role of endotoxin during thyphoid fever and tularemia in man. IV. The integrity of the endotoxin tolerance mechanisms during infection. J. Clin. Invest. 48:613, 1969.

54. Musson, R.A., Morrison, D.C. and Ulevitch, R.J.: Distribution of

endotoxin (lipopolysaccharide) in the tissues of lipopolysaccharide-responsive and -unresponsive mice. Infect. Immun. 21:448, 1978.

55. Cremer, N. and Watson, D.W.: Influence of stress on distribution of endotoxin in RES determined by fluorescein antibody technic. Proc. Soc. Exp. Biol. Med. 95:510, 1957.

56. Tanaka, N., Nishimura, T. and Yoshiyuki, T.: Histochemical studies on the cellular distribution of endotoxin *Salmonella enteritidis* in mouse tissues. Jpn. J. Microbiol. 3:191, 1959.

57. Rubenstein, H.S., Fine, J. and Coons, A.H.: Localization of endotoxin in the walls of the peripheral vascular system during lethal endotoxemia. Proc. Soc. Exp. Biol. Med. 111:458, 1962.

58. Golub, S., Groschel, D. and Nowotny, A.: Factors which affect the reticuloendothelial system uptake of bacterial endotoxins. J. Reticuloendothel. Soc. 5:324, 1968.

59. Ulevitch, R.J.: The preparation and characterization of a radio-iodinated bacterial lipopolysaccharide. Immunochemistry 15:157, 1978.

60. Mathison, J.C. and Ulevitch, R.J.: The clearance, tissue distribution and cellular localization of lipopolysaccharide (LPS) in rabbits. J. Immunol. 123:2133, 1979.

61. Ulevitch, R.J. and Johnston, A.R.: The modification of biophysical and endotoxic properties of bacterial lipopolysaccharides by serum. J. Clin. Invest. 62:1313, 1978.

62. Skarnes, R.C.: In vivo interaction of endotoxin with a plasma lipoprotein having esterase activity. J. Bacteriol. 95:2031, 1968.

63. Mathison, J.C. and Ulevitch, R.J.: Physiologic effects of bacterial lipopolysaccharide (LPS)-lipoprotein complexes. Fed. Proc. 39:674, 1980.

64. Ulevitch, R.J., Johnston, A.R. and Weinstein, D.B.: New function for high density lipoproteins. Their participation in intravascular reactions of bacteral lipopolysaccharides. J. Clin. Invest. 64:1516, 1979.

65. Ulevitch, R.J., Johnston, A.R. and Weinstein, D.B.: New function for high density lipoproteins (HDL). II. Isolation and characterization of a bacterial lipopolysaccharide-HDL complex formed in rabbit plasma. J. Clin. Invest. 67:827, 1981.

A Unidirectional Pathway of Lymphocyte-Instructed Macrophage and Monocyte Function Characterized by the Generation of Procoagulant Monokines

Thomas S. Edgington, M.D., Gary A. Levy, M.D.,
Bradford S. Schwartz, M.D. and Daryl S. Fair, Ph.D.

One of the most elementary functional elements of biological organisms is the capacity to recognize and respond appropriately to specific stimuli. Survival of higher organisms requires recognition of infectious agents, deviant cells and trauma, as well as organization of an appropriate and effective host response. It is reasonable to suggest that selectional pressures during evolution have led to cellular and molecular mechanisms that preserve biological fidelity through well-regulated and effective biological responses. Indeed, host response mechanisms such as the antibody response, the generation of cytolytic T cells or macrophages, and the complex interactions of the proteins of the complement and coagulation systems posess both discriminating recognitive molecules capable of initiating functions, sophisticated regulatory circuits and highly evolved effectors. Only with the preservation of biological fidelity of these systems by both specific recognition

Thomas S. Edgington, M.D., Gary A. Levy, M.D., Bradford S. Schwartz, M.D. and Daryl S. Fair, Ph.D., Department of Molecular Immunology, Scripps Clinic and Research Foundation, La Jolla, Calif.

This is publication No. 2395 from the Immunology Departments, Scripps Clinic and Research Foundation. This work was supported by NIH research grants CA-28166, HL-16411 and HL-07195. G.A.L. is a fellow of the Medical Research Council, Canada.

of stimuli and effective regulatory networks can host defense mechanisms serve appropriate biological roles, rather than violation of the survival of the host by misdirection.

A major component of the host defense network is embodied in the cells of the monocyte-macrophage series. Not only do these cells serve as phagocytic effectors, but they may be induced by lymphocyte products to differentiate to cyto-lytic cells [1, 2] or by appropriate stimuli to secrete media-tors [3-5]. Whereas some responses of cells of monocyte or macrophage differentiation, such as phagocytosis, appear to be a direct response to stimuli [6], other responses have been observed to require either the effects of lymphokines [1, 2, 7, 8] or direct cellular collaboration [9, 10]. These latter re-sponses, in which the recognitive functions of the T lymphocyte are first invoked and subsequently lead to the production of initiators of the coagulation system, have been only partially characterized [9-12] and are the subject of this paper. The specific response of monocytes to be addressed involves the synthesis and biological expression of at least two initiators of the coagulation pathways.

The products of the coagulation network serve as partici-pants in immunologic tissue lesions and as modifiers of the function of cells of the immune system. A participatory role of the monocyte-macrophage in initiating the coagulation path-ways is well illustrated by the studies of Colvin and col-leagues [13]. They demonstrated that the induration in classical delayed hypersensitivity reactions is a direct result of local fibrin deposition. This interpretation has been further docu-mented by the absence of induration in the delayed cutaneous hypersensitivity reactions in hereditary afibrinogenemic indi-viduals [14].

The preclusion of cellular infiltration in experimental serum sickness glomerulonephritis by anti-macrophage antisera [15] and the attenuation of glomerular disease in this model by defibrinogenation [16] provide evidence not only for a direct causal role of the monocyte but also the direct participation c fibrin formation in the mediation of injury. In another settin attenuation of tumor growth and metastasis has been observed in defibrinogenated animals [17], suggesting that products of the coagulation system participate in tumor biology. Dvorak et al [18] have suggested that fibrin formed at the surface of tumor cells may serve as a barrier to effective cellular immune attack. Initation of coagulation pathways during the active phase of immunologic diseases is supported by the observations in systemic lupus erythematosus, where the increase of plasma fibrinopeptide A is related to disease activity [19]. Furthermore, the high mortality of BXSB mice, an autoimmune-immune complex disease mouse strain, due to coronary artery thrombosis illustrates the initiation of coagulation in immune processes [20]. Although pathogenetic implications will require further analysis, the possibility exists that the procoagulant pathways evoked by products of the immune response may serve effector functions as well as modify the responses of the lymphoid system [21, 22].

Among mechanisms that may account for the association of immunologic responses with activation of the coagulation pathways are observations that a number of immunologically relevant stimuli can evoke procoagulant activity (PCA) in human peripheral blood mononuclear cells (PBM) in vitro. Stimuli such as bacterial lipopolysaccharide [9, 23, 24], allogeneic cells [25], immune complexes and aggregated IgG [10, 26] have evoked marked increases of cellular PCA; and based on the effects of anticoagulation on antigen-induced delayed cutaneous hypersensitivity reactions [27, 28], it would appear that antigen stimulation may also provoke this pathway.

The present study addresses the cellular pathways responsible for generation of procoagulant monokines, drawing from observation of the responses of murine and human cells elicited by selected stimuli in vitro. From these data we suggest the existence of a common unidirectional pathway by which T lymphocytes can be triggered directly by a variety of stimuli, and by which these triggered T cells rapidly induce monocytes or macrophages to selectively produce one of two cell-membrane-associated procoagulant monokines. This pathway embodies features distinct from the previously defined lympho-kine-mediated pathway and may play a significant role in the pathogenesis of immunologic tissue lesions.

Induction of Procoagulant Activity
in Lymphoid Cells

Peripheral blood mononuclear cells of murine or of human origin were used in the following studies as representative of migratory cells that serve as the source of cellular infiltrates in immunologic tissue lesions. Two selected stimuli are representative: (1) bacterial lipopolysaccharide (LPS) derived from *E. coli* 0111:B4, and (2) soluble immune complexes of human serum albumin and purified specific antibody. LPS was optimally stimulatory to PBM in culture at about 0.01 μg/ml in the absence of serum or 10 μg/ml in 10% fetal bovine serum. The difference in dose is assumed to be due to the binding of LPS by serum high-density lipoproteins [29]. Soluble immune complexes were used at 70 to 100 μg/ml, a maximally stimulatory dose. Both stimuli were explored with murine and human PBM at 1×10^6 cells/ml and incubated for 6 to 24 hours at 37°C. These stimuli and experimental conditions were used throughout to examine the cellular requirements, the kinetics and the products of this lymphoid pathway.

Splenic lymphoid cells and PBM, when immediately isolated, exhibited little measurable PCA when viable cells were assayed. A low but greater basal level was observed when the cells were disrupted, indicating that most endogenous or basal PCA is present within the cells, with little expressed at the cell surface. The assay of PCA involved mixing viable or disrupted cells with normal plasma. Then addition of calcium chloride initiated coagulation, and the time required for clot formation was proportional to PCA from a standard curve derived from assay of known quantities of rabbit brain thromboplastin. In Table 1 the procoagulant activity of viable and of disrupted

Table 1. Stimulation of Human and Murine Lymphoid Cell Procoagulant Activity

Cell Population*	Stimulus†	Viable Cells (mU PCA/10⁶)	Disrupted Cells (mU PCA/10⁶)	Stimulation Index‡
Murine PBM	LPS	488 ± 44	2,417 ± 30	22.0
Murine PBM	Ag:Ab	684 ± 28	3,150 ± 132	15.0
Human PBM	LPS	562 ± 60	3,150 ± 400	17.5
Human PBM	Ag:Ab	905 ± 56	3,850 ± 300	22.0

*Isolated over Ficoll-Hypaque, and cultivated at 1×10^6 cells/ml in the presence of stimulus for six hours.

†LPS at 10 μg/ml and Ag:Ab at 70-100 μg/ml.

‡Ratio of six-hour-stimulated total cellular PCA of disrupted cells to the zero-hour control of disrupted cells.

human and murine PBM is given, as well as the relative degree of stimulation compared to the zero-time basal cell concentration of PCA. Stimulation was maximal within 4 to 6 hours and remained relatively constant for 24 hours. Thus, for these studies we used a six-hour incubation. There was a 15- to 22-fold stimulation of cellular PCA. The level of induced PCA was comparable for both species and stimuli.

PCA-Positive Cell Populations

Following stimulation of PBM the cellular locus of PCA has been identified by assay of lymphocytes and of monocytes which had been isolated by adherence. In experiments representative of which are those in Table 2, it was apparent that virtually all PCA induced by either LPS or Ag:Ab complexes was resident in the adherent cell population, which was 98% to 99% monocytes by cytology as well as by reference to nonspecific esterase. Although consistent with localization to monocytes, the possibility that the PCA-positive cell might be a novel cell, or represent a minor subpopulation of monocytes, was resolved by a cytologic assay [9] in which the cells were suspended in plasma-agarose. PCA-positive cells were identified by reference to the pericellular deposition of fine strands of fibrin. Whereas unstimulated populations of cells had very few if any PCA-positive cells, most if not all monocytes from stimulated PBM were PCA positive and a few lymphocytes (1%

Table 2. Cellular Localization of Procoagulant Activity in Stimulated Human Peripheral Blood Mononuclear Cells

| | LPS | | Ag:Ab | |
| | | Stimulation | | Stimulation |
Cell Subpopulation	$mU/10^6$ Cells	Index	$mU/10^6$ Cells	Index‡
PBM	3,250 ± 350	13.0	3,600 ± 300	10.3
Lymphocytes*	370 ± 42	1.2	410 ± 53	1.1
Monocytes †	27,083 ± 1,667	9.3	30,000 ± 1,875	9.0

*Lymphocytes (<2% esterase positive) isolated from stimulated PBM by nonadherence to plastic.

†Monocytes (>98% esterase positive) isolated from stimulated PBM by adherence to plastic.

‡Stimulation index is the ratio of stimulated cell PCA at six hours to control cellular PCA at six hours.

to 10%) appeared weakly PCA positive as well. These observations demonstrate that virtually all monocytes can be induced to produce PCA and account for most if not all of the increment in PCA that is induced. It was, however, impossible to assess the quantitative contribution of individual monocytes to the total PCA expressed by viable cells or in respect to their content, since the cytological assay is qualitative rather than quantitative. Thus, it is possible that a minor subset of monocyte might contribute the majority of observed PCA. Observations were similar with human and murine cells for a variety of stimuli, including LPS and immune complexes.

Cellular Collaboration for Induction of PCA

Although the stimuli were capable of inducing PCA in whole PBM, attempts at direct stimulation of isolated lymphocytes or of adherent monocytes led to no increase of cellular PCA (Table 3), even when incubated for as long as 24 hours. When the two cell populations were mixed at the original cellular ratio, e.g. 8:1 lymphocytes to monocytes, the response of both murine PBM and human PBM to the stimuli was recapitulated. This was not observed when ultracentrifugally clarified medium from stimulated lymphocytes was added to monocytes, in contrast to a report by Edwards and Rickles using a lectin-stimulated response [12].

In separate experiments the cellular stoichiometry of collaboration was examined. Isolated lymphocytes were stimulated

Table 3. Isolated Lymphocytes and Monocytes Do Not
Produce Procoagulant Activity
Upon Direct Stimulation by LPS or Ag:Ab Complexes

Cell Population	LPS‡		Ag:Ab §	
	$mU/10^6$ Cells	Stimulation Index	$mU/10^6$ Cells	Stimulation Index
PBM	3,100 ± 250	6.9	1,575 ± 37	4.1
Lymphocytes*	551 ± 284	1.1	39 ± 1.4	1.1
Monocytes†	3,750 ± 208	1.4	3,550 ± 232	1.0

*<1% esterase positive.
†>98% esterase positive.
‡Six-hour incubation with E. coli 0111:B4 LPS at 10 μg/ml.
§Six-hour incubation with 100 μg Ag:Ab.

directly for six hours, washed and added to the monocytes. After an additional six-hour interval at 37°C the cells were harvested and assayed for total cellular PCA. At ratios of 2:1 lymphocytes to monocytes or higher, induction of PCA was observed (Fig. 1). The cellular ratios were similar for different stimuli and species, and the cellular collaboration appeared to be mediated by direct contact or by a short-lived mediator since viable lymphocytes were required. Addition of ultracentrifugally clarified medium from lymphocytes four to six hours after stimulation, homogenates of stimulated lymphocytes or lymphocytes flash-fixed for five minutes at 0°C with 0.15% glutaraldehyde was without effect. Evidence consistent with a direct-contact-mediated collaboration follows from observations that neither cycloheximide or actinomycin D, at concentrations sufficient to abolish protein and RNA synthesis, respectively, attenuated the triggering of lymphocytes by LPS or Ag:Ab. Similarly, these inhibitors had no effect on the capacity of the

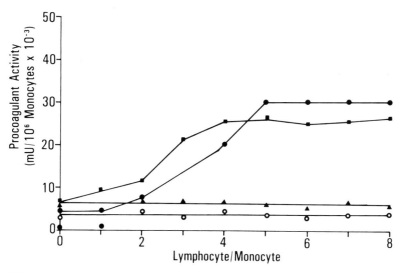

FIG. 1. Lymphocyte requirements for the generation of monocyte procoagulant activity. Human lymphocytes were triggered with LPS (■———■) or Ag:Ab (●———●), washed and added in increasing numbers to 1 × 10⁵ monocytes. Monocytes were washed and assayed for PCA. Monocytes were stimulated with LPS or Ag:Ab (▲———▲) and assayed for PCA. Untriggered lymphocytes were added in increasing numbers to 1 × 10⁵ monocytes (○———○) and monocytes were assayed for PCA activity.

triggered lymphocytes to induce PCA when added to monocytes. This effectively argues against newly synthesized lymphokines but does not preclude release of preformed labile
mediators from the lymphocytes.

Kinetics and Metabolic Requirements
of the Response

The kinetics of the PCA response has been examined in
detail with both human and murine cells. The results have been
comparable and the observations in Figure 2 are representative.
When LPS-triggered lymphocytes were added in excess to
monocytes, and the latter cells assayed, it was observed that
after about two hours PCA increased in the monocytes and
reached a maximum within four to six hours (Fig. 2A). This
concentration of PCA was equivalent to the presence of greater
than 90% PCA-positive monocytes by cytologic assay. Further
studies demonstrated that incubation of the monocytes alone in
the presence of $10\mu g$ actinomycin D per milliliter or 10 μg
cycloheximide per milliliter prevented the increase of PCA.
These data suggest that the PCA is probably newly synthesized
in the monocyte and requires newly transcribed RNA.

In contrast, when lymphocytes were exposed for variable
time periods to LPS, washed and added to monocytes for 6
hours, significant triggering of lymphocytes occurred within 15
minutes and was maximal within 30 minutes (Fig. 2B). Adding
either LPS or Ag:Ab to the monocytes did not induce the
response directly. Furthermore, subsequent addition of untriggered lymphocytes to the stimulated and washed monocytes did
not result in triggering of the lymphocytes. Thus the pathway
appeared unidirectional, as illustrated in Figure 3 (i.e. stimulus → lymphocyte → monocyte) and seems to represent a new
cellular sequence. The possibility that the monocytes may also
be susceptible to lymphokine induction [12] is not dismissed.
Presentation of antigen to T lymphocytes by macrophages in
the immune response [30] is a well-known pathway that
functions in the reverse direction, and can serve to induce
secondary macrophage responses as well [31].

Two additional kinetic details of the collaborative response
are of significance. The first is the unusually rapid induction of

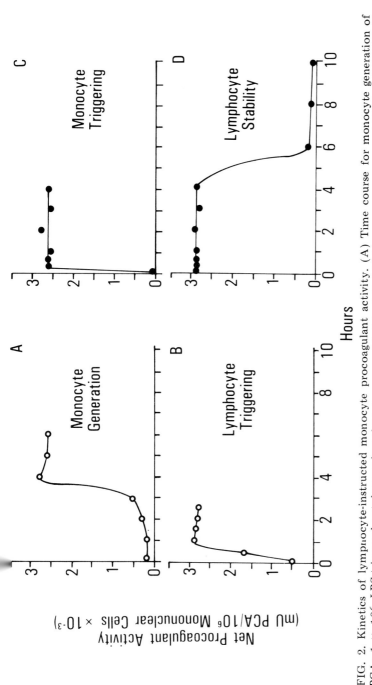

FIG. 2. Kinetics of lymphocyte-instructed monocyte procoagulant activity. (A) Time course for monocyte generation of PCA: 1×10^6 LPS-triggered autologous lymphocytes were added to 1×10^5 human monocytes, and PCA was assayed at various time intervals. (B) Time course of triggering of lymphocytes by LPS. Lymphocytes, 1×10^6 in 1 ml, were incubated with 10 μg LPS for the indicated intervals. They were then washed and added to 1×10^5 monocytes for six hours. Monocytes were then assayed for total PCA. (C) Temporal requirement for triggering of monocytes. LPS-triggered lymphocytes were washed and added to autologous monocytes for intervals of ten minutes to four hours. They were subsequently removed and the monocytes were incubated for an additional six hours and assayed for total PCA. (D) Stability of the triggered state of lymphocytes. Lymphocytes were triggered for 30 minutes with LPS, washed and held in culture for periods of 15 minutes to 10 hours. They were then assayed for their ability to trigger monocytes. The lymphocytes and monocytes were admixed and six hours later the cells were assayed for PCA.

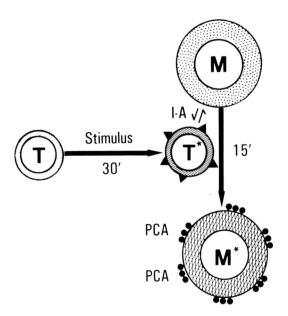

FIG. 3. Schematic depiction of the rapid T cell-instructed pathway for the induction of monocyte procoagulant molecules. Induced T cells (T) are stimulated within 30 minutes to the "triggered" state (T*). These cells induce monocytes/macrophages (M) via an *I-A*-dependent collaboration within 15 minutes to enter into RNA and protein synthesis, which within four to six hours culminates in full expression of procoagulant activity (PCA). One of two types of PCA is induced, either tissue factor or a monocyte prothrombinase. Expression of PCA persists from 24 to 72 hours following induction.

monocytes by triggered lymphocytes (Fig. 2C). When LPS-triggered lymphocytes were added to adherent monocytes for intervals of 10 minutes to 4 hours, removed and the monocytes assayed 6 hours later, it was apparent that within 15 minutes of mixing the monocytes had been fully induced to produce PCA. Partial induction was observed within ten minutes. This further supports a direct-contact-mediated event of a transient nature. Further, triggered lymphocytes could be recovered from the first set of monocytes and retained full capacity to repeatedly trigger new monocytes; thus the system embodies amplification. Finally, lymphocytes once triggered by stimulus remained in a triggered state for about four hours, after which they rapidly lost the ability to induce monocyte PCA (Fig. 2D). They apparently return to the prior basal state and are not refractory, since these same lymphocytes could again be triggered by the same stimulus.

The metabolic requirements of the lymphocyte appeared minimal. The ability to trigger lymphocytes as well as the ability of triggered lymphocytes to induce monocytes was not affected by inhibitors of protein synthesis or RNA synthesis. This is consistent with the hypothesis that triggering of lymphocytes may involve no more than a topographical realignment of lymphocyte surface structures.

The kinetic data have been integrated into the cellular scheme proposed in Figure 3 and suggest that in vivo this system might take place in an anatomically dispersed fashion. Lymphocytes could encounter appropriate stimuli at one site A, resulting in triggering of the lymphocyte. This cell could encounter monocytes at site B and induce the monocyte. The production of PCA might yet occur at site C some hours later. Such responses are consistent with the features of disseminated intravascular coagulation in which products of the coagulation pathways, such as fibrin, are deposited in multiple sites, or with coronary thrombosis in BXSB mice with generalized immune complex disease [20].

Collaborative Restriction

Genetic restriction of collaboration between triggered lymphocytes and monocytes appears to exist and to be rigorous. Whether lymphocytes and monocytes were first admixed, or the lymphocytes were first triggered by appropriate stimuli and then added to monocytes, there was no induction of monocyte PCA when the lymphocytes and monocytes were of different H-2 haplotype. This requirement was apparent also when human lymphocytes and monocytes from different random individuals were mixed, since there was no amplification of PCA following stimulation. By using recombinant mice of defined H-2 haplotype, it has been possible to delineate the genetic requirements for collaboration. When splenic or peripheral blood lymphoid cells from various strains were separated into lymphocytes and monocytes/macrophages, then mixed and stimulated by LPS, normal PCA responses were observed only when both cell classes shared *I-A* loci of the same haplotype (Table 4). No other histocompatibility requirements were essential for the collaborative induction of the PCA response. Limited compatibility at only *K* and *I-A* for the mixing of C3H and B10.A(4R) cells was sufficient to generate a full response, although compatibility at *K* alone, as for the cross between A.TL and B10.S(7R) cells, was ineffective.

Such histocompatibility restriction is particularly intriguing in light of the Ia positivity of a high proportion of circulating monocytes and the requirement for Ia-positive monocytes/macrophages in the presentation of antigen to T helper cells in the immune response [30]. Whether the I-A gene product must be present on both lymphocyte and monocyte/macrophage is not yet known; however, these data indicate that *I-A* compatibility can mediate communication in both directions.

Characteristics of the Lymphocyte

The class and subclass of the collaborating lymphocyte has been partially defined for human cells. Monocyte-depleted lymphocytes were rosetted with neuraminidase-treated sheep erythrocytes (nE), and nE$^+$ (T cells) and nE$^-$ cells (non-T cells)

Table 4. Genetic Restriction of Cellular Collaboration
Required for Induction of Procoagulant Monokines

| Mouse Strain | | MHC Compatibility | | | | | | | | PCA Induction |
Lymphocyte*	Macrophage*	K	IA	IB	IJ	IE	IC	S	D	by LPS
BALB/c	BALB/c	▪	▪	▪	▪	▪	▪	▪	▪	+
A	C3H	▪	▪	▪	▪	▪				+
A	BALB/c						▪	▪	▪	0
A.TL	A		▪	▪	▪	▪			▪	+
A.TL	C3H		▪	▪	▪	▪	▪	▪		+
A.TL	BALB/c								▪	0
A.TL	B10.S(7R)	▪							▪	0
B10.A(4R)	C3H	▪	▪							+
B10.A(4R)	C57BL/6			▪	▪	▪	▪	▪	▪	0
B10.A(5R)	C3H				▪	▪				0
B10.A(5R)	C57BL/6	▪	▪	▪						+

*All collaborations operational in both directions.

were isolated by centrifugation over Ficoll-Hypaque. Following triggering with LPS or Ag:Ab complexes, only the nE^+ (T cells) cells were capable of inducing isolated monocytes to produce PCA (Table 5). These T cells were separated into T_M, T_G and T_{NULL} by reference to the presence of receptors for IgM, IgG or neither, as described by Moretta et al [32]. Such cell fractions are by no means homogeneous, but do represent a functional separation of helper T cells (T_M) and suppressor T cells (T_G) for in vitro pokeweed mitogen-driven immuno-globulin synthesis by human PBM. Only LPS-triggered T_M induced monocyte PCA. The quantity of PCA was consistently higher than observed for induction by LPS-triggered whole T cells, suggesting the existence of suppressor cells. This has recently been confirmed and the suppressors are recovered in the T_G subclass, as observed for pokeweed mitogen-driven immunoglobulin synthesis. Whether these same sets of cells serve identical functions for Ag:Ab complex stimulation and viral stimulation remains to be determined.

Initial studies of the collaborating murine lymphocyte have identified it as a θ^+ cell using complement-dependent cytolysis with monoclonal anti-θ. Apparently postthymic T cells are required since spleen cells from homozygous nude mice (nu/nu) on a BALB/c background did not respond.

The characteristics of T cell subsets required for the rapid induction of monocyte PCA indicate that a differentiated cell of the T series is required and further support the possibility that a direct cell-cell contact mechanism may mediate collabora-

Table 5. Induction of Monocyte PCA by
LPS-Stimulated Human Lymphocyte Classes and Subclasses

Lymphocyte Class	Markers	LPS-Induced PCA $(mU/10^6 \; cells)$*
T	nE^+	3,140
Non-T	nE^-	280
T_M	nE^+, $Fc\mu^+$	4,170
T_G	nE^+, $Fc\gamma^+$	270
T_{NULL}	nE^+, $Fc\mu^-$, $Fc\gamma^-$	220

*Lymphocytes were triggered with 10 μg/ml LPS for thirty minutes, washed and added at a 5.5:1 ratio to autologous monocytes. Six hours later the cells were washed, disrupted and assayed for PCA.

tion. The pathway appears quite different from that involved in LPS-stimulated B cell proliferation in mice. Indeed, the C3H/HeJ strain of mice that lack the gene required to respond proliferatively to LPS did respond normally to induction of monocyte PCA [33].

Characteristics of Monocyte Procoagulant Activity

The characteristics of monocyte procoagulant activity were examined first, using congenital coagulation factor-deficient plasmas. As evident from the data in Table 6, both Ag:Ab complex- and LPS-stimulated human mononuclear cells expressed full procoagulant activity in factor VIII- or IX-deficient plasmas, but were unable to induce coagulation in factor X-, VII- or prothrombin-deficient plasmas. The specificity was confirmed for factor X-, VII- and prothrombin-deficient plasmas by the addition of purified factor X, VII or prothrombin, respectively, with full reconstitution of the ability of the induced human monocyte to rapidly induce fibrin formation. These data are characteristic of induction of blood coagulation by tissue factor, a cell membrane phospholipoprotein that activates factor VII, and is fully consistent with the previous observation of tissue factor induction in human PBM by LPS as described by Rickles and Rick [34].

Table 6. Characteristics of PCA Induced in Human and
Murine Monocytes by Selected Stimuli

Species PBM	Stimulus	Normal Plasma	Total PCA $(mU/10^6 PBM)$ Factor-Deficient Plasma				
			VIII	IX	VII	X	Prothrombin
Human	LPS*	2,950	2,850	3,000	200	150	25
Human	Ag:Ab†	3,100	2,800	3,000	100	150	25
Mouse	LPS*	1,800	1,700	1,650	1,500	1,200	25
Mouse	Ag:Ab†	1,750	1,800	1,700	1,650	1,100	25
Mouse	MHV‡	3,000	2,200	2,400	2,950	2,750	25

*LPS at 10 μg/ml.
†Ag:Ab at 4:1 ratio in antigen excess at 100 μg/ml.
‡Murine hepatitis virus (MHV-3) at 10^3 PFU with C3H PBM.

In contrast, the initiation of fibrin formation by murine monocytes following stimulation with LPS or Ag:Ab complexes differed [35, 36]. The murine monocyte PCA induced significant fibrin formation in all factor-deficient plasmas except those deficient in prothrombin (Table 6). The clotting of prothrombin-deficient plasmas was completely reconstituted by the addition of purified human prothrombin to reconstitute the plasma to 80 μg/ml. Evidence for direct prothrombin cleavage to a functional enzyme similar or identical to thrombin was confirmed by use of a simple two-protein clotting assay consisting of purified prothrombin and fibrinogen. Following the additon of an equal volume of induced murine monocyte suspension, there was efficient clotting which was comparable in rate to that of whole plasma. To confirm the implication that murine monocytes, when induced by LPS- or Ag:Ab complex-triggered lymphocytes, responded by synthesis of a direct prothrombinase, we examined prothrombin cleavage by SDS polyacrylamide gel electrophoresis. Cleavage of ^{125}I-prothrombin was examined after addition of disrupted human or mouse monocytes. Only with the induced murine monocytes was there limited proteolytic cleavage of ^{125}I-prothrombin to yield thrombin or at least thrombin-like cleavage products. On the basis of cleavage or by functional clotting assay, the production of monocyte prothrombinase was at least to a degree equivalent to that produced indirectly by tissue factor generation by human monocytes.

The inducible monocyte prothrombinase was not consistent with conventional activated factor X (Xa), based on inhibitor profiles and molecular weight. The enzyme was DFP sensitive and required calcium ions and phospholipid. It differed from human factor Xa with respect to the lower concentrations of DFP and higher concentration of PMSF required for inhibition. It was insensitive to Trasylol, in contrast to plasmin. Membrane-rich fractions of induced murine monocytes were analyzed by SDS gel electrophoresis. The gel was sliced, the enzyme eluted and renatured in Triton X-100. The specific activity was recovered at a molecular weight of approximately 90,000, considerably larger than purified factor Xa protein (48,000).

More recent studies have indicated that there is a human monocyte counterpart to the murine monocyte prothrombinase. This has been induced by high-density and by intermediate-density plasma lipoproteins [37]. In this system lymphocyte collaboration is required as well [38]. Subsequent studies indicate that certain other stimuli, such as purified human hepatitis B virus 22-nm particles, can induce the monocyte prothrombinase in cells of immune individuals. In Table 7 the types of PCA induced by selected stimuli are tabulated. The genetically restricted recognition of murine hepatitis virus (MHV-3) by murine PBM or splenic cells both in vitro and in vivo is equivalent and initiates the production of monocyte prothrombinase. The pathogenetic associations for many of these stimuli will require detailed exploration.

A Genetic Restriction for Viral Induction of PCA

When LPS or Ag:Ab complexes were employed as probes for genetic restrictions of the PCA response, very little difference was seen between healthy mice of normal strains, with little variaton within a single strain. The only restriction observed was the necessity for *I-A* compatibility between T lymphocyte and monocyte or splenic macrophage.

In contrast, when murine blood mononuclear cells were exposed in vitro to MHV-3 there was a clear strain-dependent

Table 7. Monocyte Procoagulant Activity Associated with Various Agents
In Vitro and In Vivo

Species	Siimulus	Setting	Type of PCA
Human	LPS	In vitro	Tissue factor
Human	Ag:Ab	In vitro	Tissue factor
Human	Viral heaptitis type B	In vivo	Monocyte prothrombinase
Human	HB$_S$Ag*	In vitro	Monocyte prothrombinase
Mouse	LPS	In vitro	Monocyte prothrombinase
Mouse	Ag:Ab	In vitro	Monocyte prothrombinase
Mouse	MHV-3†	In vitro	Monocyte prothrombinaae
Mouse	MHV-3†	In vivo	Monocyte prothrombinase
Mouse	MRL/l strain autoimmune disease	In vivo	Monocyte prothrombinase

*Human hepatitis B virus, 22-nm particles.
†Plaque-purified murine hepatitis virus.

difference in the magnitude of the PCA response (Table 8). Whereas A strain mice were unresponsive to this single-strand RNA coronavirus, the C3H mouse responded to a degree comparable for LPS. This latter strain develops a significant degree of acute viral hepatitis and hepatic injury continues, progressing to chronic hepatitis. However, when PBM from BALB/c mice were exposed to MHV-3 a response of unparalleled magnitude was observed. This strain is also most highly susceptible to the virus, infection with 100 PFU consistently resulting in death in six to seven days as a result of acute fulminant hepatitis [39]. Of interest is the close parallel observed between the in vitro PCA response and the viral disease. When these mice were infected in vivo and their PBM and spleen cells assayed ½ to 24 hours later for PCA, the activation of monocyte PCA in vivo preceded the onset of histologically or biochemically documented hepatic injury. This introduces a number of intriguing speculations, including the role of fibrin deposition in the resultant lesions.

Of particular interest, these observations with MHV-3 suggest a restriction of the PCA response similar to that described for immune responses, i.e. the Ir gene restrictions [30]. Only limited data with recombinant mice are thus

Table 8. Murine Hepatitis Virus Induction of PCA

| | In Vitro | | | In Vivo | | | |
| | PCA (mU/10^6 cells) | | | PCA (mU/10^6 cells) | | | Histo- |
Species	Control	LPS*	MHV-3†	Control	LPS‡	MHV-3§	pathology
BALB/c strain mouse	780	3,850	74,560	250	3,700	41,500	Fulminant hepatic necrosis
C3H strain mouse	810	4,100	2,850	180	4,250	3,100	Chronic hepatitis
A strain mouse	940	4,250	740	220	3,900	150	No pathology
Human	680	3,250	800				

*PBM assayed for PCA 24 hours after exposure to LPS at 10 μg/ml.

†LPS, 10 μg intraperitoneally. PBM isolated and assayed for PCA 24 hours later.

‡MHV-3, 10^6 PFU/ml. PBM analyzed 24 hours after exposure to MHV-3 in vitro.

§MHV-3, 10^6 PFU intraperitoneally, PBM isolated 12 hours later and analyzed directly for PCA.

far available for the genetic restriction of the PCA response in mice. Recognition seems species-restricted, since human cells do not respond to MHV-3. This is in contrast as well to what might be expected if triggering resulted from a simple lipid exchange or a relatively nonspecific interaction. Within the murine system the strain specificity is of interest in that A and BALB/c are compatible within *H-2* to the right of *I-E*, yet they differ profoundly in this response. The *H-2* incompatibility between these two strains falls within *K* through I-E, the *Ir* gene region. This is consistent, but is still inadequate to assign the effect to this group of genetic loci. Notably, A and C3H strains are *H-2* compatible for *K* through *I-E*, yet they also differ in the degree of the PCA response and severity of disease. These observations suggest that either more than one genetic locus influences the response or the genetic restriction is prescribed by a gene locus outside *H-2*. These data suggest a restriction other than I-A and there does appear to be an additional restriction in the response outlined in Figure 3. Whether the incompletely localized genes specifying infectivity of mouse macrophages [39] are identical to these specifying the PCA response or are independent will require analysis with currently available recombinant mouse strains.

Cellular Pathway of T Cell-Instructed Generation of Procoagulant Monokines

The pathway described here has been developed from the original observations of Rapaport and Hjort [40] and Lerner et al [41] that endotoxin could induce procoagulant activity in blood leukocytes. We further extend these observations to include a variety of stimuli and demonstrate that the pathway appears to have many common features in at least two species. This pathway draws upon the role of certain T lymphocytes as recognitive units. T lymphocytes are generally perceived as the discriminating recognitive element for the initiation of a variety of humoral and cellular immune responses. In the pathway described here, T cells are demonstrated to have a broader recognitive role. In contrast to the requirement for macrophage presentation of antigen to the lymphocyte in conventional immune responses, the pathway for PCA induction does ot exhibit evidence for such a role on the part of the macrophage/

monocyte. Rather, the lymphocyte functions as the accessory cell and the monocyte/macrophage as the effector cell. In this system, a helper T cell-enriched fraction recognizes at least two disparate stimuli, e.g. LPS and Ag:Ab complexes, and can subsequently instruct monocytes or macrophages to generate procoagulant activity. This communication appears to be unidirectional, extremely rapid and I-A restricted for collaboration, as schematically depicted in Figure 3. Interestingly, the T cell exhibits requirements for neither protein nor RNA synthesis to accomplish its task.

These studies have led to the discovery and characterization of a new pathway of initiation of the coagulation system. The monocyte/macrophage prothrombinase is induced by different stimuli in mouse as contrasted to human cells, but can be produced by either species. The alternative procoagulant activity results from generation and cell surface expression of tissue factor, the initiator of the extrinsic coagulation pathway (Fig. 4).

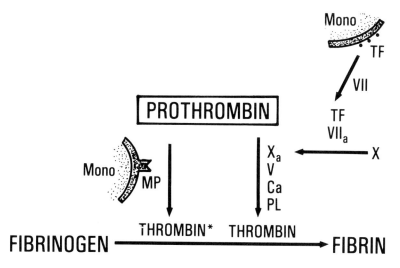

FIG. 4. Initiation of coagulation by monocytes and macrophages. Monocytes can activate the coagulation system either through the extrinsic pathway of activation with the expression of tissue factor (TF) or by direct cleavage of prothrombin with the monocyte prothrombinase (MP). In both mechanisms functional thrombin is produced which converts fibrinogen to fibrin.

Early evidence suggests the presence of not only inducer T cells but also suppressor T cells. Thus, this pathway exhibits elements of classical circuit design common to immune responses. In addition, the initial evidence for genetic restrictions in the response to stimuli such as murine hepatitis virus may be similar to the Ir gene restrictions of the immune response. It is proposed that this cellular pathway may be distinct from lymphokine activation of monocytes and macrophages in respect to generation of procoagulant monokines as well as other forms of macrophage activation.

Pathogenetic Significance

The pathogenetic implications of the PCA response remain to be fully explored. A variety of observations establish correlations between the features of a number of immunologic tissue lesions and the generation of lymphoid procoagulant activity by either direct cellular collaboration or a proposed lymphokine-mediated pathway [42].

Fibrin is commonly deposited in immunologic tissue lesions. Not only has it been established that the induration characteristic of the delayed cutaneous hypersensitivity reaction is a result of local deposition of fibrin [13, 43], such that these lesions in afibrinogenemic individuals lack induration [14], but defibrinogenation of experimental animals precludes glomerular injury and proteinuria due to experimental immune complex glomerulonephritis [16]. Fibrin deposited at the site of immunologic tissue lesions may have a variety of effects. Not only may it interfere with effective cellular attack of neoplastic cells [18] or infected cells, but if occurring in blood vessels, it may also induce platelet activation, microthrombi, vascular injury and ischemia. The effects of fibrin deposition and subsequent fibrinolysis have only been partially explored; however, discrete peptides released from fibrin by fibrinolysis suppress lymphocyte function [21, 22] and induce local increased vascular permeability [44].

The role of the monocyte and macrophage in basic host defense mechanisms has long been described and appreciated. Due to the functional diversity, or potential for diversity, it has been difficult to narrowly define the function of these cells as encountered in various types of tissue lesions. As long suspected, the specifically induced macrophage or monocyte is clearly a source of procoagulant activity, which for the first time is recognized to result from the synthesis of either of two molecules and pathways, as outlined schematically in Figure 4. What other functions may also be induced in a linked manner remain to be defined. However, the increasing delineation of these cells at the forefront of the host defense and the evidence for activation of this pathway in vivo in a variety of diseases offer the promise of more cogent delineation of the participants in the pathogenesis of a variety of diseases.

Acknowledgments

The authors appreciate the dedicated assistance of Patsy Larson and Mary Gortmaker in preparation of the manuscript, the provision of purified bacterial lipopolysaccharides by Dr. David Morrison (Department of Microbiology and Immunology, Emory University, Atlanta, Ga.), and the provision of human hepatitis B virus particles by Dr. John Gerin (Department of Microbiology and Immunology, Georgetown University, Washington, D.C.).

References

1. Piesseus, W.F., Churchill, W.H. and David, J.R.: Macrophages activated *in vitro* with lymphocyte mediators kill neoplastic but not normal cells. J. Immunol. 114:293, 1975.
2. Nathan, C.F. and Root, R.K.: Hydrogen peroxide release from mouse peritoneal macrophages. Dependence on sequential activation and triggering. J. Exp. Med. 146:1648, 1977.
3. Unkeless, J.C., Gordon, S. and Reich, E.: Secretion of plasminogen activator by stimulated macrophages. J. Exp. Med. 139:834, 1974.
4. Werb, Z. and Gordon, S.: Secretion of a specific collagenase by stimulated macrophages. J. Exp. Med. 142:346, 1975.
5. Werb, Z. and Gordon, S.: Elastase secretion by stimulated macrophages. Characterization and regulation. J. Exp. Med. 142:361, 1975.
6. Schnyder, J. and Baggiolini, M.: Role of phagocytosis in the activation of macrophages. J. Exp. Med. 148:1449, 1978.
7. Nathan, C.F., Karnovsky, M.L. and David, J.R.: Alterations of macrophage functions by mediators from lymphocytes. J. Exp. Med. 133:1356, 1971.
8. Buchmuller, Y. and Manuel, J.: Studies on the mechanisms of

macrophage activation. II. Parasite destruction in macrophages activated by supernates from concanavalin A-stimulated lymphocytes. J. Exp. Med. 150:359, 1979.

9. Levy, G.A. and Edgington, T.S.: Lymphocyte cooperation is required for amplification of macrophage procoagulant activity. J. Exp. Med. 151:1232, 1980.

10. Schwartz, B.S. and Edgington, T.S.: Lymphocyte collaboration is required for induction of murine monocyte procoagulant activity by immune complexes. (J. Immunol., submitted 1981.)

11. Edwards, R.L. and Rickles, F.R.: On the origin of leukocyte procoagulant activity. Thromb. Res. 13:307, 1978.

12. Edwards, R.L. and Rickles, F.R.: The role of human T cells and T cell products for monocyte tissue factor generation. J. Immunol. 125:606, 1980.

13. Colvin, R.B., Johnson, R.A., Mihn, M.C. and Dvorak, H.F.: Role of the clotting system in cell mediated hypersensitivity. J. Exp. Med. 138:686, 1973.

14. Colvin, R.B., Mossesson, M.W. and Dvorak, H.F.: Delayed-type hypersensitivity skin reactions in congenital afibrinogenemia lack fibrin deposition and induration. J. Clin. Invest. 63:1302, 1979.

15. Holdsworth, S.R., Neale, T.J. and Wilson, C.B.: Abrogation of immune glomerulonephritis (GN) in rabbits by anti-macrophage (M) serum. Kidney Int. (In press.)

16. Holdworth, S.R., Thomson, N.M., Glasgow, E.F. and Atkins, R.C.: The effect of defibrination on macrophage participation in rabbit nephrotoxic nephritis: Studies using glomerular culture and electron microscopy. Clin. Exp. Immunol. 37:38-43, 1979.

17. Chmielewska, J., Poggi, A., Janik, P. et al: Effect of defibrination with batroxobin on growth and metastases of JW sarcoma in mice. Eur. J. Cancer 16:919, 1980.

18. Dvorak, H.F., Orenstein, N.S., Carvalho, A.C. et al: Induction of a fibrin-gel investment: An early event in line 10 hepatocarcinoma growth mediated by tumor-secreted products. J. Immunol. 122:166, 1979.

19. Cronlund, M., Hardin, J., Burton, J. et al: Fibrinopeptide A in plasma of normal subjects and patients with disseminated intravascular coagulation and systemic lupus erythematosus. J. Clin. Invest. 58:142, 1976.

20. Accinni, L. and Dixon, F.J.: Degenerative vascular disease and myocardial infarction in mice with lupus-like syndrome. Am. J. Pathol. 96:477, 1979.

21. Girmann, G., Rees, H., Schwarze, G. and Scheurlen, P.G.: Immunosuppression by micromolecular fibrinogen degradation products in cancer. Nature 59:399, 1975.

22. Edgington, T.S., Curtiss, L.K. and Plow, E.F.: The immunosuppressive activity of plasmic degradation products of human fibrinogen. Thromb. Haemost. 38:170, 1977.

23. Niemetz, J. and Fani, K.: Role of leukocytes in blood coagulation and

the generalized Schwartzman reaction. Nature New Biol. 232:247, 1971.

24. Rickles, F.R., Levin, J., Hardin, J.A. et al: Tissue factor generation by human mononuclear cells: Effects of endotoxin and dissociation of tissue factor generation from mitogenic response. J. Lab. Clin. Med. 89:792, 1977.

25. Rothberger, H., Zimmerman, T.S. and Vaughan, J.H.: Increased production and expression of tissue thromboplastin-like procoagulant activity *in vitro* by allogenically stimulated human leukocytes. J. Clin. Invest. 62:649, 1978.

26. Rothberger, H., Zimmerman, T.S., Spiegelberg, H.L. and Vaughan, J.H.: Leukocyte procoagulant activity. Enhancement of production *in vitro* by IgG and antigen-antibody complexes. J. Clin. Invest. 59:549, 1977.

27. Cohen, S., Benacerraf, B., McCluskey, R.T. and Ovary, Z.: Effect of anticoagulants on delayed hypersensitivity reactions. J. Immunol. 98:351, 1967.

28. Edwards, R.L. and Rickles, F.R.: Delayed hypersensitivity in man: Effects of systemic anticoagulation. Science 200:541, 1978.

29. Ulevitch, R.J., Johnston, A.R. and Weinstein, D.B.: New function for high density lipoproteins. Their participation in intravascular reactions of bacterial lipopolysaccharides. J. Clin. Invest. 64:1516, 1979.

30. Benacerraf, B. and Germain, R.N.: The immune response genes of the major histocompatibility complex. Immunol. Rev. 38:70, 1978.

31. Farr, A.G., Wechter, W.J., Kiely, J.-M. and Unanue, E.R.: Induction of cytocidal macrophages following *in vitro* interactions between Listeria-immune T cells and macrophages — Role of H-2. J. Immunol. 122:2405, 1979.

32. Moretta, L., Webb, S.R., Grossi, G.E. et al: Functional analysis of two human T cell subpopulations: Help and suppression of B cell responses by T cells bearing receptors for IgM and IgG. J. Exp. Med. 146:184, 1977.

33. Levy, G.A. and Edgington, T.S.: Lymphoid procoagulant activity and mitogenesis in the C3H/HeJ mouse: Discordant response to LPS (lipopolysaccharide) stimulation. J. Immunol. 124:2665, 1980.

34. Rickles, F.R. and Rick, P.D.: Structural features of Salmonella typhimurium lipopolyssacharide required for activation of tissue factor in human mononuclear cells. J. Clin. Invest. 59:1188, 1977.

35. Schwartz, B.S., Levy, G.A., Fair, D.S. and Edgington, T.S.: Murine monocytes produce a novel prothrombin activator in response to Ag:Ab or LPS stimulated lymphocytes. Fed. Proc. (In press.)

36. Schwartz, B.S., Levy, G.A., Fair, D.S. et al: A novel prothrombin activator is expressed by human circulating monocytes exposed to certain plasma lipoproteins. Circulation 62:279, 1980.

37. Schwartz, B.S., Levy, G.A., Fair, D.S. et al: Plasma lipoprotein induction and suppression of the generation of cellular procoagulant activity *in vitro*. I. Two procoagulant activities are produced by peripheral blood mononuclear cells. J. Clin. Invest. (In press.)

38. Levy, G.A., Schwartz, B.S., Curtiss, L.K. and Edgington, T.S.: Plasma
    lipoprotein induction and suppression of the generation of cellular
    procoagulant activity *in vitro*. II. The requirement for cellular
    collaboration. J. Clin. Invest. (In press.)
39. Bang, F.B. and Warwick, A.: Mouse macrophages as host cells for the
    mouse hepatitis virus and the genetic basis of their susceptibility.
    Proc. Natl. Acad. Sci. (U.S.A.) 46:1065, 1960.
40. Rapaport, S.I. and Hjort, P.F.: The blood clotting properties of rabbit
    peritoneal leukocytes *in vitro*. Thromb. Diath. Haemmorrh. 17:222,
    1967.
41. Lerner, R.G., Goldstein, R. and Cummings, G.: Stimulation of human
    leukocyte thromboplastic activibity by endotoxin. Proc. Soc. Exp.
    Biol. Med. 138:145, 1971.
42. Edwards, R.L. and Rickles, F.R.: The role of monocyte tissue factor
    in the immune response. Lymphokine Rep. 1:181, 1980.
43. Colvin, R.B. and Dvorak, H.F.: Role of the clotting system in cell
    mediated hypersensitivity. II. Kinetics of fibrinogen/fibrin accumula-
    tion and vascular permeability changes in tuberculin and cutaneous
    basophil hypersensitivity reactions. J. Immunol. 14:377, 1975.
44. Gerdin, B. and Saldeen, T.: Effect of fibrin degradation products on
    microvascular permeability. Thromb. Res. 13:995, 1978.

Murine SLE — Its Implications for Human Diseases of Autoimmunity

Frank J. Dixon, M.D.

Introduction

It is now abundantly clear that immunologic self recognition, i.e. autoimmune responses, is neither rare nor invariably disease-producing, but rather that it plays a variety of roles — sometimes essential, often incidental and occasionally pathogenic. The normal operation of the immune system itself depends to a large extent upon self recognition. The cooperative interaction of immunocytes and macrophages in the course of an immune response involves the mutual recognition of cell surface self markers determined by genes of the major histocompatibility complex. Also, the normal response to certain antibodies (idiotypes) is the formation of anti-idiotypic antibodies, which presumably play a vital role in regulation of the immunologic network. In addition to these examples of autoimmunity that are essential to normal function, there are numerous instances of autoantibodies or autoimmune responses with no clear-cut etiologic relationship to any essential function or to any disease.

If autoimmune responses per se are not pathogenic, what then determines the development and course of autoimmune disease? If there is any generalized, consistent predisposition to known spontaneous autoimmune disease, it is the lifelong B cell

Frank J. Dixon, M.D., Member, Department of Immunopathology, Scripps Clinic and Research Foundation, La Jolla, Calif.

This is publication No. 2317 from the Department of Immunopathology, Scripps Clinic and Research Foundation. Supported in part by USPHS grants AI-07007, CA-16600, AG-01743 and the Green Endowment.

polyclonal hyperactivity detectable even before birth in conditions such as murine SLE. The precise relationship of this spontaneous lymphoid hyperactivity to autoimmune disease remains to be determined. Beyond this the immunologic specificity of the autoimmune responses — or, looked at another way, the nature of the autoantigenic target — is an important factor since, if the target antigen is essential to normal function and if it is vulnerable to an autoimmune attack, such an attack will affect function and produce disease. Also, if the antigen by its localization and/or its physicochemical character forms, upon reaction with autoantibodies or self-reactive cells, a phlogogenic stimulus, inflammation and disease will result. No doubt, there are additional quantitative and qualitative aspects of the autoimmune response itself that determine pathogenicity, for example the apparently greater pathogenic potential of IgG than IgM autoantibodies. Thus, the basis of autoimmune disease may depend more upon a limited number of genetically determined, specific and particularly pathogenic autoimmune responses, perhaps enhanced by pre-existing lymphoid hyperactivity, than upon any across-the-board defects in immune regulation, as has been postulated.

I would like to consider in depth one spontaneous animal autoimmune disease, murine SLE, and attempt to describe its pathogenesis, define the critical autoimmune responses involved, evaluate the immunologic characteristics of the host and identify some of the factors, genetic and environmental, which seem to play an etiologic role. Murine SLE is a desirable subject since in most respects it closely mimics human SLE, the prototype autoimmune disease, and since it has been the subject of intensive investigation in many laboratories. Although the analysis of murine SLE is complicated by multiple autoimmune responses, it does have the advantage of being spontaneous in origin so that its etiologic factors are likely to be more relevant to clinical disease than are those of the various experimentally induced autoimmune diseases.

Until recently the study of murine SLE was limited to NZB and (NZB $\times$ NZW)F_1 (NZB $\times$ W) mice. These studies of NZ mice have been handicapped by a number of these animals' unique immunologic, virologic and genetic features that have attracted much attention but are not necessarily important aspects of their disease. However, it is clear from these studies that the disease is multigenic in nature and that a number of secondary factors influence the expression of its essential autoimmune processes. In the past few years two new murine strains (BXSB and MRL — *lpr/lpr*) which develop spontaneous SLE have been described by Murphy and Roths [1, 2]. The availability of many, quite different kinds of mice, each of which develops SLE, allows the determination of essential common denominators of the disease wherever it develops.

Derivation and Mortality Rate of SLE-Prone Murine Strains

The derivations of the SLE-prone murine strains are given in Table 1. It has been estimated from the breeding history that the composite genome of the MRL mice is derived 75.0% from LG, 12.6% AKR, 12.1% C3H and 0.3% C57BL/6. In the 12th generation of the MRL inbreeding, due to a spontaneous autosomal recessive mutation, *lpr* (lymphoproliferation) gene, the MRL strain was subdivided into two substrains, one with the *lpr* gene and the other without. The *lpr* gene has been transferred to substrain MRL/n by cross-intercross matings producing the congenic inbred strains MRL/Mp — *lpr/lpr* and +/+. The development of BXSB/Mp strain has been detailed

Table 1. Derivation of SLE Mice and Genetic Markers

Strain	Derivation	H-2	Lymphocyte Surface Alloantigens	IgG Allotype
NZB		$H\text{-}2^d$	Thy 1.2, Ly 1.2, Ly 2.2, Ly 3.2, $Qa\text{-}1^a$, Mls^a	e
	Inbred for color from stock of undefined background			
NZW		$H\text{-}2^z$	Thy 1.2	e
BXSB	Derived from (C57BL/6J × SB/Le) F_1	$H\text{-}2^b$	Thy 1.2, TL⁻, Ly 1.2, Ly 2.2, Ly 3.2, $Qa\text{-}1^b$	b
MRL/l	Genome = 75% LG, 13% AKR, 12% C3H and 0.3% C57BL/6	$H\text{-}2^k$	Thy 1.2, TL⁻, Ly 1.2, Ly 2.1, Ly 3.1, $Qa\text{-}1^b$	a

elsewhere by Murphy and Roths [3]. This recombinant inbred strain was derived from a single cross between a C57BL/6 female and an SB/Le mouse homozygous for the linked mutant genes satin (*sa*) and beige (*bg*). The development of the NZB, NZW and NZB X W mice has been described elsewhere [4].

NZB mice of both sexes have a 50% mortality by 16 to 17 months of age. In the NZB X W mice, the disease appears first in the female at about 6 months of age, with 50% mortality at 8.5 months, while in the male 50% mortality is reached at 15 months. The MRL/Mp — *lpr/lpr* substrain (MRL/l) manifests early disease with 50% mortality in the females and males at about 5 and 6 months, respectively; whereas the MRL/Mp — +/+ (MRL/n), which lacks the *lpr* gene, has delayed disease with 50% mortality at 17 and 23 months for female and male, respectively. In contrast to NZB X W, the male BXSB/Mp (BXSB) is affected much earlier than the female, with a 50% mortality for the male at around 6 months and for the female at 15 months.

Histoimmunopathologic and Serologic Features

Immunopathologic features of these mice [5, 6] are summarized in Table 2. Immune complex (IC) glomerulonephritis is a histopathologic feature of all of these autoimmune mice and is the major cause of death. Granular glomerular deposits of IgG and C3 and sometimes DNA and gp70 retroviral envelope antigens are present. Early thymic atrophy, primarily of the cortex, is seen in all of these mice. However, the degree of lymph node hyperplasia varies considerably, ranging from normal to 2 to 3 times enlarged in NZB X W females, 10 to 20 times above normal size in BXSB males, and up to 100 times enlarged in MRL/l mice. The proliferating cells in BXSB are of B type and those in MRL/l mice of T cell type (see below). Attempts to transplant enlarged lymph nodes to find evidence of malignancy in MRL/l mice have failed. Fifteen to thirty percent of mice in each SLE strain have acute and/or old myocardial infarction [6]. Moreover, medium and small arteries and arterioles of hearts with and without infarcts have focal degenerative lesions consisting of PAS-positive or eosinophilic deposits in the intima and to a lesser extent in the media, without accompanying cellular inflammation. Granular deposits

Table 2. Histoimmunopathologic and Serologic Characteristics
of SLE-Mice

		Histopathologic Features			
Strain	IC-GN	Thymic Atrophy	Lymphoid Hyperplasia	Arteritis	Arthritis
NZB	+	+	+	0	0
NZB × W	+++	+	+	0	0
MRL/1	+++	+	+++	+	+
BXSB	+++	+	++	0	0

Serologic Features

Common = Hypergammaglobulinemia, ANA, anti-dsDNA, anti-ssDNA, anti-hapten antibodies, high levels of gp70, immune complexes, reduced complement levels (NZB is C5-deficient)

Uncommon = Anti-Sm (MRL/n, MRL/1), IgG = IgM RF (MRL/1) anti-erythrocyte (NZB, NZB × W), NTA (NZB, NZB × W, BXSB)

of mouse Ig, C3 and occasionally gp70 may be present in the walls of medium and small arteries, arterioles and venules of myocardium. Apart from the degenerative vascular disease found in all strains, over half of MRL/1 mice uniquely develop acute and/or necrotizing polyarteritis, most frequently involving renal and coronary arteries. About 25% of old, sick MRL/1 mice also have swollen joints of the hind feet and lower legs. There is destruction of articular cartilage, proliferation of synovium, pannus formation and at times joint effusions, which together present a picture not unlike that of rheumatoid arthritis.

Of the serologic abnormalities in SLE mice, some are common to all strains and others are not [5, 7-11] (Table 2). The common primary serologic abnormalities include very early polyclonal B cell hyperactivity manifest by elevated concentrations of serum Ig frequently associated with monoclonal γ-globulins, antinuclear antibodies, and anti-ds and ss-DNA antibodies. Additionally, all autoimmune mice at 2 to 4 weeks of age spontaneously produce four to six times more anti-hapten antibody-forming cells in spleens and have greater concentrations of anti-hapten antibodies in sera than age-matched, immunologically normal strains of mice [7]. Significant levels of retroviral gp70 are also observed in all kinds of autoimmune mice, being highest in NZB and followed by NZB × W, MRL/l and BXSB mice [5]. However, similar levels of retroviral gp70 are observed in sera of some immunologically normal mice (NZW, LG/J, 129/J, SM/J, DBA/2). Concentrations of serum gp70 do not increase with the autoimmune disease nor do they correlate with levels of anti-DNA and anti-hapten antibodies. Uncommon primary serologic abnormalities are as follows:

1. Anti-erythrocyte antibodies occur frequently in the NZB and NZB × W (80%), but infrequently in MRL/l (11%) and BXSB (18%) mice.

2. Antibodies against the nuclear glycoprotein Sm [9] occur exclusively in older MRL/n (35% males, 45% females) and MRL/l mice (37% males, 10% females).

3. Rheumatoid factors of both the IgM and IgG variety are present in sera of two thirds of older MRL/l mice only [5, 8, 11]. This finding is in accord with the arthritis occasionally observed in these mice and suggests that this strain may be a valuable animal model for the study of rheumatoid arthritis as well.

4. Natural thymocytotoxic antibodies (NTA) are present in high levels and incidence in NZB and NZB × W mice, low in BXSB, very low or absent in MRL/l and MRL/n mice.

A comprehensive survey [10] showed similar incidences and serum titers of NTA in some immunologically normal strains (RF, SN, NC, 129-GIX+, 129-GIX−) as compared to NZ mice. Although the fine specificities of NTAs in the various murine strains remain to be determined, we may conclude that NTAs are neither necessary nor probably unique to SLE mice and that their mere presence does not indict the individual to become autoimmune. In fact, hereditarily asplenic (Dh/+) NZB mice develop autoimmune disease in the absence of NTA [12], and NTAs could be expressed in recombinant NZB inbred strains in the absence of other types of autoantibodies or, conversely, anti-DNA and anti-erythrocyte antibodies could be expressed in the absence of NTAs [13]. Common secondary serologic features in all SLE strains are the appearance of circulating immune complexes (ICs) and a decrease in hemolytic complement as the disease progresses. Interestingly, the NZB strain is genetically C5-deficient.

Nature of Immune Complexes in Sera

Studies conducted to determine the nature of ICs detected by the Raji cell radioimmunoassay in sera of SLE-prone murine strains have demonstrated the presence of retroviral gp70-anti-gp70 complexes [14]. The sera of all older autoimmune murine strains, but not sera from several normal strains, are characterized by a rapidly sedimenting heavy form of gp70 (7-19S), in addition to 5S gp70 (Fig. 1). This heavy form of gp70, but not the 5S type, is specifically adsorbed with anti-mouse IgG antibody or *Staphylococcus aureus*, strongly suggesting that the heavy gp70 in serum is in the form of ICs. Immunoprecipitation analysis with anti-mouse IgG or adsorption to *Staphylococcus aureus* indicates that approximately one fifth to one half of the

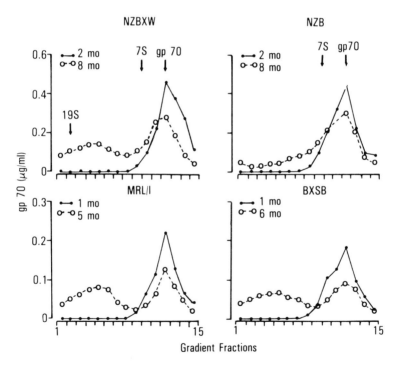

FIG. 1. Sedimentation rate of serum gp70 from SLE-prone mice at various ages, analyzed by sucrose density gradient centrifugation. The concentration of gp70 was determined by a radioimmunoassay with anti-FeLV antiserum and ^{125}I-Rauscher MuLV gp70. The position of markers is indicated by the arrows.

total serum gp70 in sera of older autoimmune mice is associated
with IgG. The amount of gp70-related ICs increases with age in
the SLE-susceptible strains, paralleling the progress of renal
disease. IgG-complexed gp70 is also found in renal eluates from
the diseased kidneys of adult mice but not those from
2-month-old mice.

Since multiple immunologically related gp70s are produced
in every mouse [15], it is important to know what kind of
retroviral gp70 is involved in the formation of ICs. Although the
primary serum gp70 in all mice is similar to that found in the
NZB xenotropic virus [15], the lack of antibody formation
against serum gp70 in normal mice raised the possibility that
SLE mice might express a unique type of retroviral gp70 in
their sera. However, immunochemical and tryptic peptide
mapping analysis of the gp70 isolated from the circulating ICs
revealed its xenotropic origin [16]. Moreover, studies of the
immunologic specificity of isolated anti-gp70 antibodies from
the ICs clearly showed that anti-gp70 antibodies have an
affinity for NZB xenotropic viral gp70 approximately ten times
higher than that for AKR ecotropic viral gp70, indicating that
the antibody involved is directed primarily to NZB xenotropic
viral gp70. This is compatible with the fact that the presence of
anti-AKR ecotropic gp70 antibodies in sera of mice does not
correlate with formation of gp70-associated ICs [14]. Thus, it
appears that mice which develop SLE do not have a unique kind
of gp70 but, instead, have the unique ability to develop an
antibody response to multiple available antigens, among them
gp70, perhaps as a result of their immunologic dysfunction.

In addition to gp70-anti-gp70 complexes, sera of older
MRL/l mice contained C-fixing IgG-IgG RF ICs of an intermediate sedimentation rate [11]. The role of this type of
complex in the pathogenesis of this strain's arthritis and
polyarteritis is not yet known. Part of the IgG RF-complexed
IgG is anti-DNA antibody, apparently without associated DNA
antigen [8].

Lymphocyte Subsets in Autoimmune Mice
and Surface Characteristics of Their B Cells

Each strain of lupus mouse has some variations from the
normal cellular distributions, but in no two of the strains are

the abnormalities the same [17]. To summarize: (1) Older NZ mice have low frequencies and absolute numbers of sIg⁺ cells, male BXSB mice have a moderate proliferation of sIg⁺ cells, male BXSB mice have a moderate proliferation of sIg⁺ cells and MRL/l mice have reduced frequencies but not absolute numbers of sIg⁺ cells. (2) B cells of older NZB, NZB × W and BXSB mice are more mature than B cells of normal mice (high frequency of complement receptor-bearing cells, loss of sIg and high ratio of sIgM:sIgD-bearing cells with age. (3) The developmental Ig-isotype diversity in autoimmune mice is normal, with sIgM⁺ cells present on spleen cells obtained immediately after birth, and sIgD⁺ cells appearing for the first time three days after birth. (4) There is a reduction of IgG FcR⁺ cells in older autoimmune mice. (5) There is a decline of T cells in NZB and NZB × W mice, normal levels of T cells in BXSB and an overwhelming T cell proliferation in older MRL/l mice. (6) The proliferating T cell in MRL/l mice is a Thy 1.2⁺, Ly "null" or weakly Ly 1⁺ cell. (7) MRL/l and BXSB mice have numerically a normal content of I-J alloantigen-bearing T cells (suppressor cells).

Further surface characterization of B cells from SLE-prone mice indicates [18]: (a) B cells from newborn SLE-prone mice, like B cells of normal strains, do not reexpress sIg after modulation with F(ab')₂ anti-Ig. (b) The rate of sIg-anti-Ig complex endocytosis and of sIg capping in autoimmune mice is similar to that of normal strains. (c) At 2 months of age, B cells of autoimmune strains, like those of normal strains, can be stimulated mitogenically with IgG anti-μ as well as F(ab')₂ anti-μ.

Functional Characteristics of B Cells

The murine SLE syndrome is marked by early B lympho-cyte hyperactivity manifested by hypergammaglobulinemia, spontaneous polyclonal antibody production and secretion of various autoantibodies [19]. Studies of in vitro magnitude and nature of the spontaneous and mitogen-induced secretion of Ig by splenic lymphocytes from these autoimmune mice indicate that all of the autoimmune murine strains do in fact have an increased frequency of mature, Ig-secreting (IgSC) or -contain-ing B cells in their spleens at one time or another, as compared to age-matched, immunologically normal strains (Fig. 2) [20]. In the NZB and NZB × W mice, the high frequency of splenic IgSC was detectable as early as 1 month of age and increased thereafter. In contrast, in BXSB male and MRL/l female mice the high frequency of IgSC was first observed at 2 to 3 months, somewhat before the clinical onset of the disease. Spleen cells from young mice of all autoimmune strains secreted predominantly IgM, but with aging and the appearance of disease, the cells switched to IgG secretion predominantly. Approximately 6% to 7% of the total spleen cells in the autoimmune mice vs. 1% in normal mice stained for intracytoplasmic Ig. With advanced clinical disease, NZ mice had 5- to 10-fold and MRL/l mice had 30-fold higher numbers of Ig-containing cells than younger, syngeneic animals. Spleen cells from 1-month-old NZB and NZB × W mice stimulated with low doses of LPS had five- to ten-fold higher frequency of IgSC than spleen cells from the two other autoimmune strains (MRL/l, BXSB) or several normal strains. It is not known whether this finding is due to an increased frequency of LPS-responding B cells in the NZ mice or increased numbers or affinity of LPS receptors on their

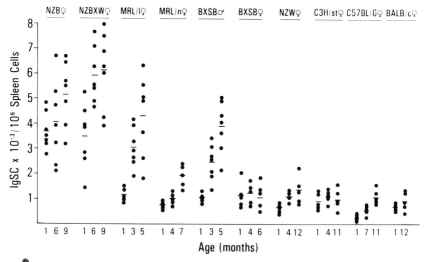

FIG. 2. Spontaneous IgSC in spleens of autoimmune and normal murine strains at various ages. IgSC were identified by a reverse hemolytic plaque assay.

splenocytes. Certainly, this finding raises the possibility that the enhanced B cell maturity in NZ mice may result from the presence of low levels of endogenous polyclonal B cell activators. The frequency of IgSC generated by LPS was greatly reduced in autoimmune mice of older age as compared to young autoimmune and young and old normal mice. This finding also indicates enhanced B cell maturity in older autoimmune mice since it suggests recruitment and differentiation of virtually all potentially LPS-reactive B cells such that few B cells are available to generate antibody when challenged in vitro with this polyclonal B cell activator.

The early and advanced generalized maturity of the B cells in autoimmune mice was also shown by studying the frequency of anti-trinitrophenyl (TNP) plaque-forming cells in the spleens of these animals [7]. The results summarized in Figure 3 indicate that all SLE strains, in contrast to normal strains, contained more PFC against TNP-SRBC than did those of normal mice. Significant elevations occurred in the majority of

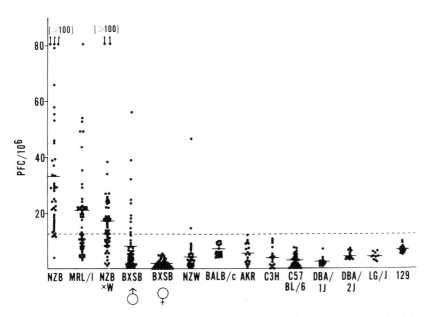

FIG. 3. Spontaneous spleen PFC against TNP-SRBC in 1- to 2-month-old SLE and normal strains. The dotted line indicates the normal mean ± 3 SD.

NZB mice at 2 weeks of age, whereas in the other three autoimmune strains (NZB × W, MRL/l, BXSB) the increase occurred at around 4 weeks of age. Further studies indicated that (a) increased polyclonal activation of B cells in spleens preceded the appearance of anti-DNP and anti-ssDNA antibodies in serum, and (b) anti-ssDNA antibodies appeared in serum at the same time as anti-DNP antibodies. Additional studies have shown an increased frequency of B cell colony-forming cells in spleens of all SLE strains as compared to normals (approximately 3000 colonies per 10^6 cells in auto-immune mice vs. $1000/10^6$ cells in normal strains). All these results on Ig secretion, polyclonal antibody production and B cell colony formation strongly indicate that there is an early generalized B cell activation in all mice with autoimmune syndromes. Similar conclusions have been reached by others with NZ mice [21-25].

Functional Characteristics of T Cells

Suppressor and Helper T Cells

The cause of the generalized B cell hyperactivity of SLE mice might be a defect or a combination of defects, such as primary B cell malfunction, the presence of endogenous or exogenous B cell activators, the lack of a negative influence by suppressor T cells, an enhanced positive influence by helper T cells, defects in subsets of intra-T regulatory cells (i.e. Ly $1,2,3^+$) or defects in other elements of the immune system such as macrophages. Evidence for functional or numerical in-adequacies in antigen-nonspecific suppressor T cells [26, 27], lack of regulatory T cells [28, 29] and lack of acceptor sites for suppressor messages on the surfaces of B cells [30] has been reported in one or another of the susceptible strains. However, others have shown that thymocyte-mediated antigen-nonspecific supression is not lost with age in autoimmune hereditarily asplenic (Dh/+) NZB mice [12] or in conventional NZB mice [24, 30]. Moreover, suppressor cells, as defined with Ly 2,3 alloantigen-expressing cells in NZB mice [28] or *I-J* subregion-controlled alloantigens in MRL/l mice [17] are normal or elevated in numbers.

Antigen-Specific Suppression. Normal antigen-specific sup-pressive mechanisms in young and old intact mice and in suppressor T cells from these mice after adoptive transfers into syngeneic recipients have been observed [31]. Suppressor cells were induced by intravenous injection of urea-denatured ovalbumin (UD-OVA) into ovalbumin (OVA)-primed mice. All mice analyzed, whether autoimmune or normal and irrespective of age, developed unmistakable OVA-specific suppressive activities that diminished IgG and IgE antibody production. To confirm the responsible cell type, T lymphocytes were isolated from the spleens of UD-OVA-treated donors by passage over nylon wool, cultured for 18 hours with UD-OVA and then transferred into naive, syngeneic young recipients. Despite some strain variability in magnitude of suppressor T cell activity, clearly all of the autoimmune mice generated suppressor T lymphocytes that adoptively suppressed both IgG and IgE antibody responses.

Antigen-Nonspecific Suppression. Con A-activated spleen cells from normal mice have been found to suppress polyclonal responses induced by several B cell mitogens, including LPS [32]. However, it has been reported that Con A-treated spleen cells from old NZB and NZB × W mice lack the ability to suppress polyclonal B cell mitogen-induced Ig secretion [26]. As shown in Figure 4, Con A effectively suppressed LPS-induced Ig synthesis by splenic cells not only from young and old normal mice but also from young and old autoimmune mice, including the NZB and NZB × W strains [20]. These results were reassessed by incubating spleen cells from young and old mice with varying doses of Con A, and then adding them to fresh syngeneic cells, derived from both young and old animals, to which a standard amount of LPS was added. After three days, the cocultures were examined for the frequency of IgSC. Spleen cells from both young and old autoimmune animals generated Con A-induced suppressor cell activity, and LPS-responding B cells of young and old syngeneic animals were equally receptive to suppressor messages. The combined results on antigen-specific and antigen-nonspecific suppression suggest that a generalized defect of suppressor T cells is not the cause of murine SLE. However, these experiments do not exclude the presence of defects on subsets of immunoregulatory T cells that control responses to specific autoantigens.

Antigen-Nonspecific Help. Because Ig hypersecretion might, at least in part, result from heightened T helper activity, the degree of help provided by increasing numbers of isolated T

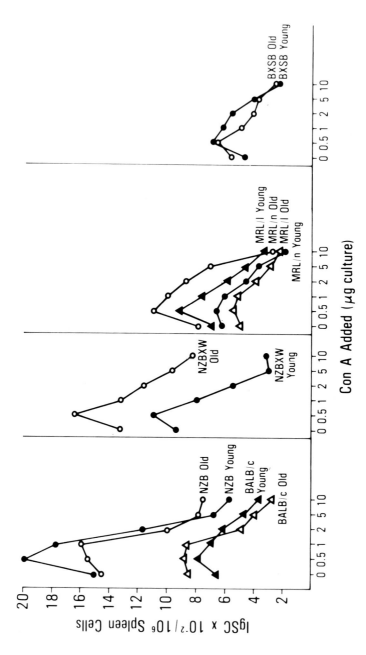

FIG. 4. Direct suppression of LPS-induced IgSC by Con A. Cells from the indicated strains were cultured in the presence of a standard amount of LPS (20 μg/culture) and increasing concentrations of Con A. IgSC were assessed three days later.

cells from SLE mice to a standard number of LPS-stimulated syngeneic and allogeneic but *H-2* identical B cells isolated from spleens of young animals was examined [20]. Increments of T cells from young and old NZB and BXSB autoimmune mice added to a standard number of B cells from syngeneic young mice provided — at all doses and at both ages — equal help in enhancing the frequency of IgSC after LPS stimulation (Fig. 5). Moreover, the help provided by T cells from these two autoimmune strains to their own B cells was not significantly different from that provided by T cells from young and old normal mice of the same *H-2* haplotype (BALB/c for NZB, C57BL/6 for BXSB). Similarly, in the reverse situation, when T

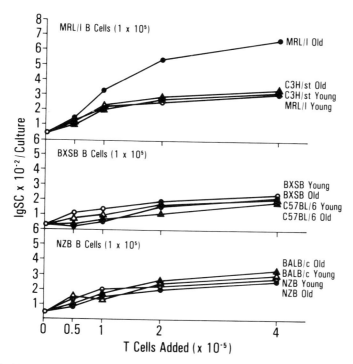

FIG. 5. Antigen-nonspecific helper activity. Frequency of IgSC in B cell-enriched spleen cell populations obtained from 1-month-old SLE mice to which increments of isolated T cells from syngeneic and allogeneic but *H-2* identical young (1-month-old) and old (4- to 7-month-old) animals were added together with LPS.

cells from young and old NZB and BXSB mice were added to B cells from young, normal counterparts, the help was not significantly greater than that from T cells of the normal strains. The only notable exception was the MRL/l strain in which T cell-enriched populations from old animals added at a 4:1 ratio to B cells from syngeneic young animals provided two to three times the help offered by equal numbers of T cells of young syngeneic animals or T cells from young and old normal mice of the same *H-2* haplotype (C3H/S5) (Fig. 5). As we have demonstrated [17], the ratio of T to B cells in MRL/l mice is significantly greater in vivo (10:1 in spleen and 30:1 in lymph nodes) than the maximal ratio employed in these experiments in vitro. Therefore, one might well expect the helper activity observed in vitro to be greatly magnified in the intact animal. Thus, our experiments and those of others [33] suggest that the hyperactivity of the older MRL/l's B cells may be the result of a heightened helper T cell activity exerted by the proliferating Ly 1^+ T cells.

T Cell-Mediated Immune Responsiveness

Several reports have described an age-dependent decline in certain T cell functions, such as allograft rejection, graft vs. host reaction, in vitro responses to phytohemagglutinin or Con A and killer cell activity against allogeneic tumor cells [reviewed in 34]. Therefore, we assessed the age-dependent capacity of NZB, NZB × W and various normal strains to generate T cell-mediated immune responses against alloantigens and virus-infected target cells as well as cell-mediated immune protection against *Listeria monocytogenes* after systemic infection [34]. The results can be summarized as follows: (a) No obvious hyper- or hypo-responsiveness was detectable when NZ and other mouse strains were tested for the generation of a cytotoxic T cell response against alloantigens in mixed lympho-cyte cultures in vitro. (b) The virus-specific cytolytic activity generated in NZ mice acutely infected with vaccinia virus was in no way different from that seen with similarly infected normal strains. (c) The kinetics and the extent of the development of footpad swelling after lymphocytic choriomeningitis virus infec-tion (a T-dependent phenomenon) were comparable in NZ strains to those of normal strains. (d) Recovery from *Listeria* infection, which is known to be dependent on generation of specific T cells that activate macrophages directly or via released lymphokines to increased bactericidal activity [35], was not different between NZ mice and other normal strains. We then similarly studied young and old BXSB and MRL/l mice and found no difference in the kinetics of appearance or relative activity of cytotoxic T cells against alloantigens and viral antigens per spleen as compared to normal strains [36]. Thus, overall cell-mediated immunity of SLE-prone mice, as assessed in these functional models, is within normal limits.

Cytolytic Reactions Against H-2 Compatible and Incompatible Allogeneic Cells

Recently, Botzenhardt et al [37] described the development of significant unidirectional primary T cell-mediated lympholytic (CML) reactions by lymphoid cells of NZB mice against H-2 identical allogeneic cells. These investigators speculated that such CML reactions represented an abnormality of NZB mice possibly associated with the pathogenesis of autoimmunity. Subsequently, studies performed by ourselves [38] and Rich et al [39] confirmed the findings of Botzenhardt et al in regard to the NZB mouse, but we failed to observe similar activity with lymphoid cells obtained from MRL/l and BXSB mice.

Tolerance Susceptibility

It has been demonstrated that 6- to 8-week-old NZB and NZB X W mice are relatively resistant to induction of tolerance by bovine gamma globulin (BGG) and human gamma globulin (HGG), compared with many normal strains of mice [40-43]. This resistance to tolerance is probably another reflection of the generalized B cell hyperactivity seen in NZ mice. Extension of these tolerance-induction experiments to the other SLE mice showed that at 5 weeks of age, MRL/l and male BXSB mice also exhibited resistance to induction of tolerance to DHGG. Of interest, MRL/n and female BXSB, which are relatively immunologically normal compared with MRL/l and male BXSB, were readily tolerized. Therefore, it appears that resistance to tolerance induction is a common feature of all autoimmune mice. In contrast, only SJL mice, among several non-SLE strains similarly tested, were found to be resistant to tolerance induction. However, one should note that SJL mice are known to exhibit certain immunologic abnormalities [44].

Role of Thymus

It has been claimed that progressive imbalances in T cell function occur in NZ mice due to diminished production of thymic hormones. Administration of thymic hormones (i.e. extract of thymic tissue) [45] to NZB mice or transplantation of thymuses from young NZB mice to old mice [46] may temporarily prevent some of the immunologic defects and delay the onset of autoimmunity. In addition, it has been reported that adult NZB mice lack a serum activity thought to be a thymic hormone [47]. Previous studies of thymic histology in NZ mice have also disclosed premature thymic involution with prominent degeneration and vacuolization of epithelial cells [48]. Moreover, significant age-dependent losses of both functional and morphologic characteristics of NZ thymic epithelial cells cultured in vitro have been observed [49]. Others have found that neonatal thymectomy inhibited the disease in NZB × W female mice but accelerated the disease in males [50].

The disparity in the time of disease onset between the congenic MRL/l and MRL/n mice permits transplantation of thymuses between these mice in order to determine whether there is an inherent thymic defect that contributes to the early appearance of SLE in this strain [51]. As indicated in Figure 6, MRL/l mice thymectomized when 1 day old and transplanted at 1 month of age with MRL/n thymus retained the disease phenotype of the unmanipulated MRL/l mice, including lymphoproliferation and a 60% mortality at 6 months of age. Similarly, thymectomized MRL/n mice transplanted with MRL/l thymus had a 50% mortality at 17 months of age like the unmanipulated MRL/n controls. In contrast, MRL/l mice thymectomized when newborn but not transplanted with thymus did not develop lymphoid hyperplasia and autoimmune disease and 60% of them were alive by the 11th month of age (time of termination of the experiment), a point well beyond the 90% death rate of control unmanipulated mice (9 months of age). Serologically, the MRL/l recipients of MRL/n thymus

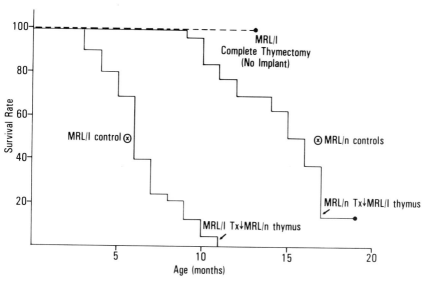

FIG. 6. Survival rates of MRL/l mice thymectomized when newborn but not transplanted, MRL/l mice thymectomized and transplanted at 1 month of age with MRL/n thymus, and MRL/n mice thymectomized and transplanted at 1 month of age with MRL/l thymus. The ⊗ depicts the time of 50% survival for control, unmanipulated MRL/l and MRL/n mice.

behave like the unmanipulated MRL/l animals with hypergammaglobulinemia and high levels of autoantibodies. In contrast, MRL/l thymectomized but not transplanted had greatly reduced levels of serum IgG and background levels of anti-DNA antibodies.

These results indicate that (a) T cell differentiation in the thymus is a necessary component in the MRL/l phenotype, (b) the genotype of the thymic microenvironment where differentiation occurs is irrelevant, and (c) the differentiation of MRL/n T cells in a thymic microenvironment that possesses *lpr* genotype does not lead to abnormal T cell differentiation and early autoimmunity.

Transfer of Autoimmune Disease

Transfer of autoimmune disease by specific tissue or tissue extracts derived from strains of mice having a genetic predisposition to autoimmunity into nonautoimmune recipients may be one of the most useful approaches in defining the humoral, cellular, microenvironmental and viral factors that influence and determine the development of autoimmunity. Others have reported the transfer of the NZB and NZB × W disease, as manifested by some autoantibody production, into lethally irradiated normal murine strains [52, 53]. However, the results have been inconclusive and sometimes difficult to interpret due to the use of normal recipients that are not congenic for NZ mice. The availability of the BXSB mice, the males and females of which differ substantially in mortality and expression of the disease, and of the MRL mice, with like differences between the congenic MRL/l and MRL/n substrains, makes possible the performance of histocompatible cell transfer experiments.

The failure to modify the male accelerated disease in BXSB mice by castration [54] suggests that the male dominance of the BXSB autoimmune syndrome is not hormonally controlled. Further, genetic studies have indicated that this male-dominant effect is linked to the Y chromosome, since the autoimmune phenotype is transmitted as a dominant trait to F_1 hybrids with an accelerated autoimmunity in male offsprings of BXSB fathers and mothers of other autoimmune strains. We have investigated the cellular basis of this male effect by transferring male and female bone marrow cells from 1-month-old mice into male and female lethally irradiated BXSB recipients of the same age [55]. As shown in Figure 7, the disease transfer is dependent not on the sex of the recipient, but on the sex of the donor cells — with male bone marrow inducing early disease (glomerulonephritis and death) in both male and female recipients and female marrow inducing late disease in both male and female recipients. Similar results were obtained by transferring spleen cells from 4-month-old donors to 2-month-old lethally irradiated recipients. Also, the recipients expressed serologic markers similar to those seen in the donor strains; i.e., recipients of male bone marrow and spleen cells had higher IgG and anti-DNA antibodies than the recipients of female bone marrow or spleen cells, and developed gp70-anti-gp70 complexes in their sera.

These results suggest that the male-specific effect that accelerates autoimmune disease in the BXSB is not hormonally or environmentally mediated, but rather is expressed in the

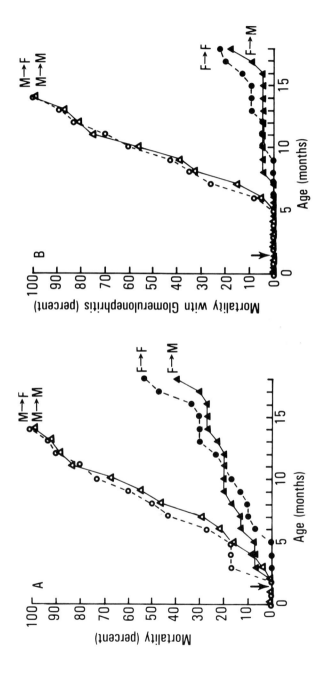

FIG. 7. (A) Mortality from all causes in BXSB bone marrow chimeras. Recipients were lethally irradiated (850 rads) and infused with donor bone marrow (5 × 10⁷ cells) at 6 weeks of age, as shown by the arrow. Male recipients are depicted by triangles; females by circles. Male bone marrow is shown by open symbols; female by closed symbols. In summary, (△———△) M→M; (○----○) M→F; (▲———▲) F→M; and (●----●) F→F. (B) Mortality from documented glomerulonephritis in BXSB bone marrow sex chimeras.

hematopoietic/lymphoid stem cell populations. Moreover, since transfer of spleen cells obtained from old male mice that already had manifest disease did not produce disease in the recipients any faster than transfer of bone marrow from premorbid mice, it can be suggested that (a) the active cell being transferred is the stem cell and not differentiated autoantibody-secreting B cells, and (b) the development of BXSB disease does not appear to be the result of an accumulation of defects at the stem cell level; i.e., stem cells from male BXSB of any age are at the same stage of abnormality.

Genetic Studies

The genetic analysis of SLE seen in NZB and NZB $\times$ W mice has revealed complex and as yet poorly understood genetic elements [56]. It is clear that this disease is multigenic in nature and that a number of secondary factors influence the expression of its autoimmune traits. Recently, two new approaches are shedding light on the genetics of this disease. The first compares the F_1 and F_2 hybrids resulting from crosses between the several SLE-prone strains, in search for common genetic denominators in this disease [19]. The second approach employs recombinant inbred strains to allow analysis of the interrelationships among individual immunopathologic traits related to SLE [13] (R. Riblet, personal communication).

In view of the different origins, MHC, allotypes and other immunogenetic aspects of the various SLE mice, it is clear that several quite different genetic backgrounds are compatible with the disease. The disease seen in each of these strains consists of, or is associated with, numerous abnormal immunologic traits, some common to all strains and others found only in some. Such multifactorial and variable pathogeneses make definitive genetic analysis of all disease components extremely difficult, if not impossible. Since some members of each variety of SLE mouse, i.e. female BXSB, male NZB $\times$ W and MRL/n, develop a late-life disease (50% mortality from 14 to 20 months) and others, i.e. male BXSB, female NZB $\times$ W and MRL/l, develop an early acute disease (50% mortality at 5 to 9 months), this natural division in the pace of disease can be used as a convenient phenotypic marker for genetic analysis and the gene or genes determining either late-life or early disease can be considered as two separate genetic units.

Late-Life SLE

There appear to be multiple autoimmune traits which can be important elements of late-life SLE. That the particular assortment or constellation of such traits varies from one strain of SLE mouse to another is clear from the immunopathologic features of the SLE in each [5, 19] and from the differences in the genetic interactions of SLE mice at the F_1 hybrid generation, as seen in Table 3. In these crosses BXSB females are used since they carry only the late-life SLE traits, and the MRL/1 can be used since the *lpr* accelerator gene is known to be recessive [3] and will not be expressed in F_1 hybrids, leaving only the late-life traits to interact. BXSB × MRL/1 hybrids of both sexes are relatively healthy, having 50% mortalities at nearly 2 years and developing only a moderate glomerulonephritis, which suggests little complementarity between the genetic backgrounds of the late-life SLE in these two strains. On the other hand, BXSB × NZB and BXSB × NZW develop a severe SLE, with early deaths from full-blown glomerulonephritis in the female. The character and timing of the SLE in BXSB × NZB or NZW hybrids are very similar to those seen in the classical NZB × W. Thus, it would appear that the BXSB late-life SLE background can either complement or add to the

Table 3. F_1 Hybrid Crosses of Late-Life SLE Mice

Crosses		50% Mortality (Months)	
F	M	Female	Male
BXSB	× MRL/1	22	>24
BXSB	× NZB	10	21
BXSB	× NZW	9	16
NZB	× NZW	9	14
BXSB	× BALB/c	>24	>24
MRL/1	× NZB	12	20
NZB	× MRL/1	17	>24
MRL/1	× NZW	16	>24
NZW	× MRL/1	19	18
MRL/1	× C578L/6	>24*	>24*

*Amyloid.

NZB and NZW backgrounds in order to produce a typical SLE appearing early in the female. That being the case, the BXSB should carry the equivalent of the genetic contributions of both NZB and NZW to the NZB × W SLE. Whether this BXSB contribution is qualitatively the same as that of the NZB and NZW or only quantitatively similar is not yet known. When the BXSB female is crossed with a normal strain such as the BALB/c, little or no disease is seen in the F_1, irrespective of the sex of the offspring. Taken together, these data indicate X-linked recessive trait complementation between BXSB and NZB or NZW, similar to what may occur between NZB and NZW and to a lesser degree, NZB and MRL/l.

Crosses of the MRL/l with other SLE mice result, in general, in either late-life or no SLE; the only possible exception is the MRL/l × NZB cross where significant disease in the first year of life is seen in the female. One possible explanation for the lack of disease in MRL/l F_1 hybrids could be that the SLE in the MRL/l is determined by homozygous recessive autoimmune traits, the expression of which is lost in the F_1 hybrid of crosses with SLE strains lacking the same recessive genes.

Accelerating Factors — Early SLE

It seems clear that in each kind of SLE mouse there may be superimposed on the late-life SLE background a distinct, but in each case different, accelerating factor capable of changing the late-life disease to an early, acute form. While these accelerating factors are not completely understood, it appears that they are relatively straightforward, direct influences which can alter the course of a predetermined disease. In the BXSB mouse the accelerating factor is Y-linked and is both transmitted and expressed by the male [3]. In the MRL/l mouse the factor is determined by a recessive, autosomal gene *lpr* for lympho-proliferation [3]. In the NZB × W the accelerating effect is apparently mediated by female hormones [57]. In Table 4 is shown the expression of the BXSB Y-linked accelerating factor in various F_1 hybrids. Most striking is the appearance of early, acute disease quite similar to that seen in the BXSB male in the F_1 males of all BXSB male crosses with SLE mice. Thus, the late-life SLE backgrounds of all SLE mice were accelerated by, or allowed the expression of, the BXSB Y-linked trait. This was true even with the MRL/l and MRL/n mice which did not complement the late-life SLE backgrounds of the BXSB female. As would be expected, the F_1 females of these crosses with male BXSB had a disease similar to that seen in the F_1 offspring of the crosses with female BXSB, since the Y chromosome was not involved in these situations. In the crosses with normal strains (C3H, BALB/c, C57BL/6), since there was no disease to accelerate, there was little effect of the Y-linked factor.

A potentially useful finding was the occurrence of early SLE in both males and females of the F_1 crosses of BXSB males with NZB or NZW. In terms of clinical characteristics and timing, the disease observed in the females was quite similar to that in the NZB × W cross. In addition, an even earlier SLE occurred in the male offspring. Whether this disease is the same as that occurring in the BXSB male is being determined, but these crosses offer the opportunity to study early SLE in both sexes, which is not possible in the NZB × W. In addition, degenerative coronary disease and/or myocardial infarcts develop in the course of disease in approximately 80% of (NZW × BXSB)F_1 offspring, making these mice excellent models of spontaneous coronary disease.

Because *lpr* is a recessive gene, it is not possible to observe its accelerating effect in hybrids. However, E. D. Murphy and J. B. Roths are establishing this gene in a homozygous state on a variety of murine strains where its effect can be observed (personal communication). Their results indicate that *lpr/lpr* induces lymphoproliferation and accelerates onset and course of SLE in both MRL/n (50% mortality from 17 to 5 months) and

Table 4. BXSB Y-Linked Accelerating Factor

Crosses		50% Mortality (Months)	
F	M	Female F_1	Male F_1
MRL/l	× BXSB	16	6
MRL/n	× BXSB	22	7
NZB	× BXSB	8	6
NZW	× BXSB	9	5
C3H	× BXSB	>24	16
BALB	× BXSB	>24	>24
C57BL	× BXSB	>24	15

NZB (50% mortality from 16 months to <5 months), in keeping with the expression of the BXSB accelerator trait in multiple SLE strains. But in spite of inducing lymphoproliferation, *lpr/lpr* causes no early SLE in C3H or AKR mice in which there is no SLE background to influence.

The acceleration of SLE in female NZB × W, presumably by female hormones, has been demonstrated by Talal and associates [57]. Early castration together with androgens given to females retarded the disease, while early castration plus estrogen administration accelerated the disease in males. That female hormones do not operate similarly in MRL/l and BXSB mice is evident, although there is a slightly earlier disease in MRL/l females than males. Interestingly, the male-first disease of the BXSB does not appear to be gonad- or hormone-dependent, as shown by castration [54] and cell transfer experiments [55].

Another kind of accelerating factor of murine SLE is chronic viral infection. LCM [58], polyoma [58] and retrovirus [59, 60] infections have all been observed to induce or elevate antinuclear antibodies and in the case of LCM and polyoma a SLE-like disease was associated. While these viruses may act in part by causing virus-anti-virus immune complexes, their stimulation of antinuclear and other autoantibody formation must be considered as enhancement of SLE. In the case of neonatal LCM infection the 50% mortality from SLE-like disease was changed from 15 to <5 months in NZB, from <24 to <6 months in NZW, from 9 months to 5 months in the female NZB × W, from 20 to 9 months in the female BXSB and from 18 to 12 months in the MRL/n. In normal mice, such as the C3H and SWR/J, with neonatal LCM infection no fatal SLE-like disease develops during the first two years of life.

SLE in F_2 Hybrids and Segregation of Disease Traits

Eight crosses between SLE and normal mice (BXSB × C3H, C3H × BXSB, BXSB × C57BL/6, C57BL/6 × BXSB, MRL/l × C3H, C3H × MRL/l, MRL/l × C57BL/6 and C57BL/6 × MRL/l) were carried to the F_2 generation to observe occurrence of SLE and segregation of various traits with each other and with disease. Only 26% of the F_2 males but no females of the C57BL/6 × BXSB and 12% of all offspring from both MRL/l crosses with C57BL/6 had early-life SLE, whereas F_2 offspring derived from the other six crosses listed above had no significant SLE. The overall low incidence or absence of SLE in most crosses suggests that the expression of disease must depend upon a critical number of genes which are reduced below the disease-producing level in F_2 offspring. There was no convincing or consistent correlation between the amount of any one of the immunologic or virologic parameters observed (IgM, anti-ssDNA, gp70 and lymphoproliferation) and the severity of disease as measured by the degree of glomerulonephritis at autopsy or by the age of death. Similarly, there was relatively little correlation among the various immunologic or virologic abnormalities themselves. However, as might have been anticipated, the occurrences of the consequences of immune complex deposition, glomerulonephritis, vascular disease and myocardial infarction were well correlated. The lack of any correlation among most of the immunologic features indicates an independent segregation of their responsible genetic factors. In addition, the failure of any of these traits to segregate convincingly with severity of disease suggests that disease is dependent upon the expression of multiple abnormal immunologic traits and that expression of various combinations of a critical number can cause disease, while expression of only a few of these same traits does not produce disease.

These results are compatible with those of others who analyzed a number of recombinant inbred strains derived from NZB crosses with DNA/2, ALN and C58J [13] (R. Riblet, personal communication). These investigators found that the production of anti-erythrocyte, anti-thymocyte and anti-ssDNA antibodies; syngeneic mixed leukocyte reactions; and hyperdiploidy segregate separately and independently. Further, it appears that most if not all of these traits are determined by a single gene, sometimes dominant as in the case of anti-erythrocyte and anti-DNA antibodies, and sometimes recessive as in the case of the syngeneic mixed leukocyte reactions. These studies clearly indicate the independence of the various immunologic abnormalities in murine SLE, at least as seen in the NZB. Further, they give no indication of any genetically determined across-the-board predisposition to autoimmune disease, as has been suggested [61].

Conclusion

The autoimmune disease murine SLE appears to occur in strains of mice with polyclonal hyperactivity of B lymphocytes detectable early in life and apparently unassociated with defects of regulatory T cells. This hyperactivity antedates any signs of autoimmune disease by months, and its precise relationship to the disease is still uncertain.

Murine SLE, while a reasonably well-defined clinical entity, comparable in homogeneity to human SLE, may be associated with several different assortments or constellations of auto-immune traits. Differences in the autoimmune traits operating in the several strains of SLE mice are demonstrated by the immunopathologic variations from strain to strain and the different genetic interactions of the various SLE backgrounds at the F_1 hybrid generation, indicating different genetic bases for the disease in the several strains.

Further, the individual autoimmune traits found in murine SLE appear to be entirely genetically independent, having no association with each other in the F_2 generation of hybrids of SLE mice or in the recombinant inbred strains derived from NZB and normal mouse crosses. This suggests that the basis of SLE is — in addition to whatever role the early lymphoid hyperactivity may have — the presence of a minimum, critical number of independently segregating genes, each determining a single pathogenic autoimmune trait. If this is so, then whatever the processes leading to pathogenic autoimmune responses, they must operate at the level of individual responses, i.e. either abnormal regulation of a particular clone of responding cells or primary abnormalities of the responding clone itself.

The action of intrinsic and possibly extrinsic (e.g. viral infections) accelerating factors in SLE is important in the development of early, severe disease. Interestingly, at least two intrinsic and several extrinsic accelerating factors can influence most, if not all, of the SLE backgrounds, even those with which they are not normally associated, but have little or no expression in hosts without a predisposition to SLE. This suggests that the accelerating factors are not an integral part of the SLE predisposition they enhance, but there must be an SLE background to allow their expression.

Finally, regardless of the particular constellation of auto-immune traits underlying SLE, the individual autoantibodies interact with their target autoantigens, forming immune complexes either in the circulation or in anatomic sites of fixed antigen. These immune complexes, interacting with humoral phlogogens such as complement or with effector cells, are responsible for the inflammatory and destructive lesions which characterize the disease. Thus, a variety of different combinations of autoantibody responses can in an appropriate host produce a rather similar disease, particularly if they operate via the formation of circulating immune complexes.

References

1. Murphy, E.D. and Roths, J.B.: A single gene model for massive lymphoproliferation with immune complex disease in new mouse strain MRL. Excerpta Medica International Congress Series No. 415, Topics in Hematology, Proceedings of the 16th International Congress of Hematology, Kyoto, Japan, September 5-11, 1976, pp. 69.

2. Murphy, E.D. and Roths, J.B.: A single gene model for massive lymphoproliferation with autoimmunity in new mouse strain MRL. Fed. Proc. 36:1246, 1977.

3. Murphy, E.D. and Roths, J.B.: Autoimmunity and lymphoprolifera-tion: Induction by mutant gene lpr, and acceleration by a male-associated factor in strain BXSB mice. In Rose, N.R., Bigazzi, P.E. and Warner, N.L. (eds.): Genetic Control of Autoimmune Disease. Amsterdam:Elsevier, 1979, p. 207.

4. Beilschowsky, M. and Goodall, C.M.: Origin of inbred NZ mouse strains. Cancer Res. 30:834, 1970.

5. Andrews, B.S., Eisenberg, R.A., Theofilopoulos, A.N. et al: Spontaneous murine lupus-like syndromes. Clinical and immunopatho-logical manifestations in several strains. J. Exp. Med. 148:1198, 1978.

6. Accinni, L. and Dixon, F.J.: Degenerative vascular disease and myocardial infarction in mice with lupus-like syndrome. Am. J. Pathol. 96:477, 1979.

7. Izui, S., McConahey, P.J. and Dixon, F.J.: Increased spontaneous polyclonal activation of B lymphocytes in mice with spontaneous autoimmune disease. J. Immunol. 121:2213, 1978.

8. Izui, S. and Eisenberg, R.A.: Circulating anti-DNA-rheumatoid factor complexes in MRL/l mice. Clin. Immunol. Immunopathol. 15:536, 1980.

9. Eisenberg, R.A., Tan, E.M. and Dixon, F.J.: Presence of anti-Sm reactivity in autoimmune mouse strains. J. Exp. Med. 147:582, 1978.

10. Eisenberg, R.A., Theofilopoulos, A.N., Andrews, B.S. et al: Natural thymocytotoxic autoantibodies in autoimmune and normal mice. J. Immunol. 122:2272, 1979.
11. Eisenberg, R.A., Thor, L.J. and Dixon, F.J.: Serum-serum interactions in autoimmune mice. Arthritis Rheum. 22:1074, 1979.
12. Gershwin, M.E., Castles, J.J., Ikeda, R.M. et al: Studies of congenitally immunologic mutant New Zealand mice. I. Autoimmune features of hereditarily asplenic (Dh/+) NZB mice: Reduction of naturally occurring thymocytotoxic antibody and normal suppressor function. J. Immunol. 122:710, 1979.
13. Raveche, S., Brown, L.J., Novotny, E.A. et al: Separable genetic traits in NZB mice, abstracted. Arthritis Rheum. 23:735, 1980.
14. Izui, S., McConahey, P.J., Theofilopoulos, A.N. and Dixon, F.J.: Association of circulating retroviral gp70-anti-gp70 immune complexes with murine systemic lupus erythematosus. J. Exp. Med. 149:1099, 1979.
15. Elder, J.H., Jensen, F.C., Bryant, M.L. and Lerner, R.A.: Polymorphism of the major envelope glycoprotein (gp70) of murine C-type viruses: Virion associated and differentiation antigens encoded by a multi-gene family. Nature 267:23, 1977.
16. Clagett, J.A. and Weigle, W.O.: Roles of T and B lymphocytes in the termination of unresponsiveness to autologous thyroglobulin in mice. J. Exp. Med. 139:643, 1974.
17. Theofilopoulos, A.N., Eisenberg, R.A., Bourdon, M. et al: Distribution of lymphocytes identified by surface markers in murine strains with SLE-like syndromes. J. Exp. Med. 149:516, 1979.
18. Cohen, I.R. and Wekerle, H.: The immune activation and specific inhibition of self-recognizing thymus-derived lymphocytes. J. Exp. Med. 137:224, 1973.
19. Theofilopoulos, A.N., McConahey, P.J., Izui, S. et al: A comparative immunologic analysis of several murine strains with autoimmune manifestations. Clin. Immunol. Immunopathol. 15:258, 1980.
20. Theofilopoulos, A.N., Shawler, D.L., Eisenberg, R.A. and Dixon, F.J.: Splenic immunoglobulin-secreting cells and their regulation in autoimmune mice. J. Exp. Med. 151:446, 1980.
21. Ohsugi, Y. and Gershwin, E.: Studies of congenitally immunologic mutant New Zealand mice. III. Growth of B lymphocyte clones in congenitally athymic (nude) and hereditarily asplenic (Dh/+) NZB mice: A primary B cell defect. J. Immunol. 123:1260, 1979.
22. Kincade, P.W., Lee, G., Fernandes, G. et al: Abnormalities in clonable B lymphocytes and myeloid progenitors in autoimmune NZB mice. Proc. Natl. Acad. Sci. U.S.A. 76:3464, 1979.
23. Moutsopulos, M.H., Boehm-Truitt, M., Kassan, S.S. and Chused, T.N.: Demonstration of activation of B lymphocytes in New Zealand black mice at birth by an immunoradiometric assay. J. Immunol. 119:1639, 1977.
24. Manny, N., Datta, S.K. and Schwartz, R.S.: Synthesis of IgM by cells of NZB and SWR mice and their crosses. J. Immunol. 122:1220, 1979.

25. Tourog, J.D., Moutsopoulos, H.M., Rosenberg, Y.J. et al: CBA/N X-linked B cell defect prevents NZB B-cell hyperactivity in F_1 mice. J. Exp. Med. 150:31, 1979.

26. Krakauer, R.S., Waldmann, T.A. and Strober, W.: Loss of suppressor T cells in adult NZB/NZW mice. J. Exp. Med. 144:662, 1976.

27. Barthold, D.R., Kysela, S. and Steinberg, A.D.: Decline in suppressor T cell function with age in female NZB mice. J. Immunol. 112:9, 1974.

28. Cantor, H., McVay-Boudreau, L., Hugenberger, J. et al: Immunoregulatory circuits among T cell sets. II. Physiologic role of feedback inhibition *in vivo*: Absence in NZB mice. J. Exp. Med. 147:1116, 1978.

29. Cantor, H. and Gershon, R.K.: Immunological circuits: Cellular composition. Fed. Proc. 38:2058, 1979.

30. Primi, D., Hammarstrom, L. and Smith, C.I.E.: Genetic control of lymphocyte suppression. I. Lack of suppression in aged NZB mice is due to a B cell defect. J. Immunol. 121:2241, 1978.

31. Creighton, W.D., Katz, D.H. and Dixon, F.J.: Antigen-specific immunocompetency, B cell function and regulatory helper and suppressor T cell activities in spontaneously autoimmune mice. J. Immunol. 123:2627, 1979.

32. Primi, D., Hammarstrom, L. and Smith, C.I.E.: Regulation of thymus-independent responses by concanavalin A-activated spleen cells. Cell. Immunol. 42:40, 1979.

33. Sawada, S. and Talal, N.: Evidence for a helper cell promoting anti-DNA antibody production in murine lupus, abstracted. Arthritis Rheum. 22:655, 1979.

34. Zinkernagel, R.M. and Dixon, F.J.: Comparison of T cell-mediated immune responsiveness of NZB, (NZB × NZW)F_1 hybrid and other murine strains. Clin. Exp. Immunol. 29:110, 1977.

35. Mackaness, G.B.: The influence of immunologically committed lymphoid cells on macrophage activity *in vivo*. J. Exp. Med. 129:973, 1969.

36. Creighton, W.D., Zinkernagel, R.M. and Dixon, F.J.: T cell-mediated immune responses of lupus-prone BXSB mice and other murine strains. Clin. Exp. Immunol. 37:181, 1979.

37. Botzenhardt, V., Klein, J. and Ziff, M.: Cytotoxic reactions of NZB spleen cells with lymphocytes of MHC identical strains. J. Exp. Med. 147:1435, 1978.

38. Theofilopoulos, A.N., Shawler, D.L., Katz, D.H. and Dixon, F.J.: Patterns of immune reactivity in autoimmune murine strains. II. Cell-mediated immune responses induced by H-2 identical and H-2 incompatible stimulator cells. J. Immunol. 122:2319, 1979.

39. Rich, R.R., Sedberry, D.A., Kastner, D.L. and Chu, L.: Primary *in vitro* cytotoxic response of NZB spleen cells to Qa-1γ-associated antigenic determinants. J. Exp. Med. 150:1555, 1979.

40. Staples, P.J. and Talal, N.: Relative inability to induce tolerance in adult NZB and NZB/NZW F_1 mice. J. Exp. Med. 129:123, 1969.

41. Golub, E.S. and Weigle, W.O.: Studies on the induction of immuno-

logic unresponsiveness. III. Antigen form and mouse strain variation. J. Immunol. 102:389, 1979.

42. Cerottini, J.C., Lambert, P.H. and Dixon, F.J.: Comparison of the immune responsiveness of NZB and NZB × NZW F$_1$ hybrid mice with that of other strains of mice. J. Exp. Med. 130:1093, 1969.

43. Parks, D.E., Doyle, M.V. and Weigle, W.O.: Induction and mode of action of suppressor cells generated against human gamma globulin. I. An immunologic unresponsive state devoid of demonstrable suppressor cells. J. Exp. Med. 148:625, 1978.

44. Fujiwara, M. and Cinader, N.: Cellular aspects of tolerance. VI. The effect of age on responsiveness and tolerance inducibililty of SJL mice. Cell. Immunol. 12:205, 1974.

45. Dauphinee, M.J., Talal, N., Golstein, A.L. and White, A.: Thymosin corrects the abnormal DNA synthetic response of NZB mouse thymocytes. Proc. Natl. Acad. Sci. U.S.A. 71:2637, 1974.

46. Steinberg, A.D., Law, L.D. and Talal, N.: The role of NZB/NZ F$_1$ thymus in experimental tolerance and autoimmunity. Arthritis Rheum. 13:369, 1970.

47. Bach, J.F., Dardenne, M. and Salomon, J.C.: Studies on thymus products. IV. Absence of serum thymic activity in adult NZB and (NZB × NZW)F$_1$ mice. Clin. Exp. Immunol. 14:247, 1973.

48. De Vries, M.J. and Higmans, W.: Pathological changes of the thymic epithelial cells and autoimmune disease in NZB, NZW and (NZW × NZW)F$_1$ mice. Immunology 12:179, 1967.

49. Gershwin, M.E., Ikeda, R.M., Kruse, W.L. et al: Age-dependent loss in New Zealand mice of morphological and functional characteristics of thymic epithelial cells. J. Immunol. 120:971, 1978.

50. Roubinian, J.R., Papoian, R. and Talal, N.: Effects of neonatal thymectomy and splenectomy on survival and regulation of autoantibody formation in NZB/NZW F$_1$ mice. J. Immunol. 118:1524, 1977.

51. Wigzell, H.: Positive autoimmunity. In Talal, N. (ed.): Autoimmunity. New York:Academic Press, 1977, p. 693.

52. Morton, J.I. and Siegel, B.V.: Transplantation of autoimmune potential. I. Development of antinuclear antibodies in H-2 histocompatible recipients of bone marrow from New Zealand Black mice. Proc. Natl. Acad. Sci. U.S.A. 71:2162, 1974.

53. Akizuki, M., Reeves, J.P. and Steinberg, A.D.: Expression of autoimmunity by NZB/NZW marrow. Clin. Immunol. Immunopathol. 10:247, 1978.

54. Eisenberg, R.A., Lee, S. and Dixon, F.J.: Effect of castration on male-determined acceleration of autoimmune disease in BXSB mice. (J. Immunol., submitted 1980.)

55. Eisenberg, R.A., Izui, S., McConahey, P.J. et al: Male determined accelerated autoimmune disease in BXSB mice: Transfer by bone marrow and spleen cells. J. Immunol. (In press.)

56. Warner, N.L.: Genetic aspects of autoimmune disease in animals. In Talal, N. (ed.): Autoimmunity. New York:Academic Press, 1977, p. 33.

57. Roubinian, J.R., Talal, N., Greenspan, J.S. et al: Effect of castration and sex hormone treatment on survival, anti-nucleic acid antibodies, and glomerulonephritis in NZB/NZW F_1 mice. J. Exp. Med. 147:1568, 1978.
58. Tonietti, G., Oldstone, M.B.A. and Dixon, F.J.: The effect of induced chronic viral infections on the immunologic diseases of New Zealand mice. J. Exp. Med. 132:89, 1970.
59. Cannat, A. and Varet, B.: Induction of antinuclear antibodies in mice inoculated with Rauscher leukemogenic virus: Possible role of genetic factors in non-New Zealand strains. Immunol. Commun. 2:257, 1973.
60. Croker, B.P., Del Villano, B.C., Jensen, F.C. et al: Immunopathogenicity and oncogenicity of murine leukemia viruses. I. Induction of immunologic disease and lymphoma in (BALB/c × NZB)F_1 mice by Scripps leukemia virus. J. Exp. Med. 140:1028, 1974.
61. Miller, K.B. and Schwartz, R.S.: Familial abnormalities of suppressor-cell function in systemic lupus erythematosus. N. Engl. J. Med. 301:803, 1979.

Tissue-Fixed Antigens
in Immune Renal Injury

Curtis B. Wilson, M.D.

It is the purpose of this chapter to present some of our recent findings in renal immunopathology. The work of Frank Dixon, summarized in a classic editorial of 1968 [1], defined two basic mechanisms of antibody-induced renal injury. In one, antibodies react directly with the glomerular basement membrane (GBM) [2, 3]; in the other, antibodies combine with circulating antigens to form immune complexes that are subsequently trapped nonspecifically in the glomerulus [4-6]. In this presentation, I will expand upon the first mechanism to describe new observations of other fixed glomerular antigens that can undergo direct nephritogenic antibody attack [7-9]. I will also review the updated information about anti-GBM disease gained since Dixon's work in the late 1960s.

The humoral mechanisms of immunologic renal injury are summarized in Table 1. For ease in understanding, the mechanisms are classified on the basis of the antigens involved; namely, insoluble (kidney-fixed) antigens and soluble antigens in the circulating or extravascular fluids. The reaction of the latter antigens with antibody leads to immune complex formation and, potentially, the associated disorders, either systemically or locally. Circulating immune complexes can form involving exogenous antigens, generally from infectious agents, or endogenous antigens, such as nuclear materials or tumor-associated antigens [reviewed in 10]. Circulating immune complexes can attain

Curtis B. Wilson, M.D., Member, Department of Immunopathology, Scripps Clinic and Research Foundation, La Jolla, California.

This is publication No. 2340 from the Department of Immunopathology, Scripps Clinic and Research Foundation. This work was supported in part by USPHS grants AM-20043, AM-18626 and AI-07007; and Biomedical Research Support Grant RRO-5514.

Table 1. Categorization of Antibody-Induced Renal Injury
Based on the Solubility and Location of the Antigens Involved

Antibodies reactive with soluble antigens
    Soluble antigens in the circulation
        Circulating immune complex disease
            Exogenous antigens – drugs, microbial antigens, etc.
            Endogenous antigens – nuclear proteins, tumor antigens, etc.
    Soluble antigens in the extravascular fluids
        Extravascular immune complex disease
            Experimental models – Arthus reaction, tubular antigens

Antibodies reactive with insoluble or tissue-fixed antigens
    Structural antigens of the kidney
        Classic basement membrane antigens
            GBM antigens
            TBM antigens
        Other, nonclassical glomerular capillary wall antigens
            Experimental models – glomerular antigens in rats (Heymann nephritis), rabbits

Exogenous or endogenous antigens trapped or "planted" in the kidney
    Experimental models – immunoglobulins, immune complexes, mesangial deposits, lectins, ? bacterial products, ? DNA, etc.

widespread vascular deposition or their localization may be confined primarily to the glomerulus, which appears to be a particularly susceptible site. Immune complex formation also occurs locally, as in experimental thyroiditis [11] and in the Arthus reaction [12]. There are now some renal tubulointerstitial diseases in which tubular antigens, including Tamm-Horsfall protein, have been implicated in local immune complex formation [13, 14].

Nephritogenic Tissue-Fixed Antigens

Tissue-fixed antigens (Table 1) may be either structural components of the kidney, such as the GBM, other nonglomerular capillary wall materials, or substances from some extrarenal source that are trapped or planted within the glomerulus or potentially other vascular or tubular structures within the tissue for subsequent interaction with antibody.

Once an immune reaction has occurred and antibody has deposited in the glomerulus or extraglomerular renal tissue [15, 16], mediation systems are brought into play, leading to tissue injury. Depletion studies have clearly shown a role for complement and polymorphonuclear leukocytes in certain stages of glomerular damage in experimental animals [17, 18]. Additionally, several other systems are potentially involved, as reviewed by other authors in this volume. Within the last two or three years, we and others have had an interest in monocytes and macrophages as mediators of immune renal injury [19]. Monocytes accumulate in animals' glomeruli during experimental anti-GBM antibody-induced glomerulonephritis, particularly in the later stages, and also when excessive damage has occurred, leading to extraglomerular proliferation and crescent formation within Bowman's space. Accordingly, radiation of rats to deplete macrophages in anti-GBM antibody-induced glomerulonephritis modifies the lesion [20]. In some recent experiments, we have shown that the monocyte/macrophage is a prominent infiltrating cell in experimental serum sickness glomerulonephritis of rabbits [21]. After administration of anti-macrophage serum to rabbits with acute serum sickness or a passive autologous-phase model of anti-GBM antibody nephritis, it is quite clear that prevention of glomerular monocyte and macrophage accumulation almost completely protects the animal from developing histologic and clinical manifestations of either disorder [22]. In thinking about mechanisms of renal injury, it would also be appropriate to consider the possibility of nonimmunologic activation of mediator systems. Nephritic factor, an immunoconglutinin with reactivity for C3 convertase of the alternative complement pathway, is observed in certain forms of hypocomplementemic membranoproliferative glomerulonephritis [reviewed in 23]. The antibody seems to stabilize and enhance the activity of C3 convertase, leading to profound hypocomplementemia. Although present in the circulations of these patients and in certain patients with partial lipodystrophy prior to the onset of hypocomplementemic membranoproliferative glomerulonephritis, this material has no proven immunopathologic role. Coagulation proteins may also be activated in certain forms of disseminated intravascular coagulation and, in turn, lead to glomerular injury. Again, there may be no clear-cut immunologic cause for the induction of coagulation.

Of tissue-fixed antigens that react deleteriously with antibody (Table 1), the GBM has been recognized as a nephritogenic antigen from experiments dating back through the work of Masugi in the 1930s to the original observation of Lindemann in

1900, who showed the nephrotoxicity of heterologous anti-kidney antisera. More recently, the tubular basement membrane (TBM) has been shown to be the nephritogenic antigen in certain forms of tubulointerstitial nephritis [10, 24]. One can expand this category of immunologic reactions by adding a number of structural components of the glomerular wall other than the classic GBM antigens with which antibodies can react (Table 1). Planted antigens, that is, materials not related to the kidney but trapped there for physiologic or physicochemical reasons, can participate in subsequent immune reactions [7, 8].

Basement Membrane Antigens

Experimentally, anti-basement membrane antibody disease has been studied for about 80 years. Heterologous anti-GBM antibody disease occurs in two phases. The first is an immediate phase, determined when a sufficient amount of antibody is administered. In the rat, this takes about 75 μg of antibody per gram of kidney, or by making some assumptions, 1.2×10^{10} molecules per glomerulus [25]. Sheep are more susceptible to injury than rats and require only about 5 μg per gram[26]. Seven to ten days after administration of the antibody, a second, autologous or delayed phase occurs when the host makes an immune response to the foreign or planted immunoglobulin that is bound to its glomerulus [27]. This phase of injury is the classic example of a planted antigen leading to glomerular injury. The roles of complement and polymorphonuclear leukocytes as mediators have been delineated in such models, with certain anti-GBM antibodies shown to be complement- and polymorphonuclear leukocyte-dependent, although avian anti-GBM antibodies and certain mammalian anti-GBM antibodies can produce injury in the absence of detectable complement or polymorphonuclear leukocytes [18, 28]. In recent micropuncture physiology studies to evaluate the dynamics of filtration through the glomerulus, anti-GBM antibodies have been shown to produce acute complement-dependent reductions in glomerular plasma flow and complement-independent decreases in the coefficient of glomerular filtration (determined by glomerular permeability and total glomerular filtration area [29, 30]. Endothelial cell abnormalities which persist even after complement depletion are presumed to contribute to the decreased ultrafiltration of water and small molecules. Increased permeability of the glomerular capillary wall to proteins may relate to structural damage, and breaks in continuity or other as yet unexplained physiologic disturbances in the glomerular filtration barrier, such as diminished fixed anionic charges, which could be an important factor in repelling anionic materials with the molecular weight of albumin [31].

Several models of both anti-GBM and anti-TBM antibody-induced diseases have been produced in experimental animals by active immunization with GBM, GBM-like antigens isolated from the urine, or TBM [reviewed in 10]. For example, sheep immunized with GBM in adjuvant develop a fulminant proliferative glomerulonephritis, with immunologic evidence of anti-GBM antibodies bound to the GBM [32]. Furthermore, anti-GBM antibodies recovered from their circulations transfer the disease to normal sheep [26]. The sheep model was useful in the study of spontaneous anti-basement membrane antibody diseases of man.

Anti-Basement Membrane Antibody Diseases in Man. In 1967, Dixon and associates clearly demonstrated the immunopathologic role of anti-GBM antibodies in a series of patients with glomerulonephritis and linear deposits of IgG and C3 along their GBMs [3]. Anti-GBM antibodies, either obtained from the circulations of these patients or dissociated from the GBM of their renal homogenates by elution in acid pH, were capable of transferring glomerulonephritis to subhuman primates. The immunopathogenicity of anti-GBM antibodies in human glomerulonephritis was further confirmed when glomerular injury was accidentally induced in a renal transplant placed in one of these patients who had demonstrable circulating anti-GBM antibodies. We have maintained an intense interest in this disease [33] and, with the help of many collaborators located around the United States and abroad, have been able to identify almost 700 patients with anti-GBM antibodies. As the series grows, an increasingly larger spectrum of clinical manifestations emerges (Table 2). About 65% of the patients have a condition called Goodpasture syndrome, consisting of pulmonary hemorrhage and glomerulonephritis. Most of the remaining 35% have glomerulonephritis alone, except for a few patients whose clinical disease is confined to the lung [34]. Glomerulonephritis is often rapidly progressive but may be milder and self-remitting. Anti-TBM antibodies accompany the anti-GBM antibodies in about 70% of instances [16]. At least two types of anti-TBM antibodies

Table 2. Anti-Basement Membrane Antibody Diseases in Man

Anti-GBM antibodies are associated with:
  Combined pulmonary hemorrhage and glomerulonephritis (Goodpasture
    syndrome)
  Severe, often rapidly progressive glomerulonephritis
  Occasionally milder, sometimes remitting forms of glomerulonephritis
  Pulmonary hemorrhage presenting as idiopathic hemosiderosis
  Recurrent or de novo glomerulonephritis after transplantation

Anti-TBM antibodies are associated with:
  Tubulointerstitial nephritis
    Complicating anti-GBM glomerulonephritis
    Complicating immune complex glomerulonephritis
    Some drug-associated tubulointerstitial nephritis
    Rarely primary tubulointerstitial nephritis
    Recurrent or de novo tubulointerstitial nephritis after transplantation

Other anti-basement membrane antibodies may be responsible for:
  Choroid plexus injury
  Intestinal injury

are associated with anti-GBM disease, one reacting with only a few tubules and the other diffusely reactive with the TBMs of all cortical nephrons. Anti-TBM antibodies also occasionally complicate immune complex disease and have been induced by drugs, for example, in association with methicillin-related tubulointerstitial nephritis [35]. There are also a few patients who may have primary tubulointerstitial anti-TBM disease [reviewed in 10, 24]. The choroid plexus basement membrane is an occasional additional site for the reaction of anti-basement membrane antibodies [10]. We have seen one patient with intractable diarrhea and nephrotic syndrome who had anti-basement membrane antibodies that reacted with the basement membrane of the jejunum in addition to the TBM [10]. Even transplanted kidneys may provide a reactive site, and a complication of this surgical procedure is the recurrence or de novo production of both anti-GBM and anti-TBM antibodies.

Anti-basement membrane antibodies are detected in tissue by immunofluorescence (Fig. 1) These antibodies react with antigenic sites spread diffusely along the basement membranes so that immunofluorescent staining assumes a smooth linear pattern, as opposed to the irregular staining of granular antibody accumulations associated with immune complex deposition.

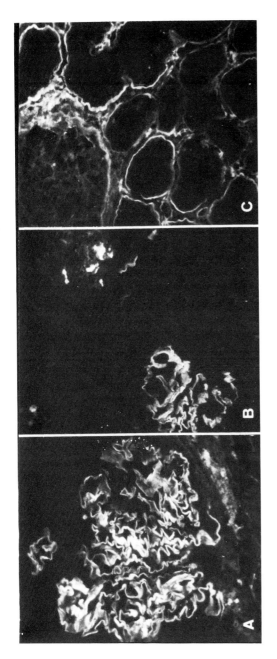

FIG. 1. The immunofluorescent findings of anti-basement membrane antibodies fixed to renal basement membranes are shown. (A) Smooth linear deposits of IgG outline the GBM of a glomerulus early in the course of anti-GBM anti-induced Goodpasture syndrome. The distortion of the renal glomerular architecture is produced by a proliferative response in Bowman's space (crescent formation). (B) In later stages of anti-GBM antibody-induced glomerulonephritis, the pattern of antibody fixation to the GBM corresponds with structural glomerular damage. Linear deposits are still visible in a less damaged glomerulus (lower left), but only minimal deposits remain in the sclerosed glomeruli (upper right). (C) Circumferential linear deposits of IgG typical of anti-TBM antibodies are seen. Note that the anti-TBM antibody has no reaction with the GBM of the glomerulus in the upper left. (Fluorescein isothiocyanate-conjugated anti-human IgG; original magnification A and C, × 250; B, × 160.)

Recently, the nephritogenic GBM antigens have been suggested to be concentrated along the subendothelial aspect of the GBM [36]. The corresponding anti-GBM antibodies are almost always of the IgG class, with no strict subclass restriction, although occasionally IgA or IgM antibodies are also present [33]. By immunofluorescence, C3 and other complement components are found accompanying the IgG in about three fourths of patients with the related disease [33].

Very little is known about the stimuli that initiate spontaneous autoimmune antiGBM antibody responses (Table 3). Since the anti-GBM antibody response is usually transient, the stimulus may also be short-lived. Although no obvious stimulus has been identified as common to an appreciable number of the known patients, some possible stimuli, such as influenza A2 infection, hydrocarbon solvents, drugs and renal injury, are associated temporally with the onset of disease, at least in some patients [33, 35, 37, 38]. Occasionally, immunologic renal injury can precede the formation of anti-GBM antibodies, as in membranous glomerulonephritis [39] or systemic lupus erythematosus [10], observed by radioimmunoassay. Very interestingly, we have three or four patients in our series who have developed the antibody after treatment for Hodgkin disease or other lymphomas. Others have also noted this association [40], which is of interest because the crude anti-lymphocyte globulin preparations used in immunosuppressive regimens for renal transplantation years ago were frequently contaminated with anti-GBM antibodies thought to be induced by inclusion of lymphoid stroma within the inoculum [41]. It may be that stroma of the lymph node, particlarly after treatment with radiation for lymphoma,

Table 3. Events Associated with the Induction of
Anti-Basement Membrane Antibodies in Man

Temporal associations
Infections − influenza A2
Toxic exposure − hydrocarbons, drugs
Renal injury − immunologic, ischemic
Neoplasia − Hodgkin disease
Neoantigens − Alport syndrome
Endogenous GBM antigens − urine, serum, kidney

may in some way induce anti-GBM antibodies in occasional patients. Differences in basement membrane antigens also occur between individuals, which, as will be discussed later, may contribute to the formation of anti-GBM and/or anti-TBM antibodies after renal transplantation [42]. Basement membrane antigens are also present in the urine (and serum) and, when concentrated and reinjected, can induce nephritogenic anti-GBM antibodies in experimental animals [43, 44]. Similar antigens conceivably could lead to induction of anti-basement membrane antibodies in man.

Several years ago, a radioimmunoassay for anti-basement membrane antibodies was developed in our laboratory [45], using as an antigen a collagenase-solubilized GBM preparation. Additional assays are available for the same purpose but involve somewhat different methods of GBM antigen solubilization [reviewed in 10]. The antigen used in our radioimmunoassay detects all the anti-GBM antibodies that we have identified by other immunopathologic means. Moreover, the collagenase-solubilized GBM antigen blocks the reaction of antibodies with basement membranes detectable by indirect immunofluorescence and is nephritogenic in animal studies. These findings suggest that the antigenic mixture used in the assay contains most, if not all, of the relevant nephritogenic GBM antigens. The reactive antigen can be characterized by polyacrylamide gel electrophoresis (PAGE). When the immune precipitates of human anti-GBM antibodies and collagenase-solubilized antigens are analyzed by the PAGE technique, two peaks of reactivity can be seen migrating near the heavy and light chain markers and having molecular weights of approximately 54,000 and 27,000 [46]. These reactive peaks in the polyacrylamide gels have about an 80% homology on peptide map analysis, and some reactivity remains in material that does not enter the gel (Fig. 2). With immunoabsorption, it is possible to isolate the reactive antigen peaks, which have PAGE profiles similar to those of the immune precipitates shown in Figure 2. Amino acid analysis of the material purified by immunoabsorption reveals that there is no hydroxyproline or hydroxylysine, indicating the noncollagenous nature of the material with which we are dealing. The antigenic mixture has significant amino acid differences from the whole isolated GBM, having considerably more serine, glutamic acid and lysine, and less proline, valine, methionine, isoleucine, leucine, tyrosine,

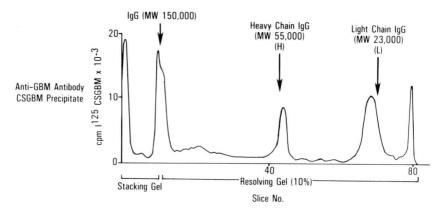

FIG. 2. The polyacrylamide gel electrophoresis (PAGE) pattern of the radiolabeled antigens in collagenase-solubilized human GBM (CSGBM) that bind to spontaneously formed human anti-GBM antibody is shown. Size markers include IgG and its light and heavy chains.

phenylalanine and arginine. Quantitative assessment of the carbohydrate content of the reactive materials suggests a heteropolysaccharide content.

By manipulating the elution characteristics of the immunoabsorbent columns, it is possible to obtain fractions that are enriched for either the 54,000- or the 27,000-MW peaks. We have tested a number of sera from patients with anti-GBM antibodies against the antigen fractions semipurified in this way. Although each serum reacts with both fractions, most sera have higher values of binding with the fraction enriched for the 54,000-MW peak. Samples from a few patients react preferentially with the fraction enriched for the 27,000-MW material, and several sera react similarly with both fractions. Thus, individuals vary somewhat in reactivity. As we progress in isolating the reactive antigens, this variation may allow for further subdivision of the anti-GBM antibody patient population.

By using the immunoabsorbent-purified GBM antigen material, it has been possible to detect anti-basement membrane antibodies in almost all patients who have other immunopathologic features of anti-basement membrane antibody disease [47]. For positive identification, serum must be obtained early in the course of disease, since antibody production is generally transient. Very occasionally, anti-GBM antibodies can be detected in patients with immunopathologic features of immune complex disease, such as membranous glomerulopathy and systemic lupus erythematosus. When present, the antibody may modify the course of the underlying glomerulonephritis [39].

There is little quantitative difference in the levels of antibody binding between patients with Goodpasture syndrome and those with antibody-induced glomerulonephritis alone, implying that the different clinical presentations are not related to the quantities of antibody produced [47]. The production of circulating anti-GBM antibody is transient in almost all patients of both groups, the antibody disappearing within a mean duration of about 15 months. We have seen only one patient who has had repeated episodes of anti-GBM antibody disease [48]. This woman had three bouts of Goodpasture syndrome over an 11-year period, with reasonable documentation of anti-GBM antibodies during the first and last episodes. Undoubtedly, there are some differences in anti-basement membrane antibodies of patients with Goodpasture syndrome and those with glomerulonephritis alone, as suggested by the relative extent of nonrenal basement membrane reactivity demonstrated some years ago by using immunofluorescence [49]. We have just completed a survey of circulating anti-lung basement membrane antibodies in 60 patients with anti-basement membrane antibody-induced Goodpasture syndrome, compared to 60 patients with clinical renal anti-basement membrane antibody involvement only. Samples from patients with Goodpasture syndrome reacted with lung basement membrane antigens, as tested by indirect immunofluorescence, much more frequently than did those from non-Goodpasture patients. Since the clinical breakdown between the two groups is rather inadequate, some of the overlap may reflect incorrect clinical classification.

The observation that antibody production is transient [33] has generated enthusiasm for hastening the decline of antibody production in these patients and removing antibody already present in their circulations. This is done with immunosuppressive regimens — including steroids, cyclophosphamide and other immunosuppressive drugs — and plasma exchange to remove 4 to 5 liters of plasma every day, replacing the plasma volume with physiologic fluids that do not contain antibody [50, 51]. Figure 3 shows the course of detectable circulating anti-GBM antibody in a patient treated with combined immunosuppression and

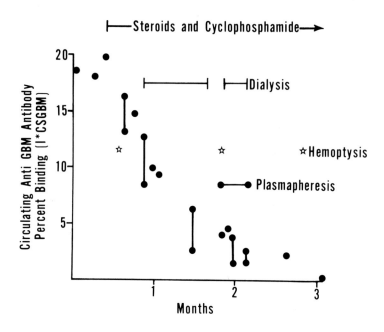

FIG. 3. The levels of circulating anti-GBM antibodies in a patient being treated by combined immunosuppression (steroids and cyclophosphamide) and plasmapheresis are shown. A decrease in binding is seen after each plasmapheresis, followed by a slight rebound as reequilibration between intra- and extra-vascular fluid occurred. Renal failure was severe enough to require periods of dialysis. Three episodes of hemoptysis, noted by stars, occurred and did not correlate with levels of circulating anti-GBM antibody. The levels of antibody detected by the radioimmune assay are expressed in percent binding of radiolabeled collagenase-solubilized GBM (CSGBM).

plasmapheresis. In this patient, the amount of circulating anti-GBM antibody was reduced with each plasma exchange, followed by an increase as reequilibration occurred between intravascular and extravascular fluids. The patient, who had sufficient renal damage to require artificial kidney dialysis for a time, became well enough so that dialysis was no longer needed. Also notable, the three episodes of hemoptysis (pulmonary hemorrhage) did not correlate well with the level of antibody present in this patient's circulation. For many patients, clinical problems such as infection and physiologic disturbances, as in fluid overload [51, 52], bring on a bout of pulmonary hemorrhage, which can be very severe and actually life-threatening, although generally short-lived.

At the moment, combined plasma exchange and plasmapheresis therapy is in favor [53]. Whether this is warranted or not will await carefully controlled clinical trials, which are in progress. In the most advanced trial, no improvement has been noted in patients treated with immunosuppressive regimens and plasmapheresis, compared with those treated with immunosuppression alone [54]. However, within the random data available to us from individual patients at many centers (patients not treated in a uniform protocol), the results look promising. In patients with only mild to moderate renal damage at the onset of therapy, about 20% who were untreated retained adequate renal function to support life without dialysis. About 40% of those treated with steroids and immunosuppressive agents alone and 70% of those treated with combined steroids, immunosuppression and plasma exchange therapy have improved initially, with maintenance of adequate renal function. We do not yet know how many of these will eventually deteriorate and lose renal function in a matter of months [55].

Often, patients who lose renal function from the activities of anti-basement membrane antibodies are faced with a decision regarding renal transplantation. As noted earlier, one of the most convincing pieces of evidence demonstrating the nephrotoxicity of human anti-GBM antibodies was the observation of recurrent glomerulonephritis in a kidney transplanted into a patient while circulating anti-basement membrane antibody was present [3]. This has been a concern of transplant teams ever since. Whenever an individual is transplanted while high levels of anti-GBM antibody remain, a significant chance of immediate recurrence of disease exists [33]. On the other hand, if transplantation is postponed until antibody has largely disappeared from the circulation, patients do not usually develop clinically severe recurrences when heavily immunosuppressed for transplant management. Whether the patient's ability to produce autoimmune anti-basement membrane antibody responses has disappeared, or whether this function is simply blunted by the immunosuppressive regimen, remains to be evaluated fully. However, in one recent instance, the question could be answered [56]. This involved a woman who had classic anti-GBM antibody-induced Goodpasture syndrome that was well documented. After she was nephrectomized, the circulating anti-GBM antibody disappeared and remained absent over a two-year period of follow-up. She was then transplanted with an identical-twin kidney, so theoretically did not require usual transplant immunosuppression. She soon redeveloped circulating anti-GBM antibody and clinical and immunopathologic evidence of recurrent anti-GBM antibody-induced glomerulonephritis. Subsequently, immunosuppression and plasma exchange terminated the antibody response, and graft function was maintained. The initial nonimmunosuppressed course allowed redevelopment of the anti-GBM antibody response, apparently stimulated by antigens in the identical-twin kidney.

We have been interested recently in the differences in nephritogenic basement membrane antigens between individuals as another potential inducer of anti-basement membrane antibody responses in the renal transplant population [42]. There are obvious strain and individual differences in basement membrane antigens in animals and in man. For example, the Brown Norway rat contains a nephritogenic TBM antigen that the Lewis rat lacks [57]. It is possible to induce anti-TBM antibodies in a Lewis rat by transplanting it with a TBM antigen-positive kidney from a Brown Norway × Lewis F_1 hybrid [58]. We have seen one similar example of anti-TBM antibodies induced in man. This individual lacked the usual nephritogenic TBM antigens in his own kidneys, and upon receiving two separate kidney grafts, each with the normal TBM antigens, developed anti-TBM antibodies both times [59].

Some kindreds of individuals with hereditary kidney disease, known as Alport syndrome, also lack the usual nephritogenic GBM antigens [60]. We have seen one individual with Alport syndrome who lacked the nephritogenic GBM antigens in his own kidney but developed anti-GBM antibodies when transplanted with a normal kidney [42]. Studies are now in progress to design quantitative assays for better assessment of the relative and absolute differences in basement membrane antigens between individuals. Researchers in England recently found that patients with anti-GBM antibody-induced Goodpasture syndrome had a high frequency of DRw2 alloantigen [61]. Whether such a genetic distribution, if confirmed, relates to the antibody response or to the distribution of GBM antigen remains to be determined.

Other Nephritogenic Glomerular
Capillary Wall Antigens

Now, to turn to some new models in which antibodies react with antigens present in the kidney (Table 1), their mechanism is no different but the antigens differ from the classical GBM antigenic systems described above. We sometimes elute antibody from human glomerulonephritic kidneys that appears to react with antigens like those from the animal models discussed later, suggesting that as time passes and methods improve we will be able to identify human counterparts of these models.

Structural Glomerular Antigens. By immunofluorescence study, 30% to 40% of older New Zealand White rabbits have evidence of glomerulonephritis [62]. Their glomerular disease is characterized by what appears to be granular deposits of immunoglobulin and complement, which on first inspection are suggestive of those seen in immune complex types of glomerular injury. When viewed by electron microscopy, their renal tissues contain electron-dense deposits along the subepithelial aspect of the GBM in the area of the immunofluorescent immune deposition. These electron-dense deposits are not as distinct and circumscribed as deposits usually associated with immune complex glomerulonephritis, for example of the serum sickness type, raising some question as to their true nature. The immunoglobulin eluted from these kidneys reacts with normal rabbit glomeruli when studied by indirect immunofluorescence. The reaction with the glomerular capillary wall is somewhat irregular, with reactive sites appearing to extend away from the epithelial aspect of the GBM. When the binding of this eluted antibody was studied at the ultrastructural level with immunoperoxide techniques, fixation was found in the areas where the epithelial cell foot processes attach to the GBM [63]. This, then, is an example of a nonclassic GBM glomerular capillary wall antigen that is involved in glomerulonephritis. The physicochemical nature of the antigen remains to be defined. A radioimmunoassay is being developed to detect the antibody in rabbits, and in turn may prove useful in extending our understanding of similar systems to man.

Another type of glomerulonephritis also seems to involve the direct reaction of antibody with glomerular capillary wall antigens. This is the model developed by Heymann and colleagues in the late 1950s, in which rats were immunized with rat kidney

suspensions in adjuvant [64]. Animals with Heymann nephritis
have immunofluorescent evidence of granular immunoglobulin
and complement deposits along the GBM and, by electron
microscopy, electron-dense material accumulated along the
subepithelial aspect of the GBM. On immunofluorescently
stained samples viewed at high magnification, the deposits are
not as round and circumscribed as those usually associated with
circulating immune complex deposits, but are rather more
geographic in nature, suggesting that they may outline structures within the glomerular capillary wall. In 1967, Edgington,
Glassock and Dixon evaluated the Heymann nephritis model in a
series of papers [65, 66]. They found that eluates from these
kidneys reacted with renal tubular brush border antigens of the
proximal renal convoluted tubule and postulated that this
disease was an autologous immune complex disease involving
formation of circulating immune complexes of antibody with
renal tubular brush border antigen, which subsequently deposit
in the glomerulus. They identified a crude extract of renal tubules
termed Fx1A, which induced the lesion, and were able to purify a
28S lipoprotein from the Fx1A, termed RTE-α-5, which could induce the illness when given in very small quantities. In 1973,
Sugisaki was able to transfer the glomerular immunofluorescence
findings of Heymann nephritis by injecting sera from affected
animals into autologous recipients [67]. In the mid-1970s, reports
began to appear describing a similar model induced by passive
administration of heterologous anti-Fx1A antibodies [68, 69].
More recent studies indicate that the glomerular binding of the
heterologous anti-Fx1A antibodies occurs as a slow buildup of
materials over several days [70]. The passive heterologous anti-
Fx1A model suggests that the glomerular deposits seen by immunofluorescence reflect either the formation of circulating immune complexes by combination of the heterologous antibodies
with circulating antigens, or the direct binding of the antibody to
antigen already present in the glomerulus. In 1978, in vivo and in
vitro perfusion studies suggested direct glomerular binding [71,
72]. In these studies of the isolated perfused kidney, antibody
was infused in such a way as to exclude the presence of circulating antigen and subsequent immune complex formation.

A question then arose regarding the nature of reactivity in
the active Heymann nephritis model. To address this issue, we
removed a large number of kidneys from rats with Heymann

nephritis. In the eluates was antibody that could bind to an antigen present within the animals' glomerular capillary walls [73]. The antibodies binding to the glomerular capillary wall were present in much lower dilutions than those also present that bound to the renal tubular brush border antigens, as had been observed earlier by Edgington et al [65, 66]. By using an immunoperoxidase electron microscopic method, it was possible to localize the reactive antigen in the glomerular wall in a scattered granular distribution concentrated along the subepithelial aspect of the GBM. Similar eluates have been passed through the isolated perfused kidney described above under circumstances in which immune complex formation is excluded. This process shows that the eluted antibody can bind directly to the glomerulus (T.J. Neale, W.G. Couser and C.B. Wilson, unpublished observations). These studies, however, neither exclude an additional role of tubular antigen-antibody complexes in this model, as suggested by Edgington [65], nor do they provide information regarding a separation, if any, between glomerular and tubular antigens and the antibody reactivities to them.

Based on the rabbit and rat models, the concept of direct antibody attack against glomerular antigens must now be expanded to include not only the GBM but at least two other glomerular capillary wall antigens (Fig. 4). These are antigens concentrated around the epithelial cell foot processes in the rabbit model and antigens present as scattered granular accumulations along the subepithelial aspect of the GBM in the Heymann nephritis model.

Planted Glomerular Antigens. Materials normally exogenous to the glomerulus may also become trapped or planted within the glomerular capillary wall for subsequent nephritogenic immune reaction. Heterologous anti-GBM antibody present in the autologous phase of experimental anti-GBM antibody nephritis serves as a classic example of a planted antigen, as mentioned earlier. In immune complex-induced glomerulonephritis, the immune complex becomes a source of planted antigen (or antibody) for continued interaction of antibody (or antigen) from the circulation. In experimental situations, it is possible to show that antibody can bind to the immune complex deposits, as done several years ago in animals with acute serum sickness [74] and more recently in the chronic serum sickness model assayed similarly in our laboratory. We have since transplanted kidneys from donors

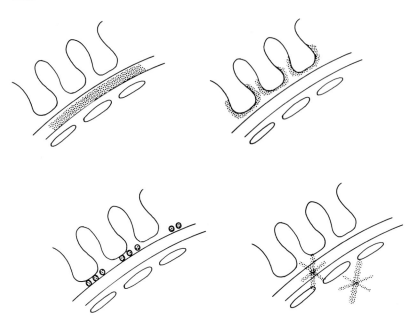

FIG. 4. The location of various nephritogenic glomerular capillary wall antigens is depicted schematically by areas of stippling. In the upper left, the classic GBM antigen(s) of anti-GBM antibody-induced glomerulonephritis is shown distributed evenly along the GBM. In the upper right, antigen concentrated around the area of epithelial foot process attachment to the GBM is tentatively identified in spontaneous glomerulonephritis in New Zealand White rabbits. In the lower left, the scattered granular subepithelial sites of antigen reactive with glomerular eluate for rats with Heymann nephritis are outlined. In the lower right, nonglomerular antigens trapped or "planted" in the glomerular capillary wall are drawn.

with chronic serum sickness into normal hosts to avoid circulating antibody and subsequent immune complex formation, and could then insert antigen into the previously deposited glomerular immune complex (D.M. Ward and C.B. Wilson, unpublished observations). Once an immune complex lesion starts, it can in theory be perpetuated by interactions of either antigen or antibody alone from the circulation, as they react with previously planted immune complexes. The most convincing evidence that materials from the circulation interact with planted immune complexes in the serum sickness models is the situation in which extreme antigen excess is created purposely; just as immune complexes are dissolved in vitro by such a manipulation, they are removed quantitatively from the glomerulus [75]. As a result, the rabbit with chronic serum sickness glomerulonephritis recovers completely if treatment begins before irreversible damage is done [76]. Extreme antigen excess treatment also rapidly terminates specific antibody production, providing another therapeutic benefit. It is possible in this situation to create glomerulonephritis, then take away the inciting mechanism, namely the immune complex deposits, and thereby cause the lesion to regress.

Other planted antigens are known or have been discussed. Material taken up in the mesangium can react with antibody and in turn can cause glomerular injury [77]. It has also been suggested that DNA may combine with the GBM for subsequent immune complex formation in situ when anti-DNA antibody is present [78, 79]. If so, this mechanism could play a part in some of the autoimmune anti-DNA diseases that are inducible with bacterial lipopolysaccharide or parasites.

Just as antigen and antibody can combine with deposited immune complexes in situ, other antibodies formed by the host to components of the immune complex deposit, for example anti-idiotypic antibody, rheumatoid factor or potentially immunoconglutinins, might add to the deposit and thus increase phlogogenicity. Once a nidus of planted antigen is present, continuing development of the inflammatory lesion is possible.

We have been interested in determining whether material that binds to the glomerular capillary wall for physicochemical reasons could serve as a nephritogenic planted antigen. For these experiments, we have used the lectin, concanavalin A, which binds to carbohydrate in the glomerular capillary wall [80]. Concanavalin A infused into the renal artery of a rat attaches to the glomerular capillary wall in a pattern that varies depending on how much is given and the time sequence of sampling, localization being rather linear early and more irregular and scattered later. Subsequently infused antibody to the concanavalin A binds to the planted antigen, which in turn incites significant glomerulonephritis [80]. In quantitative terms, about 75 μg of concanavalin A is planted in the kidney; when increasing amounts of anti-concanavalin A antibody are given, we find that glomerular injury occurs after about 75 μg of the administered antibody binds per gram of kidney. As mentioned earlier, it takes a similar amount (about 75 μg) of anti-GBM antibody per gram of kidney to induce immediate-phase anti-GBM antibody injury in the rat [25]. Concanavalin A infused into a rat previously immunized to concanavalin A also incites glomerular injury by interaction of the autologously formed antibody with the planted antigen. This lectin model clearly establishes the potential of antigens fixing to the glomerular capillary wall for any of a variety of physicochemical reasons, including charge characteristics of the polyanionic glomerular capillary wall by attracting cationic substances such as protamine, ruthenium red and other cationic dyes [81]. Some infectious organisms pathogenic for man have materials with lectin-like properties, suggesting similar potentials. Occasionally, patients have bacterial antigen localized within the glomeruli, but little or no immunoglobulin, suggesting the possibility that bacterial antigens bind directly to the glomerulus [82-84]. In addition to the participation of infectious agents in supplying antigens for circulating immune complex formation, they could also contribute as planted antigens in in situ immune complex formation within the glomerular capillary wall.

Conclusion

This discussion has focused largely on the direct binding of antibodies to antigens in or of the glomerular capillary wall, leading to nephritogenic immune reactions. The observations present herein expand the direct binding concept to include antigens in animal models in addition to the classical GBM antigens. With the identification of potentially more tissue-fixed nephritogenic antigens, the direct antibody attack mechanism may take on more importance in man. The expanded direct attack mechanism is unlikely to be as common a factor as the circulating immune complex mechanism, which is now being reevaluated and redefined in light of the possible contributions of fixed and planted antigens leading to in situ immune complex formation.

References

1. Dixon, F.J.: The pathogenesis of glomerulonephritis. Am. J. Med. 44:493-498, 1968.

2. Unanue, E.R. and Dixon, F.J.: Experimental glomerulonephritis: Immunological events and pathogenetic mechanisms. Adv. Immunol. 6:1-90, 1967.

3. Lerner, R.A., Glassock, R.J. and Dixon, F.J.: The role of anti-glomerular basement membrane antibody in the pathogenesis of human glomerulonephritis. J. Exp. Med. 126:989-1004, 1967.

4. Dixon, F.J., Vazquez, J.J., Weigle, W.O. and Cochrane, C.G.: Pathogenesis of serum sickness. Arch. Pathol. 65:18-28, 1958.

5. Dixon, F.J., Feldman, J.D. and Vazquez, J.: Experimental glomerulo-nephritis. The pathogenesis of a laboratory model resembling the spectrum of human glomerulonephritis. J. Exp. Med. 113:889-920, 1961.

6. Dixon, F.J.: The role of antigen-antibody complexes in disease. Harvey Lect. 58:21-52, 1963.

7. Wilson, C.B.: Immune reactions with antigens in or of the glomerulus. In Milgrom, F. and Albini, B.(eds.): Immunopathology. Basel:Karger, 1979, pp. 127-131.

8. Wilson, C.B. and Dixon, F.J.: Renal injury from immune reactions involving antigens in or of the kidney. In Wilson, C.B., Brenner, B.M. and Stein, J.H. (eds.): Contemporary Issues in Nephrology. New York:Churchill Livingstone, 1979, vol. 3, pp. 35-66.

9. Couser, W.G. and Salant, D.J.: In situ immune complex formation and glomerular injury, editorial. Kidney Int. 17:1-13, 1980.

10. Wilson, C.B. and Dixon, F.J.: The renal response to immunological injury. In Brenner, B.M. and Rector, F.C., Jr. (eds.): The Kidney, ed. 2. Philadelphia:W. B. Saunders, 1981, pp. 1237-1350.

11. Clagett, J.A., Wilson, C.B. and Weigle, W.O.: Interstitial immune complex thyroiditis in mice. The role of autoantibody to thyro-globulin. J. Exp. Med. 140:1439-1456, 1974.

12. Cochrane, C.G. and Janoff, A.: The Arthus reaction: A model of neutrophil and complement-mediated injury. In Zweifach, B.W., Grant, L. and McCluskey, R.T. (eds.): The Inflammatory Process, ed. 2. New York:Academic Press, 1974, vol. 3. pp. 85-162.

13. Unanue, E.R., Dixon, F.J. and Feldman, J.D.: Experimental allergic glomerulonephritis induced in the rabbit with homologous renal antigens. J. Exp. Med. 125:163-176, 1967.

14. Hoyer, J.R.: Tubulointerstitial immune complex nephritis in rats immunized with Tamm-Horsfall protein. Kidney Int. 17:284-292, 1980.

15. Brentjens, J.R., Sepulveda, M., Baliah, T. et al: Interstitial immune complex nephritis in patients with systemic lupus erythematosus. Kidney Int. 7:342-350, 1975.

16. Lehman, D.H., Wilson, C.B. and Dixon, F.J.: Extraglomerular immunoglobulin depositis in human nephritis. Am. J. Med. 58:765-786, 1975.

17. Cochrane, C.G.: Mediating systems in inflammatory disease. J. Invest. Dermatol. 71:40-48, 1978.

18. Cochrane, C.G.: Mediation systems in neutrophil-independent immunologic injury of the glomerulus. *In* Wilson, C.B., Brenner, B.M. and Stein, J.H. (eds.): Contemporary Issues in Nephrology. New York:Churchill Livingstone, 1979, vol. 3, pp. 106-121.
19. Atkins, R.C., Holdsworth, S.R., Glasgow, E.F. and Matthews, F.E.: The macrophage in human rapidly progressive glomerulonephritis. Lancet 1:830-832, 1976.
20. Schreiner, G.F., Cotran, R.S., Pardo, V. and Unanue, E.R.: A mononuclear cell component in experimental immunological glomerulonephritis. J. Exp. Med. 147:369-384, 1978.
21. Holdsworth, S.R., Neale, T.J. and Wilson, C.B.: The participation of macrophages and monocytes in experimental immune complex glomerulonephritis. Clin. Immunol. Immunopathol. 15:510-524, 1980.
22. Holdsworth, S.R., Neale, T.J. and Wilson, C.B.: Abrogation of macrophage dependent injury in experimental glomerulonephritis in the rabbit: Use of an anti-macrophage serum. J. Clin. Invest., 1981. (In press.)
23. Schreiber, R.D. and Müller-Eberhard, H.J.: Complement and renal disease. *In* Wilson, C.B., Brenner, B.M. and Stein, J.H. (eds.): Contemporary Issues in Nephrology. New York:Churchill Livingstone, 1979, vol. 3, pp. 67-105.
24. Andres, G.A. and McCluskey, R.T.: Tubular and interstitial renal disease due to immunologic mechanisms. Kidney Int. 7:271-289, 1975.
25. Unanue, E.R. and Dixon, F.J.: Experimental glomerulonephritis. V. Studies on the interaction of nephrotoxic antibodies with tissues of the rat. J. Exp. Med. 121:697-714, 1965.
26. Lerner, R.A. and Dixon, F.J.: Transfer of ovine experimental allergic glomerulonephritis (EAG) with serum. J. Exp. Med. 124:431-442, 1966.
27. Unanue, E.R. and Dixon, F.J.: Experimental glomerulonephritis. VI. The autologous phase of nephrotoxic serum nephritis. J. Exp. Med. 121:715-725, 1965.
28. Henson, P.M: Release of biologically active constituents from blood cells and its role in antibody-mediated tissue injury. *In* Amos, D.B. (ed.): Progress in Immunology. New York:Academic Press, 1971, pp. 155-171.
29. Blantz, R.C. and Wilson, C.B.: Acute effects of anti-glomerular basement membrane antibody on the precess of glomerular filtration in the rat. J. Clin. Invest. 58:899-911, 1976.
30. Blantz, R.C., Tucker, B.J. and Wilson, C.B.: The acute effects of antiglomerular basement membrane antibody upon glomerular filtration in the rat. The influence of dose and complement depletion. J. Clin. Invest. 61:910-921, 1978.
31. Blantz, R.C., Hostetter, T.H. and Brenner, B.M.: Functional adaptations of the kidney to immunological injury. *In* Wilson, C.B., Brenner, B.M. and Stein, J.H. (eds.): Contemporary Issues in Nephrology. New York:Churchill Livingstone, 1979, vol. 3, pp. 122-143.

32. Steblay, R.W.: Glomerulonephritis induced in sheep by injections of heterologous glomerular basement membrane and Freund's complete adjuvant. J. Exp. Med. 116:253-272, 1962.
33. Wilson, C.B. and Dixon, F.J.: Anti-glomerular basement membrane antibody-induced glomerulonephritis. Kidney Int. 3:74-89, 1973.
34. Wilson, C.B.: Immunologic diseases of the lung and kidney (Goodpasture's syndrome). In Fishman, A.P. (ed.): Pulmonary Diseases and Disorders. New York:McGraw-Hill, 1979, pp. 699-706.
35. Border, W.A., Lehman, D.H., Egan, J.D. et al: Antitubular basement-membrane antibodies in methicillin-associated interstitial nephritis. N. Engl. J. Med. 291:381-384, 1974.
36. Fish, A.J., Carmody, K.M. and Michael, A.F.: Spatial orientation and distribution of antigens within human glomerular basement membrane. J. Lab. Clin. Med. 94:447-457, 1979.
37. Beirne, G.J. and Brennan, J.T.: Glomerulonephritis associated with hydrocarbon solvents: Mediated by antiglomerular basement membrane antibody. Arch. Environ. Health 25:365-369, 1972.
38. Beirne, G.J., Wagnild, J.P., Zimmerman, S.W. et al: Idiopathic crescentic glomerulonephritis. Medicine 56:349-381, 1977.
39. Klassen, J., Elwood, C. Grossberg, A.L. et al: Evolution of membranous nephropathy into anti-glomerular-basement-membrane glomerulonephritis. N. Engl. J. Med. 290:1340-1344, 1974.
40. Kleinknecht, D., Morel-Maroger, L., Callard, P. et al: antiglomerular basement membrane (GBM) antibody-induced glomerulonephritis after solvent exposure, abstracted. Kidney Int. 15:450, 1979.
41. Wilson, C.B., Dixon, F.J., Fortner, J.G. and Cerilli, J.: Glomerular basement membrane-reactive antibodies in anti-lymphocyte globulin. J. Clin. Invest. 50:1525-1535, 1971.
42. Wilson, C.B.: Individual and strain differences in renal basement membrane antigens. Transplant. Proc. 12 (suppl. 1):69-73, 1980.
43. McPhaul, J.J., Jr. and Dixon, F.J.: Immunoreactive basement membrane antigens in normal human urine and serum. J. Exp. Med. 130:1395-1409, 1969.
44. Willoughby, W.F. and Dixon, F.J.: Experimental hemorrhagic pneumonitis produced by heterologous anti-lung antibody. J. Immunol. 104:28-37, 1970.
45. Wilson, C.B., Marquardt, H. and Dixon, F.J.: Radioimmunoassay (RIA) for circulating antiglomerular basement membrane (GBM) antibodies, abstracted. Kidney Int. 6:114a, 1974.
46. Holdsworth, S.R., Gclbus, S.M. and Wilson, C.B.: Characterization of collagenase solubilized human glomerular basement membrane antigens reacting with human antibodies, abstracted. Kidney Int. 16:797, 1979.
47. Wilson, C.B.: Radioimmunoassay for anti-glomerular basement membrane antibodies. In Rose, N.R. and Friedman, H. (eds.): Manual of Clinical Immunology, ed. 2. Washington, D.C.:American Society for Microbiology, 1980, pp. 376-379.
48. Dahlberg, P.J., Kurtz, S.B., Donadio, J.V., Jr. et al: Recurrent

Goodpasture's syndrome. Mayo Clin. Proc. 53:533-537, 1978.
49. McPhaul, J.J., Jr. and Dixon, F.J.: Characterization of human anti-glomerular basement membrane antibodies eluted from glomerulonephritic kidneys. J. Clin. Invest. 49:308-317, 1970.
50. Lockwood, C.M., Boulton-Jones, J.M., Lowenthal, R.M. et al: Recovery from Goodpasture's syndrome after immunosuppressive treatment and plasmapheresis. Br. Med. J. 2:252-254, 1975.
51. Johnson, J.P., Whitman, W., Briggs, W.A. and Wilson, C.B.: Plasmapheresis and immunosuppressive agents in antibasement membrane antibody-induced Goodpasture's syndrome. Am. J. Med. 64:354-359, 1978.
52. Rees, A.J., Lockwood, C.M. and Peters, D.K.: Enhanced allergic tissue injury in Goodpasture's syndrome by intercurrent bacterial infection. Br. Med. J. 2:723-726, 1977.
53. Lockwood, C.M., Pussell, B., Wilson, C.B. and Peters, D.K.: Plasma exchange in nephritis. In Hamburger, J., Crosnier, J., Grünfeld, J.-P. and Maxwell, M.H. (eds.): Advances in Nephrology. Chicago:Year Book, 1979, vol. 8, pp. 383-418.
54. Johnson, J.P., Briggs, W.A., Bohan, L. et al: The role of plasmapheresis in anti-glomerular basement membrane antibody mediated renal disease. In Schreiner, G., Winchester, W., Mattern, W. and Mendelssohn, B. (eds.): Controversies in Nephrology — 1979. Washington, D.C.:Georgetown University, 1979, vol. 1, pp. 303-312.
55. Finch, R.A., Rutsky, E.A., McGowan, E. and Wilson, C.B.: Treatment of Goodpasture's syndrome with immunosuppression and plasmapheresis. South. Med. J. 72:1288-1290, 1979.
56. Almkuist, R.D., Buckalew, V.M., Hirszel, P. et al: Recurrence of anti-glomerular basement membrane antibody mediated glomerulonephritis in an isograft. Clin. Immunol. Immunopathol. (In press.)
57. Lehman, D.H., Wilson, C.B. and Dixon, F.J.: Interstitial nephritis in rats immunized with heterologous tubular basement membrane. Kidney Int. 5:187-195, 1974.
58. Lehman, D.H., Lee, S., Wilson, C.B. and Dixon, F.J.: Induction of antitubular basement membrane antibodies in rats by renal transplantation. Transplantation 17:429-431, 1974.
59. Wilson, C.B., Lehman, D.H., McCoy, R.C. et al: Antitubular basement membrane antibodies after renal transplantation. Transplantation 18:447-452, 1974.
60. McCoy, R.C., Johnson, H.K., Stone, W.J. and Wilson, C.B.: Variation in glomerular basement membrane antigens in hereditary nephritis, abstracted. Lab. Invest. 34:325-326, 1976.
61. Rees, A.J., Peters, D.K., Compston, D.A.S. and Batchelor, J.R.: Strong association between HLA-DRW2 and antibody-mediated Goodpasture's syndrome. Lancet 1:966-968, 1978.
62. Verroust, P.J., Wilson, C.B. and Dixon, F.J.: Lack of nephritogenicity of systemic activation of the alternate complement pathway. Kidney Int. 6:157-169, 1974.
63. Neale, T.J. and Wilson, C.B.:   Non-GBM glomerular antigen in

spontaneous nephritis in rabbits, abstracted. Kidney Int. 14:715, 1978.

64. Heymann, W., Hackel, D.B., Harwood, S. et al: Production of nephrotic syndrome in rats by Freund's adjuvants and rat kidney suspensions. Proc. Soc. Exp. Biol. Med. 100:660-664, 1959.

65. Edgington, T.S., Glassock, R.J. and Dixon, F.J.: Autologous immune complex pathogenesis of experimental allergic glomerulonephritis. Science 155:1432-1434, 1967.

66. Edgington, T.S., Glassock, R.J. and Dixon, F.J.: Autologous immune complex nephritis induced with renal tubular antigen. I. Identification and isolation of the pathogenetic antigen. J. Exp Med. 127:555-572, 1968.

67. Sugisaki, T., Klassen, J., Andres, G.A. et al: Passive transfer of Heymann nephritis with serum. Kidney Int. 3:66-73, 1973.

68. Barabas, A.Z. and Lannigan, R.: Induction of an autologous immune complex glomerulonephritis in the rat by intravenous injection of heterologous anti-rat kidney tubular antibody. I. Production of chronic progressive immune-complex glomerulonephritis. Br. J. Exp. Pathol. 55:47-55, 1974.

69. Feenstra, K., van der Lee, R., Greben, H.A. et al: Experimental glomerulonephritis in the rat induced by antibodies directed against tubular antigens. I. The natural history: A histologic and immuno-histologic study at the light microscopic and ultrastructural level. Lab. Invest. 32:235-242, 1975.

70. Salant, D.J., Darby, C. and Couser, W.G.: Experimental membranous glomerulonephritis in rats. Quantitative studies of glomerular immune deposit formation in isolated glomeruli and whole animals. J. Clin. Invest. 66:71-81, 1980.

71. Couser, W.G., Steinmuller, D.R., Stilmant, M.M. et al: Experimental glomerulonephritis in the isolated perfused rat kidney. J. Clin. Invest. 62:1275-1287, 1978.

72. Van Damme, B.J.C., Fleuren, G.J., Bakker, W.W. et al: Experimental glomerulonephritis in the rat induced by antibodies directed against tubular antigens. V. Fixed glomerular antigens in the pathogenesis of heterologous immune complex glomerulonephritis. Lab. Invest. 38:502-510, 1978.

73. Neale, T.J. and Wilson, C.B.: Fixed glomerular antigen in Heymann's nephritis: Eluted antibody reactivity with normal rat glomeruli, abstracted. Kidney Int. 16:799, 1979.

74. Lambert, P.H., Brictoux, N., Salmon, J. and Miescher, P.A.: Dynamics of immune complex nephritis during antibody excess. Int. Arch. Allergy Appl. Immunol. 45:185-189, 1973.

75. Wilson, C.B. and Dixon, F.J.: Quantitation of acute and chronic serum sickness in the rabbit. J. Exp. Med. 134:7s-18s, 1971.

76. Wilson, C.B.: Immune complex glomerulonephritis. In Proceedings of the 5th International Congress of Nephrology, Mexico, 1972. Basel: Karger, 1974, vol. 1. pp. 68-74.

77. Mauer, S.M., Sutherland, D.E.R., Howard, R.J. et al: The glomerular

mesangium: III. Acute immune mesangial injury: A new model of glomerulonephritis. J. Exp. Med. 137:553-570, 1973.

78. Izui, S., Lambert, P.H. and Miescher, P.A.: In vitro demonstration of a particular affinity of glomerular basement membrane and collagen for DNA. A possible basis for a local formation of DNA-anti-DNA complexes in systemic lupus erythematosus. J. Exp. Med. 144:428-443, 1976.

79. Izui, S., Lambert, P.H., Fournie, G.J. et al: Features of systemic lupus erythematosus in mice injected with bacterial lipopolysaccharides. Identification of circulating DNA and renal localization of DNA-anti-DNA complexes. J. Exp. Med. 145:1115-1130, 1977.

80. Golbus, S.M. and Wilson, C.B.: Experimental glomerulonephritis induced by in situ formation of immune complexes in glomerular capillary wall. Kidney Int. 16:148-157, 1979.

81. Farquhar, M.G.: Structure and function in glomerular capillaries: Role of the basement membrane in glomerular filtration. In Kefalides, N.A. (ed.): Biology and Chemistry of Basement Membranes. New York: Academic Press, 1978, p. 43.

82. Treser, G., Semar, M., McVicar, M. et al: Antigenic streptococcal components in acute glomerulonephritis. Science 163:676-677, 1969.

83. Hyman, L.R., Jenis, E.H., Hill, G.S. et al: Alternate C3 pathway activation in pneumococcal glomerulonephritis. Am. J. Med. 58:810-814, 1975.

84. Pertschuk, L.P., Woda, B.A., Vuletin, J.C. et al: Glomerulonephritis due to Staphylococcus aureus antigen. Am. J. Clin. Pathol. 65:301-307, 1976.

Inflammatory Mechanisms in Lung Injury

Peter A. Ward, M.D. and Kent J. Johnson, M.D.

There is increasing evidence that, as in the kidney, a major cause of interstitial inflammatory diseases of the lung can be related to the presence of immune complex-like material in the serum, in the lung tissue or in bronchoalveolar lavage fluids from these patients. For instance, in idiopathic pulmonary fibrosis, immune complexes have been found in the serum of a high percentage of these patients and recently complement-fixing material, perhaps related to immune complexes, has been found in bronchoalveolar fluids of patients with this disease [1]. Immune complexes present in lung tissue (as defined by immunofluorescent techniques) or in serum (as defined by the RAJI assay) have also been described in patients with interstitial inflammatory lung diseases, which have been clinically classified as eosinophilic granuloma or histiocytosis X of lung [2, 3]. Increasingly, it would appear that immune complexes are becoming recognized as important factors in the causation of acute and progressive interstitial lung diseases in humans.

Our experimental studies on lung inflammatory mechanisms related to immune complexes have addressed the following questions:

1. How can acute lung reactions to immune complexes be reproducibly induced and quantitatively measured?

Peter A. Ward, M.D., Professor and Chairman; and Kent J. Johnson, M.D., Assistant Professor, Department of Pathology, The University of Michigan Medical School, Ann Arbor.

This work was supported in part from NIH grants HL-23192, HL-26809, HL-07517 and HL-00889.

2. What features of the complexes relate to their tissue-damaging activities in lung?
3. What mediators are involved in these reactions?
4. Do geographic considerations within the tissue or organ affect the outcomes of the reactions produced by these mediators?

The Experimental Model

In an attempt to develop a lung model that permits a reproducible pattern of injury that can be rigorously quantitated, two different models of acute immune complex-induced lung injury in the rat have been developed. The *first* represents a reversed passive type of Arthus reaction in the lung, with antibody being instilled into the airways during inspiration [4]. This is accomplished by the threading of a fine Teflon catheter through a tracheostomy incision. The catheter is passed approximately to the level of the carina, and the bolus of reagent in a volume of 0.25 ml is injected during inspiration. Following intravenous injection of antigen, the pattern of the developing injury is usually bilateral and reflects the distribution of the aspirated fluid. Immediately following airway instillation of the antibody, antigen is injected intravenously along with ^{125}I-rat albumin or IgG. The radiolabeled protein serves as a marker of lung permeability, which reflects intrapulmonary damage induced by the reactants. Ordinarily, rabbit antibody to bovine serum albumin (BSA) is employed, using the IgG fraction of hyperimmune rabbit serum containing a high level (>1000 μg antibody N per milliliter) of precipitating antibody. Usually, 100 μg N anti-BSA is used for the airway instillation. The amount of antigen (BSA) injected intravenously is not critical. Usually 10 mg is used. At the time of sacrifice (four hours after intrapulmonary instillation of antibody, unless otherwise stated), acute alveolitis develops with extensive intraalveolar hemorrhage and edema, large numbers of neutrophils and intraalveolar deposits of fibrin. Quantitation of lung injury can be accomplished by perfusion of the pulmonary vasculature with saline to remove blood-associated radioactivity. The remaining radioactivity represents an interstitial and intraalveolar leakage of the marker protein, which is a sensitive quantitative indication of lung injury. When the typical intrapulmonary reaction with acute injury occurs, there is a three- to ten-fold increase of radioactivity in the lung parenchyma as compared with values for the negative control animals (e.g. intrapulmonary instillation of antibody in the absence of antigen). The extent of permeability change varies, depending on considerations of time, amount of antibody employed, etc.

The *second* model developed in our laboratories involves the use of preformed immune complexes which can be instilled directly into the airways. If phlogistic, preformed immune complexes are used, complexes containing as little as 100 μg N anti-BSA are intensely tissue-damaging to the lung, in contrast to the kidney or dermal vessels where much larger amounts of complexes are required to achieve tissue injury. Either the lung is considerably more sensitive to the injurious effects of these complexes or the route of intrapulmonary delivery is more efficient than intravascular injection in the case of the kidney or intradermal injection in the case of the dermis. Quantitation of lung injury in the case of airway instillation of preformed immune complexes is also accomplished by measuring the leakage of a circulating radiolabeled protein, as described above.

Regardless of the form of delivery to lung of the complexes, the histopathologic picture is similar; large numbers of neutrophils accumulate in intraalveolar spaces; their presence is evident as early as 30 minutes. As the reactions intensify, intrapulmonary hemorrhage and edema develop (Fig. 1). Recent transmission electron microscopic studies reveal that type II alveolar epithelial cells are susceptible to damage in these reactions; large numbers are damaged or destroyed in the course of the immune complex-triggered reactions (Fig. 2). It is not known what is responsible for type II cell damage. Like the case of acute immune complex-induced vasculitis in the dermis, the intrapulmonary reactions are limited in their severity, probably due to the phagocytic removal by neutrophils and alveolar macrophages of the deposited complexes. There is no evidence that a single intraalveolar insult by immune complexes incites a fibrotic response in the interstitium.

Physical-Chemical Features of the Injurious Immune Complexes

Using the model of preformed immune complexes, the most intensely phlogistic and tissue-damaging complexes have two

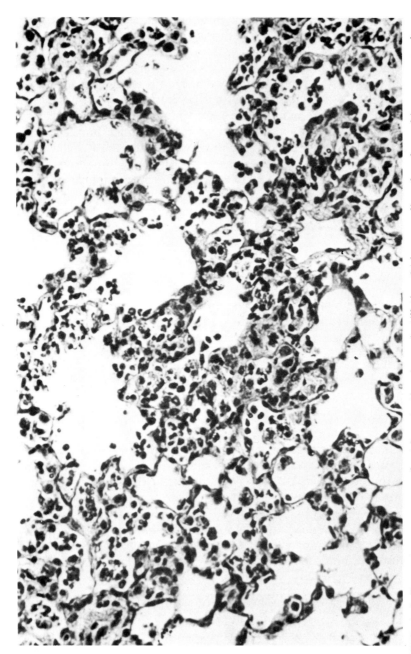

FIG. 1. Inflammatory response of rat lung to the airway instillation 24 hours earlier of preformed immune complexes containing 175 µg N anti-BSA and 35 µg N BSA. Large numbers of neutrophils are present within alveolar spaces. (Hematoxylin and eosin, × 350.) (Reprinted from Scherzer and Ward [6], © 1978, Williams & Wilkins Co, Baltimore.)

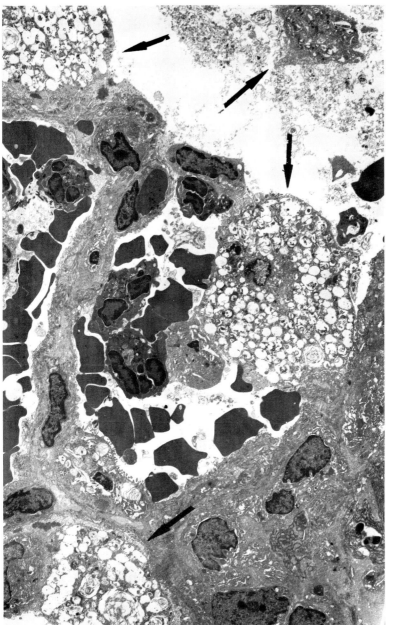

FIG. 2. Transmission electron microscopic analysis of acute immune complex injury in rat lung three hours after deposition of immune complexes (antibody instilled into airways and antigen injected intravenously). There are large numbers of neutrophils and red cells within alveolar spaces. Type II alveolar epithelial cells (*arrows*) have discharged their lamellar bodies and show evidence of damage and dissolution (× 1200.)

features that correlate directly with their lung-damaging activities: complement-fixing properties and molecular weights. In turn, as would be expected, these two parameters are related to the ratio of antigen and antibody in the preformed complexes [5, 6] using the rabbit anti-BSA-BSA system; when an amount of antigen that exceeds this ratio is present, the complement-fixing activity is rapidly lost (Fig. 3). In turn, a direct relation to molecular size, as determined by elution of the complexes from Separose 4B, is readily demonstrable (Fig. 4). These physical-chemical features can, in turn, be directly related to the lung-damaging activities of these complexes. When animals are instilled with preformed complexes containing 100 μg N anti-BSA and varying amounts of antigen, lung damage, as defined by permeability changes, is directly linked

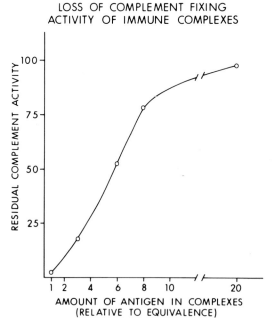

FIG. 3. Loss of complement-fixing activity as the ratio of antigen to antibody in the complexes increases. Preformed BSA-anti-BSA complexes were added to fresh rat serum and residual CH_{50} levels were measured. Details are available elsewhere. (Reprinted from Scherzer and Ward [6], © 1978 Williams & Wilkins Co., Baltimore.)

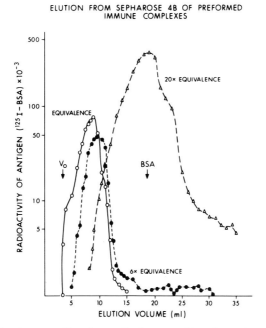

FIG. 4. Elution profile from Sepharose 4B of preformed immune complexes containing BSA and anti-BSA. Three different preparations of complexes, differing only in the amount of antigen (BSA) present, were eluted with saline. The void volume (Vo) and BSA positions are indicated by the arrows.

to the ratio of antigen to antibody in the preformed complexes (Table 1). That antigen in the aggregated form lacks phlogistic activity for the lung has been demonstrated by the inability of heat-aggregated antigen to produce lung injury (Table 1). Although increasing size of the complexes may lead to greater local retention of the complexes within lung, the essential requirement of the complexes to activate the complement system is underscored by data presented below.

Mediators Involved in Immune Complex-Induced Lung Damage

Extensive work on the mechanisms responsible for immune complex-induced damage of dermal vessels has emphasized the

Table 1. Lung Injury Produced by
Preformed Immune Complexes

Material Instilled into Airways*	Lung Injury†
Complexes at equivalence	9.4
Complexes at 2X equivalence	5.0
Complexes at 4X equivalence	4.1
Complexes at 8X equivalence	2.7
Aggregated antigen	0.8
Saline	1.0

*Complexes contained 100 μg N anti-BSA; at equivalence, 20 μg N BSA was present. Aggregated antigen consisted of 100 μg N heat-aggregated BSA. At least four rats were used in each experiment.

†Lung injury is expressed as lung permeability change relative to animals receiving airways instillation of saline four hours previously.

critical role of the complement system for the subsequent tissue injury. In reversed passive dermal Arthus reactions, prior inactivation of the complement system precludes accumulation of neutrophils. This can be explained by an inability to generate locally the essential C5-derived chemotactic peptides [7, 8]. In the lung, using either the reversed passive Arthus model or preformed immune complexes, the nonavailability of the complement system precludes the accumulation of leukocytes (neutrophils) and the development of tissue damage. This point has been proven experimentally by two entirely different approaches. On the one hand, animals have been pretreated with the C3 inactivator isolated from cobra venom. If serum C3 levels are reduced to <5% the pretreatment value (as assessed immunochemically), then >95% of the tissue damage, as measured by increases in lung permeability, is averted [4]. The second approach demonstrating the role of C5 chemotactic peptides in the pulmonary reactions triggered by the intra-pulmonary deposition of immune complexes has been to instill into the airways, along with the antibody, very small amounts of the chemotactic factor inactivator (CFI) that has been isolated from human serum [9]. The coinstillation of 10 μg CFI with the antibody completely protects the lung from the expected acute damage [10]. For instance, >90% of the lung permeability change, >90% of the hemorrhage (as measured quantitatively by the extraction of hemoglobin from lung tissue) and virtually all of the accumulation of neutrophils are prevented by this treatment. Since we know that CFI irreversibly blocks the chemotactic activity of both C5a and C5a des arg, there is a strong likelihood that the protective effects of CFI are directly related to the inactivation of C5 chemotactic peptides.

In addition to obtaining evidence that C5-related chemotactic peptides are essential chemical signals that govern the development of acute inflammatory responses of the lung to immune complexes, an additional approach has been used. This involves the direct intrapulmonary instillation of purified human C5a, followed by a qualitative and a quantitative assessment of the resulting inflammatory reaction. These experiments have been done in several species (rat, rabbit, hamster), but they have been most thoroughly studied in the hamster [11]. In this species, the airway instillation (by techniques described above) of approximately 5 μg C5a results in a rapid intrapulmonary accumulation of neutrophils. Using ^{111}In-labeled neutrophils, there is clear-cut accumulation of leukocytes within 5 minutes, with a plateau being reached within 60 minutes. It should be noted that during the course of these studies the changes in lung permeability are quite limited, stressing the lack of relation between permeability changes and neutrophil accumulation in vivo. Although calculations on the precise number of neutrophils accumulating in the lung parenchyma under these conditions are very difficult, we have estimated conservatively that within 60 minutes the instillation of 5 μg human C5a will induce the accumulation of more than threefold the entire number of neutrophils circulating in the peripheral blood vasculature of the hamster. The intrapulmonary inflammatory reaction involves neutrophils almost exclusively, and the exudate is predominantly intraalveolar (Fig. 5).

Geographic Determinants Affecting Intrapulmonary Instillation of Chemotactic Factors

As has been emphasized above, the production of chemotactic mediators related to the deposition of immune complexe$

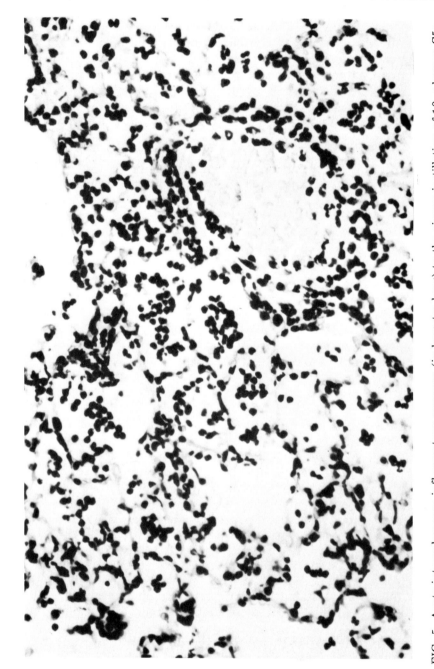

FIG. 5. Acute intrapulmonary inflammatory response (in hamster lung) to the airway instillation of 10μg human C5a three hours earlier. There is an intense intraalveolar accumulation of neutrophils. (Hematoxylin and eosin, × 300).

within alveolar spaces and alveolar septae of the lung results in an intense intrapulmonary accumulation of neutrophils within the same locales. As noted, these inflammatory reactions can be reproduced by the airway instillation of preformed chemotactic peptides (see above). It seems probable that the pathogenesis of the inflammatory reaction induced by immune complexes involves a gradient of chemotactic factor starting at highest concentration in or around the alveolar spaces and terminating in a low concentration in or around the interstitial capillaries. However, the outcome is altogether different when the gradient of chemotactic factor is reversed, with the greatest concentration of chemotactic peptide appearing within the vasculature. This situation can be reproduced by the intravascular activation of the complement system (e.g. by the intravenous injection of the C3 inactivator isolated from cobra venom) or by the direct vascular infusion of a chemotactic peptide. When either approach is used, a profound neutropenia develops as a result of the intrapulmonary, intravascular sequestration of neutrophils. Although the pulmonary vascular bed does not appear to be unique in regard to the entrapment process, its sheer mass probably predestines it as the major region of neutrophil sequestration. The pathophysiological consequences of this event are not understood, although it has been postulated that these responses place the pulmonary vasculature in jeopardy [12]. Although this broad biological question cannot be resolved, there is fairly good evidence to explain the injury as being related to the neutrophil sequestration process. This can, in large part, be explained by the fact that neutrophils from a variety of species (human, rabbit, rat, hamster) respond to contact with chemotactic factors by undergoing a series of changes that are dependent on availability of glucose, Ca^{++} and Mg^{++} and the prostaglandins' biosynthetic pathways. These events result in surface changes on neutrophils, rendering them hyperadherent to each other and, also, to other surfaces such as nylon fibers and plastic surfaces [13, 14]. In vitro these events can be easily measured in the Coulter counter, where the increase in cell aggregates ("large particles") can be demonstrated (Fig. 6). The aggregation response of human neutrophils to chemotactic peptides can also be induced by incubating neutrophils with arachidonic acid [15]. It is currently assumed

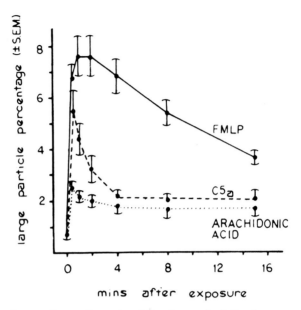

FIG. 6. Aggregation of neutrophils (human) following exposure to chemotactic factors (FMLP, N-formyl-Met-Leu-Phe and human C5a were present at 10^{-8} M). Arachidonic acid (10^{-5} M) also induced an aggregation response of neutrophils.

that the chemotactic peptides achieve their effects by activating biosynthetic pathways of arachidonic metabolism and that the critical product related to the cell aggregation may be a leukotriene produced by the lipoxygenase pathway. This putative leukotriene may act as an internal calcium ionophore. The events responsible for changes on the surfaces of leukocytes leading to their subsequent aggregation are entirely unknown, although we have demonstrated the deletion of one surface cell membrane protein and the appearance of another membrane protein in neutrophils undergoing a response to chemotactic peptides [16].

The consequences of chemotactic factor-induced, intra-vascular aggregation of neutrophils remain to be seen, although the potential exists for secretory release of lysosomal proteins and production of oxygen metabolites, such as O_2^- and H_2O_2, which have demonstrated toxic potential for a variety of cells.

References

1. Gadek, J.E., Hunninghake, G.W., Zimmerman, R. et al: Pathogenetic studies in idiopathic pulmonary fibrosis: Control of neutrophil migration by immune complexes. Chest 75 (suppl.):264S-265S, 1979.
2. Ward, P.A.: Immune complex injury of the lung. Am. J. Pathol. 97:85-91, 1979.
3. Hunninghake, G.W., Gadek, J.E., Kawanami, O. et al: Inflammatory and immune processes in the human lung in health and disease: Evaluation by bronchoalveolar lavage. Am. J. Pathol. 97:149-206, 1979.
4. Johnson, K.J. and Ward, P.A.: Acute immunologic pulmonary alveolitis. J. Clin. Invest. 54:349-352, 1974.
5. Scherzer, H. and Ward, P.A.: Lung and dermal vascular injury produced by preformed immune complexes. Am. Rev. Respir. Dis. 117:551-557, 1978.
6. Scherzer, H. and Ward, P.A.: Lung injury produced by immune complexes of varying composition. J. Immunol. 121:947-952, 1978.
7. Ward, P.A. and Cochrane, C.G.: Bound complement and immunologic injury of blood vessels. J. Exp. Med. 121:215-234, 1965.
8. Ward, P.A. and Hill, J.H.: Biological role of complement products. Complement-derived leukotactic activity extractable from lesions of immunologic vasculitis. J. Immunol. 108:1137-1145, 1972.
9. Kreutzer, D.L., Claypool, W.D., Jones, M.L. and Ward, P.A.: Isolation by hydrophobic chromatography of the chemotactic factor inactivators from human serum. Clin. Immunol. Immunopathol. 12:162-176, 1979.
10. Johnson, K.J., Anderson, T.P. and Ward, P.A.: Suppression of immune complex-induced inflammation by the chemotactic factor inactivator. J. Clin. Invest. 59:951-958, 1977.
11. Desai, U., Kreutzer, D.L., Showell, H. et al: Acute inflammatory pulmonary reactions induced by chemotactic factors. Am. J. Pathol. 96:71-86, 1979.
12. Craddock, P.R., Fehr, J., Dalmasso, A.P. et al: Hemodialysis leukopenia. Pulmonary vascular leukostasis resulting from complement activation by dialyzer cellophane membranes. J. Clin. Invest. 59:879-888, 1977.
13. O'Flaherty, J.T., Kreutzer, D.L. and Ward, P.A.: Neutrophil aggregation and swelling induced by chemotactic agents. J. Immunol. 119:232-239, 1977.
14. O'Flaherty, J.T. and Ward, P.A.: Chemotactic factors and the neutrophil. Semin. Hematol. 16:163-174, 1979.
15. O'Flaherty, J.T., Showell, H.J., Becker, E.L. and Ward, P.A.: Neutrophil aggregation and degranulation: Effect of arachidonic acid. Am. J. Pathol. 95:433-444, 1979.
16. Thrall, R.S., Phan, S.H., Showell, H.J. et al: Membrane protein alterations in the neutrophil in response to chemotactic factors. Molec. Immunol. 17:181-190, 1980.

Viral Immunopathology: Virus Persistence, Resultant Tissue Injury and Escape from Immune Surveillance

Michael B. A. Oldstone, M.D.

Introduction

My work with persistent virus infection began by using the experimental model of lymphocytic choriomeningitis virus (LCMV) infection in mice, the most illuminating and carefully studied model of virus persistence. At that time, nearly 14 years ago, it was believed that mice persistently infected with virus since birth became tolerant to the virus; that is, they did not make a specific immune response to the infecting virus. In fact, the early observations with LCMV formed a basic foundation for McFarland Burnett's hypothesis of immune tolerance. Subsequently, these LCMV persistently infected animals were found not tolerant, but rather the producers of antiviral specific immune responses [1, 2]. However, the immune responses were made in antigen (virus) excess, so no free antibody was detectable; only antibody complexed to viral antigens was apparent. Immune complexes formed in the circulations of these persistently infected mice became trapped in several bodily tissues, notably glomeruli, leading to glomerulonephritis; arteries, leading to arteritis; and the choroid plexus, leading to

Michael B. A. Oldstone, M.D., Member, Department of Immunopathology, Scripps Clinic and Research Foundation, La Jolla, Calif.

This is Publication No. 2333 from the Department of Immunopathology, Scripps Clinic and Research Foundation. This research was supported by USPHS grants NS-12428, NS-14068, AI-09484, AI-07007, and National Multiple Sclerosis Society Research Grant 1285-A-4.

271

choroid plexus disease [reviewed in 3]. Subsequent years showed that mice persistently infected with LCMV are fully competent immunologically and respond to that virus at both the B lymphocyte and T helper lymphocyte levels [4]. That is, antibodies are generated to all the known LCMV polypeptides.

Although this persistent infection with LCMV occurs in antigen excess, most persistent infections of man occur in antibody excess. Hence, chronic infections (with measles virus-subacute sclerosing panencephalitis [SSPE], herpes virus, rubella virus, etc.) endure despite vigorous immune responses by the hosts. Our theory to explain virus persistence in antibody excess as well as in antigen excess is represented schematically in Figure 1. Basically the hypothesis has two main events. First, during virus persistence the number of viral antigens expressed on the surfaces of infected cells decreases so that insufficient material is present to cause lysis by cytotoxic immune

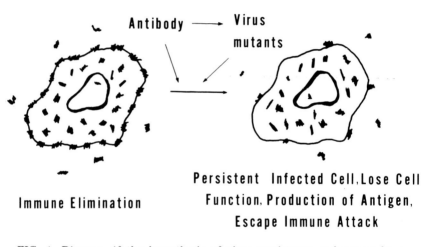

FIG. 1. Diagram of the hypothesis of virus persistence and escape from immune surveillance presented in this chapter. The cell on the left can be attacked and eliminated by the host's immune system because it expresses sufficient viral antigens on the external surface of its plasma membrane. In contrast, the cell on the right escapes immune surveillance because it lacks sufficient expression of viral antigens on its surface. Yet this cell expresses viral products in its cytoplasm and releases viral antigens into the fluid phase. It is suggested that such a cell may have a physiologic dysfunction, i.e. loss of luxury or differentiation function. Note that antibody, the generation of viral mutants alone or both in concert can shift an acute to a persistent infection.

constituents. Thereby, viral genetic information persists within the cell, yet such infected cells escape immunologic surveillance. The decrease of viral antigens expressed on the cell surface may be a function of a virus itself, perhaps by deleting that part of its genome that codes for the viral glycoproteins normally inserted and expressed on the cell's surface. Alternatively, the decrease in viral antigens expressed on the cell's surface may be a function of antibody. In this instance specific antiviral antibody binds to viral antigens on the cell's surface and strips such antigens off the plasma membrane. The second point in the hypothesis is that an infected cell devoid of viral antigens on its surface and escaping immune surveillance continues to replicate viral polypeptides, which may lead to dysfunction in the cell's biology or physiology. Inherent in this hypothesis are the notions that persistent virus infections occurring ordinarily in nature stem from noncytopathic rather than lytic viruses and that the related injury is caused, in part, by dysfunction of a differentiated cell. That is, persistent virus infection in a neuronal cell may alter its transmission and synaptic abilities; persistent infection of hormonal cells may decrease the amount of hormone made by that cell, or persistent infection of an immunocompetent lymphocyte may enhance or decrease its immunoglobulin synthesis or cytotoxic T cell activity. Further, the differentiated cell is altered physiologically without being destroyed or killed. Immune-mediated tissue injury accompanying persistent virus infection is often indirect in that viral antigens or virions are released which then elicit immune responses and cause formation of virus-antibody immune complexes, the deposition of which leads to tissue damage. The remainder of this chapter describes our work done with several colleagues over a number of years that provides the framework for the concepts cited above. Other mechanisms whereby viruses can persist and cause tissue injury do exist but are not included in this presentation.

Measles Virus: Structural Organization of Viral Polypeptides on the Surfaces of Infected Cells and Their Relationship to the Major Histocompatibility Complex

Measles virus is an RNA negative strand virus. Its natural host is man, and the virus most often causes an acute childhood illness. Infrequently measles virus causes a hyperallergic encephalitis and rarely a persistent infection called SSPE. Because SSPE combines both measles virus persistence and a vigorous host immune response, it provides a naturally occurring model for questioning how a virus can withstand immune attack.

Measles virus, per se, does not significantly shut off host-cell protein synthesis. Cell death actually results from fusion of cell membranes causing formation of giant cells and syncytia. These events are documented by the observation that removal of the fusion protein (F), one of the two viral structural glycoproteins expressed on the cell's surface, during infection prevents cell-cell fusion, cellular injury and death. In fact, cells devoid of F protein and viral hemagglutinin (HA) survive for prolonged periods in culture.

Measles virus codes six polypeptides. Of these, only the HA and F protein are found on the surfaces of infected cells; both proteins are glycosylated. HA is present on the cell surface as a dimer of 160,000 molecular weight and under reducing conditions migrates as a monomer. The F polypeptide is expressed on the cell surface as F0, denoting two disulfide-linked polypeptides, F1 (42,000 MW) and F2 (24,000 MW). One sees the F1 and F2 forms when studying the proteins under reducing conditions and finds most of this protein's carbohydrate in the F2 fragment, not in F1. The one-half turnover time for HA is nine hours and for F0 is ten hours during the course of normal infection. The remaining four polypeptides are a replicative complex composed of an L protein with a molecular weight of approximately 160,000, a phosphoprotein (P) with a molecular weight of 70,000 and a nucleocapsid protein (NC) with a molecular weight of 60,000. This replicative complex aligns under the inside of the plasma membrane by seeking the membrane or matrix (M) protein, which has a molecular weight of 36,000. All six of these polypeptides contain tyrosine and methionine residues, so they can be labled with ^{125}I and ^{35}S, respectively. Only the P, NC and M are phosphorylated viral polypeptides, and they can be labeled with ^{32}P. The polypeptides of measles virus and their mutual relationships are depicted in Figures 2, 3 and 4A, and described in Fujinami et al [5, 6].

Genes of the major histocompatibility complex code the histocompatibility antigens and also control immune responses to certain antigens. The human histocompatibility (HLA) antigens are major glycoprotein components of the plasma membrane and as such are clearly definable. When one maps HLA antigens and measles viral glycoproteins expressed on cells' plasma membranes to determine their relationship, the HLA antigens are functionally and structurally distinct from both of these measles virus glycoproteins. Moreover, these antigens cap totally independently of one another. The distinct relationship of HLA being segregated from measles virus glycoproteins is demonstrated in Figure 4B and C by Haspel et al [7].

Interaction of Antiviral Antibody with Measles Virus Antigens on the Surfaces of Infected Cells: Acute Interaction

According to the Singer-Nicholson hypothesis [8], most cell membranes have a fluid mosaic structure; their surface proteins

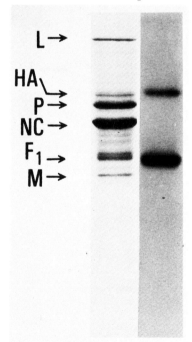

FIG. 2. The polypeptides of measles virus. The gel on the left represents viral polypeptides in the cytoplasms of infected cells as detected by ^{35}S-methionine labeling. The gel on the right represents the viral polypeptides detected with ^{125}I and restricted to the cell's surface (HA and F1). Gels run under reducing conditions. See text for details and references 5 and 6.

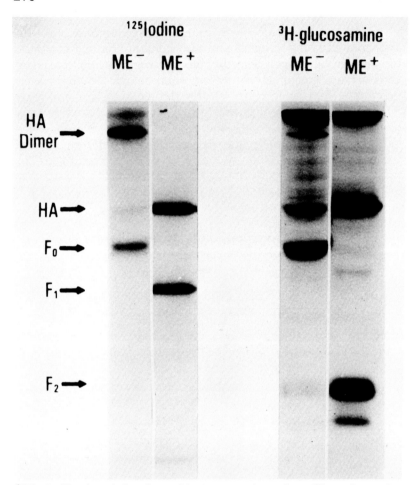

FIG. 3. Measles viral polypeptides expressed on the cell's surface using nonreduced (ME⁻) and reduced conditions (ME⁺). Note the viral hemagglutinin (HA) is a dimer and becomes reduced to a monomer, while the F0 is reduced to F1 and F2 fragments. See text and references 5 and 6 for details.

are free to diffuse in a lipid matrix and assume a random distribution over the cell's surface. Support for this hypothesis derives from several studies, including that describing the redistribution of viral antigens on a cell's surface caused by specific antiviral antibodies. In culture, measles virus antigens on the surfaces of infected cells are redistributed (capped) by antibodies specific for measles virus, but only multivalent

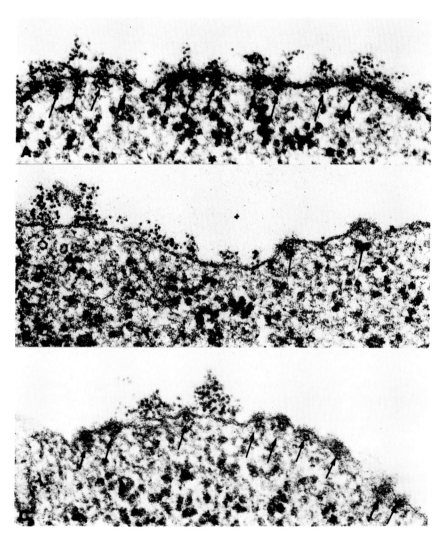

FIG. 4. Relationship of measles viral glycoproteins expressed on the cell's surface to other measles viral polypeptides inside the cell and to the major histocompatibility antigens (HLA). Panel A relates the viral glycoproteins (HA and F) to the viral nucleocapsid (arrows). Viral glycoproteins expressed on the surface of human lymphoblastoid cell RPMI-8866 are marked by ferritin-labeled antibodies against measles virus glycoproteins. Panels B and C relate viral glycoprotein (unmarked fuzz above NC) and NC (arrows) to HLA in RPMI-8866 (panel B) and WI-L2 (Panel C) human lymphoblastoid cells. In Panels B and C ferritin-labeled antibodies to HLA are used. See reference 7 for experimental details.

antibody is effective; univalent antibody is not. In these studies of a human cell line, a virus pathogenic for humans and a human antibody source, capping proceeded most efficiently at $37°C$, indicating that these events observed in vitro could also occur in vivo. In addition, capping is dependent on active cell metabolism. Capping of measles virus antigens is inhibited with oligomycin D, vinblastine sulfate, colchicine or cytocholasine B, suggesting that the production of ATP and the functions of microfilaments and microtubules are involved in the capping process [9]. Additional studies, in which immunoelectron microscopy [10] and radiolabeled antibodies [11] were used to follow the fate of virus-antibody complexes formed on the plasma membrane, strongly support the notion that these complexes are usually stripped and shed from the cell surface but only infrequently are endocytosed.

Interaction of Antiviral Antibody with Measles Virus Antigens on the Surfaces of Infected Cells: Prolonged Interactions

Antibody to measles virus removes measles virus antigens from the surfaces of infected cells not only during acute infection but also during persistent infection. In both instances, the expression of viral antigens diminishes notably by 6 hours and greatly by 12 hours after continuous exposure to measles virus antibodies. This stripping or removal of viral antigens from the cell surface has been termed antibody-induced modulation. Modulation of surface measles virus antigens can be completely reversible. For example, measles virus antigens are reexpressed on the cell's surface within 24 hours of removing antibody from the medium. However, when infected cells are cultured for prolonged periods in antimeasles virus antibody, modulation results in a population of cells devoid of surface measles virus antigens [12]. As exposure to antiviral antibody lengthens, the rate at which measles virus antigens return to the cell's surface is extended once the antibody is removed. Thus, after one day's incubation with antiviral antibody, viral antigens reappear on 50% of the cells within 24 hours. In contrast, after five days' incubation, six days pass before surface viral antigens are detected on 50% of the cells, and after six weeks of culture with antibody, it is difficult to detect any viral antigens on the cell surface after removing the antibody [12].

Three major biological events occur as a result of antibody-induced modulation of measles virus antigens. First, infected cells that are cultured in the presence of anti-measles virus antibodies survive and grow as efficiently and at the same rate as uninfected cultured cells. Thus, removal of the surface viral glycoproteins, specifically the F protein, prevents cell-to-cell fusion, and despite its continuing replication of measles virus polypeptides, the infected cell survives and grows as well as an uninfected cell. Second, the distribution of viral polypeptides, as studied by light and transmission electron microscopy, is altered during antibody-induced modulation. As noted in Figure 5, one sees little if any virus budding from the plasma

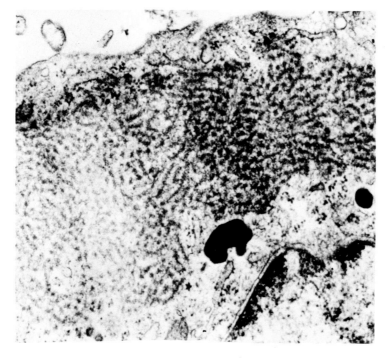

FIG. 5. The result of culturing measles virus-infected cells with anti-measles virus antibodies. Packed nucleocapsids are arranged at random in the cytoplasm and fail to align properly under the plasma membrane. Further, there is no expression of viral glycoproteins on the cell's surface (compare with Fig. 4). This picture, the result of antiviral antibody-induced modulation of measles virus-infected HeLa cells in vitro, closely resembles the picture of neuron cells seen from biopsied materials obtained from patients with chronic measles virus infection (SSPE).

membrane; yet the increased number of NC is misaligned and disarrayed in the cytoplasm. It is useful to recall that the electron micrograph in Figure 5, which was obtained by culturing measles virus-infected cells with anti-measles virus antibody, is identical to those from biopsied tissues of patients with chronic measles virus infection (SSPE). The patients' cells expressed no measles polypeptides on the surfaces; yet the number of viral NC in the cytoplasms increased dramatically. The NCs were arrayed randomly and were disoriented in relation to the inner plasma membrane.

The third important biological consequence of antibody-induced modulation is that, as their surface measles virus antigens are stripped, the virus-infected cells are no longer lysed by either antibody and complement or cytotoxic lymphocytes. Hence, the ability either of antibody and complement or of cytotoxic lymphocytes to kill measles virus-infected cells directly parallels the quantity of viral antigens expressed on the cells' surfaces. Under modulating conditions in which measles virus antigens are stripped off the cell surface, these infected cells resist immune lysis (Fig. 6). Upon removal of antibodies from the culture medium, these cells reexpress their viral antigens and are again subject to immune destruction.

But what molecular events occur during antibody-induced antigenic modulation? Robert Fujinami, currently working in my laboratory, has addressed this question. We noted that 6 hours after measles virus antibodies bound at the surfaces of cells infected with measles virus, the expression of the external polypeptide F1, as well as internal polypeptides P and M, was altered (Figs. 7 and 8). The decreases in F1, P and M viral polypeptides were specific, since only antibodies directed against the measles virus antigens expressed on the cell's surface caused the effect, not antibodies directed against nonviral surface antigens [5, 12]. The loss of F1 molecules early during antibody-induced antigenic modulation explains the lack of cell-cell fusion and giant cell formation and the survival of infected cells. The associated loss of HA molecules in conjunction with F1 molecules accounts for the resistance of virus-infected cells to immunologic assault by humoral and cell-mediated reactants. Additionally, since the P molecules or their analogs in other viral systems seem to be associated with the transcriptive complex, whereas the M proteins are associated

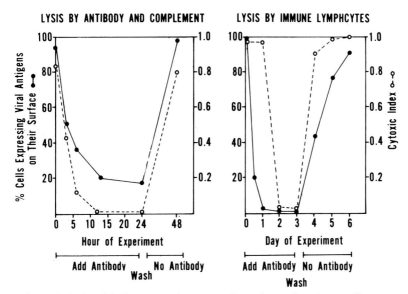

FIG. 6. Relationship between the expression of measles virus antigens on the cell's surface and the ability of cytotoxic antibody and complement or cytotoxic lymphocytes to lyse infected cells. Antibody-induced stripping of measles virus antigens off the surface of infected cells. *Left panel*: Alteration of surface expression of measles virus antigens (●———●) and the ability of measles virus antibody and complement (○— — —○) to specifically lyse persistently infected cells. *Right panel*: Alteration of surface expression of measles virus antigens (●———●) and the ability of immune lymphocytes (○— — —○) to specifically lyse persistently infected cells.

with nucleocapsid recognition and alignment at the plasma membrane, alterations in these polypeptides might well lead to aberrations in measles virus synthesis and maturation that are the hallmarks of persistent measles virus infections.

A schematic drawing of events occurring in antibody-induced antigenic modulation during measles virus infection appears in Figure 9.

Overview and Concepts of Antibody-Induced Antigenic Modulation

The loss of a specific antigen on the surfaces of cells cultured with their respective antibody was first observed by Boyse et al and termed antigenic modulation [reviewed in 13].

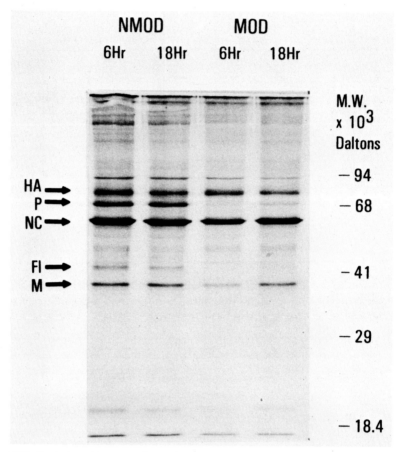

FIG. 7. Autoradiogram of measles virus polypeptides from nonmodulated (NMod) or modulated (Mod) infected cells. Cells were incubated in the absence or presence of measles virus antibody for 6 or 18 hours and then pulse-labeled with ^{35}S-methionine for two hours. Normal concentrations of P protein and F1 (fusion protein) are decreased in antibody-treated cells. Viral polypeptides are HA, hemagglutinin; P, phosphoprotein; NC, nucleocapsid; F1, fusion or hemolysin; and M, matrix or membrane proteins. See references 5 and 17 for details.

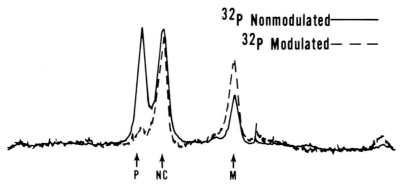

FIG. 8. Fate of measles virus phosphoproteins during antibody-induced measles virus antigen modulation. Cells infected with measles virus were incubated in the presence or absence of antibody to measles virus. Cells were pulse-labeled with ^{32}P. The ordinate represents the relative density and the abscissa, the relative migration. The three phosphorylated measles virus polypeptides seen are phosphoprotein (P), nucleocapsid (NC) and matrix or membrane protein (M). ——— = ^{32}P nonmodulated; — — — = ^{32}P modulated. See references 5 and 17 for details

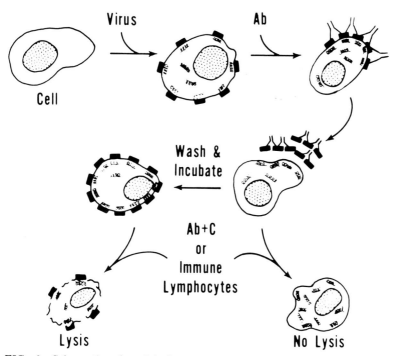

FIG. 9. Schematic of antiviral antibody-induced redistribution, capping and shedding of viral antigens off the surface of an infected cell. As long as antiviral antibody (Ab) is present, then viral antigens are not reexpressed on the cell's surface and the infected cell resists immune attack. When Ab is removed from the culture fluids, viral antigens are reexpressed and immune lysis ensues. See text for discussion.

In working with the differentiation antigen TL on normal thymus cells and leukemia cells, they noted that the phenotypic expression of TL was suppressed by TL antibodies both in vivo and in vitro. Since then, several investigators have studied a variety of retroviruses and shown comparable results [reviewed in 13]. As with the evidence for antibody-induced modulation of measles virus-infected cells presented above, others have suggested similar mechanisms for persistent herpes virus and hepatitis B virus infections. In general, antibody-induced antigenic modulation of virus-infected cells requires that the virus per se does not interfere significantly with host protein synthesis.

How well does antibody-induced antigenic modulation account for the events of persistent measles virus infection? Measles virus infection in humans usually follows an acute, self-limiting course as the patient mounts an immune response that clears the virus from his tissues. Convalescence is associated with low titers of antibody to measles virus and immune lymphocytes that remain throughout life. In contrast, in the rare instance of chronic measles virus infection, represented by SSPE, patients have high titers of anti-measles virus antibodies and effective cytotoxic lymphocytes; yet virus persists. Although the virus can be isolated from the cells of their central nervous systems and lymphoid tissues, antibody titers are simultaneously 100- to 1000-fold above normal in their sera and other body fluids; the complement system is functionally active, and cytotoxic lymphocytes present in the peripheral blood are fully effective in killing measles virus-infected targets in vitro. Experimental evidence indicates that antibody to measles virus strips viral antigens off the surface of virus-infected cells, that these cells express less viral antigens on their surfaces and thereby avoid immune lysis by humoral antibodies or cytotoxic lymphocytes. Hence, cells denuded of viral antigens escape immunologic assault but retain viral genetic information. The viral nucleocapsids accumulated inside the cells rise dramatically in number and assume a random arrangement, in vitro, resembling the scattered nucleocapsids in cells from patients with SSPE and contrasting with the rigid alignment in virus-infected cells in acute infection. Further, there are a variety of in vivo experiments indicating that antibody actually initiates virus persistence. For example,

Albrecht et al [14] showed that measles virus or SSPE virus inoculated into monkeys did not result in virus persistence unless the monkeys already had antibody to measles virus. Recently McFarland and his associates at the NIH (personal communication) used monoclonal antibody to measles virus HA to initiate a persistent infection in mice much the same way as Albrecht did. Similar findings were noted in mother hamsters immune to measles virus and nursing infected newborns [15].

Concept of Alteration of Differentiated or Luxury Functions as a Mechanism of Cellular Injury During Persistent Virus Infection

Of the many possible interactions between a virus and a cell that it infects, the outcome is largely determined by the susceptibility of the cell and the virulence of the virus concerned. Lethal cellular damage may be caused by products of a viral genome or by the cell's regulatory mechanisms. Viral-coated proteins may shut down host protein and RNA synthesis, and the result is cell death. In other instances, large numbers of viral macromolecules accumulate within cells late in the infectious cycle, and some of these products may be toxic to the cell. Viral proteins or virions may also distort cells, cause substantial swelling and probably alter membrane permeability so that subsequent leakage of lysosomal enzymes can engender autolytic digestion of the infected cells. Usually these are the activities of cytopathic viruses. In contrast, noncytopathic viruses can cause long-lasting, relatively nonpathogenic states in which cells frequently show normal growth rates and cloning efficiencies. However, the question remains as to what happens to the differentiated or luxury function of cells that are infected with noncytopathic viruses when viral polypeptides are made continuously and accumulate inside the cells.

We have noted that a relatively noncytopathic virus, LCMV, infects neuroblastoma cells, causes persistent infection and alters their specialized (luxury) function without affecting their vital functions [16]. Hence, during persistent LCMV infection of murine neuroblastoma cells, the cells' content of choline acetyltransferase and acetylcholine esterase dropped significantly. These are the enzymes that synthesize or break down acetylcholine, the major neurotransmitter. Cloning experiments showed that the loss of choline acetyltransferase and acetyl-choline esterase occurred in the majority of LCMV-infected neuroblastoma cells, not just a specific subpopulation. Nevertheless, these cells remained normal in growth rate, protein synthesis and RNA synthesis. Thus, the cells' luxury function was dampened without altering their vital functions. These persistently infected neuroblastoma cells have been cultured continuously for over six years and have maintained their deficiency in differentiated function. Certain viruses show unique tropisms for differentiated cells that make hormones (insulin, thyroid and growth hormone), cells of the immune system (thymus cells, B and T lymphocytes, macrophages) and oligodendrocytes, the cental nervous system cell responsible for production of myelin. It is the interest and task of our next several years of observations to determine whether these viruses may persist in such differentiated cells and alter their luxury functions, with the final result being disease states such as diabetes, autoimmunity, immunodeficiency or demyelination.

Acknowledgments

The work described here represents contributions by investigators in the viral immunobiology unit over the last several years. In particular the author would like to acknowledge the past input of Luc Perrin, Martin Haspel, Michael Doyle, Raymond Welsh and Patrick Sissons, and the continuing input of Robert Fujinami, Michael Buchmeier, John Huddlestone, Paolo Casali, Frank Dutko, Bengt Harfast, Robert Knobler, Peter Lampert and Antoinette Tishon in this work.

References

1. Oldstone, M.B.A. and Dixon, F.J.: Lymphocytic choriomeningitis: Production of anti-LCM antibody by "tolerant" LCM-infected mice. Science 158:1193-1194, 1967.
2. Oldstone, M.B.A. and Dixon, F.J.: Pathogenesis of chronic disease associated with persistent lymphocytic choriomeningitis viral infection. I. Relationship of antibody production to disease in neonatally infected mice. J. Exp. Med. 129:483-505, 1969.
3. Oldstone, M.B.A.: Virus neutralization and virus-induced immune complex disease: Virus-antibody union resulting in immunoprotection or immunologic injury — Two different sides of the same coin. In Melnick, J.L. (ed.): Progress in Medical Virology. Basel:S. Karger, 1975, vol. 19, pp. 84-119.

4. Buchmeier, M.J. and Oldstone, M.B.A.: Virus-induced immune complex disease: Identification of specific viral antigens and antibodies deposited in complexes during chronic lymphocytic choriomeningitis virus infection. J. Immunol. 120:1297-1304, 1978.

5. Fujinami, R.S. and Oldstone, M.B.A.: Alterations in expression of measles virus polypeptides by antibody: Molecular events in antibody-induced antigenic modulation. J. Immunol. 125:78-85, 1980.

6. Fujinami, R.S., Sissons, J.G.P. and Oldstone, M.B.A.: Characterization and turnover of measles virus polypeptides expressed on the surface of infected cells. J. Immunol. (Submitted, 1980.)

7. Haspel, M.V., Pellegrino, M.A., Lampert, P.W. and Oldstone, M.B.A.: Human histocompatibility determinants and virus antigens: Effect of measles virus infection on HLA expression. J. Exp. Med. 146:146-156, 1977.

8. Singer, S.J. and Nicholson, G.L.: The fluid mosaic model of the structure of cell membranes. Science 175:720-731, 1972.

9. Joseph, B.S. and Oldstone, M.B.A.: Antibody induced redistribution of measles virus antigens on the cell surface. J. Immunol. 113:1205-1209, 1974.

10. Lampert, P.W., Joseph, B.S. and Oldstone, M.B.A.: Antibody-induced capping of measles virus antigens on plasma membranes studied by electron microscopy. J. Virol. 15:1248-1255, 1975.

11. Perrin, L.H. and Oldstone, M.B.A.: The formation and fate of virus antigen-antibody complexes. J. Immunol. 118:316-322, 1977.

12. Joseph, B.S. and Oldstone, M.B.A.: Immunologic injury in measles virus infection. II. Suppression of immune injury through antigenic modulation. J. Exp. Med. 142:864-876, 1975.

13. Oldstone, M.B.A., Fujinami, R.S. and Lampert, P.W.: Membrane and cytoplasmic changes in virus infected cells induced by interactions of antiviral antibody with surface viral antigens. In Melnick, J.L. (ed.): Progress in Medical Virology. Basel:S. Karger, 1980, vol. 26, pp. 45-93.

14. Albrecht, P., Burnstein, T., Klutch, M. et al: Subacute sclerosing panencephalitis: Experimental infection in primates. Science 195:64-66, 1977.

15. Weir, D. and Rapp, F.: Latent measles virus infection of the hamster central nervous system. J. Immunol. 107:1593-1598, 1974.

16. Oldstone, M.B.A., Holmstoen, J. and Welsh, R.M., Jr.: Alterations of acetylcholine enzymes in neuroblastoma cells persistently infected with lymphocytic choriomeningitis virus. J. Cell. Physiol. 91:459-472, 1977.

17. Fujinami, R.S. and Oldstone, M.B.A.: Antiviral antibody reacting on the plasma membrane alters measles virus expression inside the cell. Nature 279:529-530, 1979.

Immunopathology of Protozoan Diseases

P. H. Lambert, M.D. and L. M. Rose, Ph.D.

During the last 20 years, more research has been done on the pathogenesis of rare autoimmune diseases than on the immunology of major protozoan diseases such as malaria or trypanosomiasis. However, recent estimations indicate that about 800 million people are affected by malaria and approximately 1 million African children die each year of that disease. Similarly, other protozoan infections, due to trypanosomes, leishmania or amoebae, have a considerable impact on the population in many developing countries. Therefore, there is without doubt a need to improve understanding of the pathogenesis of these diseases and to increase our efforts toward the development of potential vaccines against these infections.

In this review, we will consider some of the major immunopathological features of protozoan infections. We will refer particularly to some of our recent observations, made in man and mice infected with trypanosomiasis or malaria, which emphasize the role of the immune response of the host in the expression of the parasitic disease and the effects of the parasite itself on the host immune system.

Role of the Host Immune Response in the Pathological Expression of Protozoan Infection

Several mechanisms can be involved in the expression of a protozoan infection. The persistence of parasites in blood (e.g.

P. H. Lambert, M.D., Head, WHO Immunology Research and Training Center, Geneva/Lausanne; and L. M. Rose, Ph.D., Research Fellow, WHO Immunology Research and Training Center, Geneva, Switzerland.

This work has been supported by WHO, by the World Bank, UNDP, WHO Special Programme for Research and Training in Tropical Diseases and by the Swiss National Foundation (Grant No. 3.908.0.80).

malaria, African trypanosomes) or their localization in some tissues (e.g. *Trypanosoma cruzi* in myocardial cells or *Trypanosoma gambiense* in cerebral intertitium) represents an important source of antigens. Some of these antigens can be released from living parasites while others, only from disrupted parasites. The reaction of parasite antigens with corresponding antibodies leads to the generation of immune complexes, locally or in the general circulation, and to local or diffuse manifestations of immune complex diseases (e.g. malaria, trypanosomiasis). Immunopathology can also be due to antibody-dependent cell-mediated inflammation or to T cell-dependent inflammation (e.g. leishmaniasis). In some instances, parasite antigens which have common determinants with host proteins may induce an autoimmune response (e.g. anti-myocardial response in *T. cruzi* infections).

In mice infected with *Trypanosoma brucei*, features of both diffuse and localized immune complex lesions have been observed [1, 2]. The infection is characterized by waves of parasitemia which reflect the sequential appearance of antigenic variants of the parasite. Surface antigens are thus chronically released in the surrounding medium. Circulating immune complexes are detected in large amounts (Fig. 1) and there is a deposition of immune complexes in renal glomeruli. Trypanosomes also invade the extravascular compartment and particularly striated muscles. They can be seen in foci in the interstitial spaces in association with inflammatory cells and in the presence of immunoglobulin deposits. The lesions can progress to muscle necrosis. The development of tissue lesions in mice infected with *T. brucei* seems to be directly dependent on the host's immune response. Indeed, the infection of nude athymic BALB/c or irradiated (400 rads) or newborn mice does not lead to a similar pathological expression although there is an extensive parasite proliferation. The transfer of immunoglobulin from immunized BALB/c mice into infected nude mice triggers the development of Arthus-like inflammatory foci in striated muscles. However, in the same model, the transfer of syngeneic spleen cells or of purified T cells fully reconstitutes the lesions, as seen in infected normothymic mice [2]. These results highly suggest that associated lesions are due to the immune response of the host against parasite antigens and not to any direct pathogenic effect of the parasite itself.

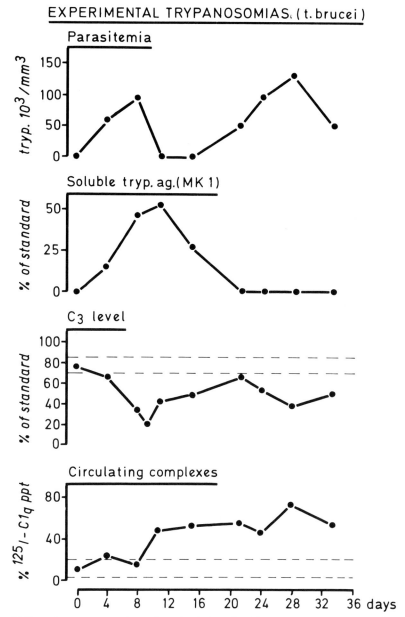

FIG. 1. Immune complexes in mice infected with *Trypanosoma brucei*. This graph shows a follow-up study of the parasitemia, the serum level of soluble variant trypanosome antigen (MK 1), the C3 level and the C1q binding activity.

In African trypanosomiasis, the invasion of the central nervous system (CNS) by parasites may also be favored by immune mechanisms. During the early stages of the disease, when mice are infected with *Trypanosoma brucei*, parasites proliferate in the blood, but are not found in the choroid plexus or in the meninges [3]. After three to four weeks, there is a simultaneous appearance of circulating immune complexes and, as seen by electron microscopy, of dense deposits within the capillary basement membrane of the choroid plexus. Trypanosomes then move across these capillaries and localize in the choroid plexus interstitium. At that stage, immunoglobulin deposits and electron-dense deposits can be demonstrated in the subependymal area. Later, the parasites cross the blood-brain barrier and move to the minenges.

In man, the invasion of the CNS by parasites is also a feature of African trypanosomiasis. The appearance of parasites in the cerebrospinal fluid (CSF) is associated with only moderate changes of the function of the blood-brain barrier, but with a marked elevation of the CSF immunoglobulin concentration [4]. This has been shown to reflect an intense intracerebral synthesis of immunoglobulins, comparable to that observed in subacute sclerosing encephalitis (Table 1). There is evidence that antibodies to trypanosome antigens and, occasionally, antibodies to neuron antigens are locally produced in the CNS. This local immune response may also account for the generation of immune complexes in the CSF. Indeed, immune complexes have been

Table 1. Human Trypanosomiasis

Stage	n	Intracerebral Synthesis of	
		IgG*	IgM
I†	3	− 5.3	0
II	3	+ 0.8	+ 3.0
III	10	+11.1	+10.5
Controls (Afr.)‡	9	− 0.9	0

*mg/100 ml CSF.
†Stages of the disease: I = hemolymphatic, II = Trypanosomes in CSF, III = encephalitis.
‡Hospitalized African patients.

detected in most CSF samples from patients at the encephalitic stage of trypanosomiasis (Fig. 2). Paired CSF-serum analysis indicates a local formation of immune complexes in CSF rather than their diffusion from serum to CSF [4].

In malaria, several immunopathological features have been recognized as important manifestations of the disease. Renal lesions occur during acute *Plasmodium falciparum* infection and in assocation with chronic *P. malariae* infections. They are characterized by a deposition of immune complexes in glomeruli, in which parasite antigens have been frequently identified [5]. Cerebral manifestations which are a major complication of acute *falciparum* malaria also appear as immunologically mediated. They are due to a plugging of cerebral vessels by heavily infected erythrocytes, to cerebral edema and to hemorrhagic foci. The le-

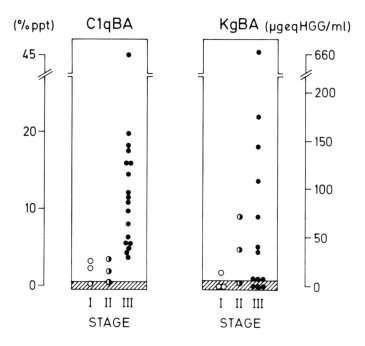

FIG. 2. Immune complexes in cerebrospinal fluid from patients with African trypanosomiasis. The complexes are measured either with a C1q binding assay (C1qBA) or with a conglutinin binding assay (KGBA). Stages are described in Table 1.

Table 2. Mouse Malaria

	Parasitemia	Cerebral Lesions	Mortality
Nu/Nu	++	0	±
Nu/+	+++	++	+++

sions do not develop in thymectomized hamsters [6] nor in nude, athymic mice (Table 2) [7, 8]. It has also been suggested that the malaria-associated hemolytic anemia is not due primarily to the invasion of erythrocytes by plasmodia but may be caused by immune complexes or by autoimmune reactions [9].

Effects of the Parasite on the Host Immune System

Many protozoan infections are known to trigger a polyclonal B cell activation and to induce immunosuppression. In mice or in man infected with trypanosomes, there is an intense activation of the B cell compartment. Mice infected with *Trypanosoma brucei* show a dramatic increase of the spleen B lymphocyte population [10] which is paralleled by a broad expression of the B cell repertoire including anti-hapten antibody-producing cells. In man, there is also a marked increase of immunoglobulin levels (IgM up to 25 mg/ml). A full expression of the B cell repertoire is reflected by the appearance of antibodies against haptens (DNP, FITC, PC, PEN), against proteins (KLH, ovalbumin, tetanus toxoid) and against autoantigens. Indeed, patients with African trypanosomiasis develop antibodies against single-stranded DNA, against IgG (RF-like), against human erythrocytes and against striated and smooth muscle. The level of rheumatoid factor is closely correlated with the IgM and seems to directly reflect the degree of polyclonal activation in individual patients.

Two *indirect consequences of polyclonal B cell activation* are (a) the nonspecific induction of immune complexes, and (b) the perturbation of idiotypic interactions. The high levels of circulating immune complexes observed in human African trypanosomiasis [4] are closely correlated with the immunoglobulin and particularly the IgM levels (Fig. 3). A similar

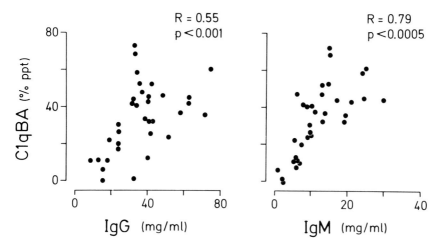

FIG. 3. Circulating immune complexes in African trypanosomiasis: correlation with the serum immunoglobulin levels.

situation exists in disseminated leishmaniasis. Immune complexes have been purified from such sera [12] and were shown to contain little or no parasite antigens, while the major constituents were 7S and 19S anti-immunoglobulin antibodies. The importance of polyclonal activation in this phenomenom has been suggested by the demonstration of immune complexes and anti-immunoglobulin antibodies in mice which were injected with LPS or dextran sulfate or PPD or poly-I-poly-C [13].

Polyclonal B cell activation during trypanosomiasis also leads to a perturbation of the idiotypic network. Indeed, it has been shown, in experimental models, that BALB/c mice infected with *Trypanosoma brucei* develop *simultaneously* anti-phosphorylcholine (PC) antibodies bearing the T15 idiotype and corresponding anti-idiotype antibodies (anti-T15) (Fig. 4). In parallel, circulating immune complexes are detected which contain anti-T15 antibodies [14]. Therefore, the full expression of the B cell repertoire is clearly associated with an increased level of interactions between complementary idiotypic and anti-idiotypic determinants. Such perturbations of the idiotypic network may play a role in the generation of immune complexes but may also be involved in the immunosuppressive effects of protozoan infections.

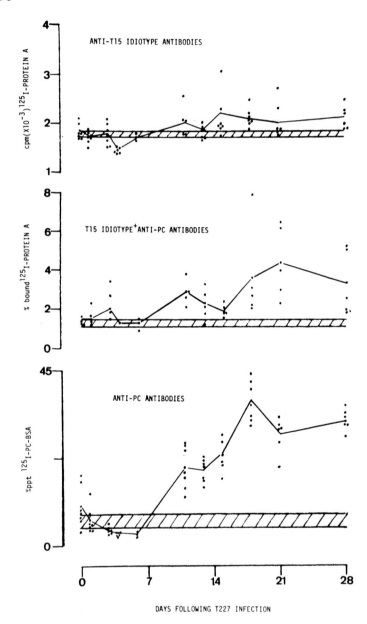

DAYS FOLLOWING T227 INFECTION

FIG. 4. Perturbation of the idiotypic network in African trypanosomiasis: simultaneous increase of (T15 +) anti-phosphorylcholine antibodies and of anti-T15 idiotype antibodies during polyclonal B cell activation.

References

1. Lambert, P.H. and Houba, V.: Immune complexes in parasitic diseases. *In* Brent, L. and Holborow, J. (eds.): Progress in Immunology. Amsterdam: North-Holland, 1974, vol. 5, p. 57.

2. Galvao-Castro, B., Hochmann, A. and Lambert, P.H.: The role of the host immune response in the development of tissue lesions associated with African trypanosomiasis in mice. Clin. Exp. Immunol. 33:12, 1978.

3. Poltera, A.A., Hochmann, A., Rudin, W. and Lambert, P.H.: Trypanosoma brucei: A model for cerebral trypanosomiasis in mice. Clin. Exp. Immunol. 40:496, 1980.

4. Lambert, P.H., Berney, M. and Kazyumba, L.: Immune complexes in serum and cerebrospinal fluid in African trypanosomiasis. J. Clin. Invest. (In press.)

5. Houba, V., Lambert, P.H., Mackey, L. and Miescher, P.A.: Immunopathology of malaria. Springer Semin. Immunopathol. 2:359, 1980.

6. Wright, D.H.: The effect of neonatal thymectomy on the survival of golden hamsters infected with Plasmodium berghei. Br. J. Exp. Pathol. 49:379, 1968.

7. Mackey, L., Hochmann, A., June C.H., et al: Immunopathological aspects of Plasmodium berghei infection in five strains of mice. Clin. Exp. Immunol. 42:412, 1980.

8. Finley, R., Mackey, L., Hochmann, A. and Lambert, P.H.: Features of malaria immunopathology in nude mice. (In preparation.)

9. Woodruf, A.W., Ansdell, V.E. and Pettitt, L.E.: Cause of anemia in malaria. Lancet 1:1055, 1979.

10. Kobayakawa, T., Louis, J., Izui, S. and Lambert, P.H.: Autoimmune response to DNA, red blood cells and thymocyte antigens in association with polyclonal antibody synthesis during experimental African trypanosomiasis. J. Immunol. 122:296, 1979.

11. Lambert, P.H., Berney, M., Kazyumba, L. and Brighouse, G.: Autoimmunity and expression of the V gene repertoire during human African trypanosomiasis. (In preparation.)

12. Casali, P. and Lambert, P.H.: Purification of soluble immune complexes from serum using PMMA beads coated with conglutinin or C1q. Clin. Exp. Immunol. 37:295, 1979.

13. Ramos-Niembro, F. and Lambert, P.H.: The generation of immune complexes during polyclonal B cell activation. (In press.)

14. Rose, L., Goldman, M. and Lambert, P.H.: Perturbation of idiotypic interactions during African trypanosomiasis. (In preparation.)

Biological Significance of Human Melanoma-Associated Antigens Defined by Xenoantisera

A. C. Morgan, Jr., Ph.D. and R. A. Reisfeld, Ph.D.

Introduction

The quest for tumor-specific antigens on human tumors has encompassed almost four decades of intensive investigations. The advent of hybridoma technology has greatly facilitated the identification and immunochemical characterization of a variety of cell surface molecules [1-3]. Our laboratory has focused on antigens shed into the culture medium of human melanoma cells. The emphasis placed on this approach was based on (1) our belief that shed molecules may be of particular importance in the elicitation and blockade of host immune responses, and (2) our data indicating spent culture medium to be a good source of soluble melanoma-associated antigens (MAA) for isolation and biochemical characterization.

Two tumor-specific glycoprotein components have, thus far, been identified in the spent culture medium of human tumor cells [4]. The first is a 240K dalton molecule shed by most human melanoma cell lines but not by various carcinoma and lymphoid cell lines. The second, a 94K dalton molecule, is shed by both melanoma and carcinoma cell lines but not by lymphoid cells [5]. Biochemical characterization of the 94K component isolated from spent culture medium of melanoma and carcinoma cells with

A.C. Morgan, Jr., Ph.D. and R.A. Reisfeld, Ph.D., Department of Molecular Immunology, Scripps Clinic and Research Foundation, La Jolla, Calif.

This is publication No. 2290 from Scripps Clinic and Research Foundation. This work was supported by grants AI 10180 and CA 28420 from the National Institutes of Health.

monoclonal antibody indicated that the 94K molecules from different tumor sources are virtually identical [6]. Information on the molecular characteristics of these tumor antigens becomes even more relevant when substantiated by data indicating their biological significance. Thus, we have directed our major efforts (1) to produce monoclonal antibodies for eventual use in radioimmunodetection and diagnosis, and (2) to establish the origin of these MAA and to determine their relation to transformation events. Results obtained in these research areas will be presented here and their implications for tumor biology will be discussed.

Production of Monoclonal Antibodies to MAA

Hybridoma antibodies represent reagents of unparalleled specificity when used for diagnosis and radioimmunodetection [7, 8] and possible therapy of tumors [9]. As a prerequisite for evaluating the usefulness of the 240K and 94K MAA in these areas, we have produced monoclonal antibodies using purified immunogens.

These immunogens were prepared from 4 M urea extracts of melanoma cells, depleted of fibronectin by adsorption with gelatin-Sepharose 4B and bound to *Lens culinaris* lectin-Sepharose 4B. The rationale for this approach was based on our previous experience in the production of rabbit anti-MAA xenoantisera that indicated a selective affinity of 240K MAA for *Lens culinaris* lectin [5, 10] and the need for removal of fibronectin, which is a dominant immunogen of tumor cells and their extracts [11]. Screening of hybridoma products was accomplished with a modified solid-phase RIA [12] that utilizes fibronectin-depleted, chemically defined, spent culture medium from melanoma cells as target antigen and polyclonal rabbit anti-mouse Ig and ^{125}I-SpA for detection of bound antibody. The assay was particularly suitable in screening for monoclonal antibodies to 240K because the chemically defined spent medium represents an enriched source of this antigen and is lacking in molecules common to lymphoid cells such as HLA-A,B and HLA-DR [12]. Polyethylene glycol-mediated fusion of antigen-sensitized mouse splenocytes and X63-AG8:653 mouse myeloma cells at a 1:1 ratio, as well as subsequent selection of hybridomas, was done according to previously established techniques [13].

The results of one screening of hybridoma supernates are shown in Figure 1. With an input of 1×10^5 cpm a maximum of 60% of ^{125}I-SpA was bound to hybridoma antibody, an amount more than 14-fold greater than background. Positive hybridomas were subsequently screened by indirect immunoprecipitation and SDS-PAGE, and those binding 240K antigen were cloned and subcloned. A typical SDS-PAGE profile of one such monoclonal antibody using ^{3}H-valine-labeled spent culture medium of melanoma cells is depicted in Figure 2B. Compared to the profile of spent culture medium immunoprecipitated with polyclonal antiserum to melanoma cells (Fig. 2A), the monoclonal antibody immunoprecipitated only a single component of 240K daltons. In addition, the monoclonal antibody bound only to melanoma cells when assayed against melanoma, carcinoma, lymphoid and fibroblast cell lines.

Thus, the efficacy of immobilized, purified MAA in the elicitation of monoclonal antibodies was clearly demonstrated. Furthermore, these techniques of immunization and screening were found more successful in yielding hybridomas to tumor-associated antigens than were procedures utilizing intact cells.

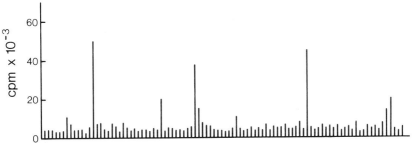

FIG. 1. Screening hybridomas to MAA by solid-phase RIA. Seventy-five microliters of hybridoma supernatant together with 25 μl of PBS + 20% chicken serum + 0.5% Tween 20 + 0.1% ovalbumin (PTOCS) is incubated in polyvinyl microtiter plates coated with 1 to 5 μg/well of fibronectin-depleted, chemically defined spent medium from M14 melanoma cells. After incubation of two hours at 4°C, plates are washed three times with PTO and then incubated with polyclonal rabbit anti-mouse Ig in PTOCS for one hour at 4°C. Plates are washed twice, 1×10^5 cpm/well of ^{125}I-SpA is added and incubation continued for an additional hour. After three further washes with PTO, wells are sliced out of the plates and counted.

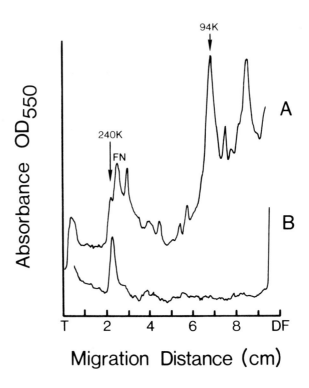

FIG. 2. Indirect immunoprecipitation with monoclonal antibody to 240K. Twenty microliters of Protein A Sepharose was incubated at 4°C for two hours with 5 μl of rabbit anti-mouse Ig. After washing twice with PTO, 100 μl of hybridoma 51.5 was added and incubation continued for two hours. The immunosorbent was washed twice and 1×10^6 cpm of ^{3}H-leucine-labeled spent medium from M14 melanoma cells was added. Following an overnight incubation at 4°C, the immunosorbent was washed four times, the last two washes without ovalbumin, and bound antigen was eluted by boiling for three minutes in the presence of 0.1 M Tris buffer, pH 6.8 with 2% 2-mercapethanol, 2% SDS, 10% glycerol and 0.001% bromophenol blue. After centrifugation, the supernate was electrophoresed on a 5% acrylamide, 0.135% bis-acrylamide slab gel.

Fetal Origin of the 94K Glycoprotein

Numerous reports of fetal antigen expression by human tumors [14-16] have given rise to a hypothesis of retrodifferentiation of neoplastic cells [17]. The availability of a cell strain of normal melanocytes derived from fetal uvea [18] allowed us to determine whether fetal and malignant melanocytes synthesize common molecules and to establish the immunochemical identity of any shared cellular products.

We first sought evidence indicating that this cell strain was of melanocyte origin. To this end, cultures were examined by transmission electron microscopy three to four days after reaching confluence. Numerous desmosomes (Fig. 3A) and melanosomes (Fig. 3B) were observed, indicative of the melanocytic origin of these cells. The melanocyte cultures were then metabolically labeled with ^{3}H-valine and ^{3}H-glucosamine and their spent culture medium and detergent lysates examined by indirect immunoprecipitation and SDS-PAGE, using both polyclonal and monoclonal antibody to MAA. Figure 4 shows the profiles of spent culture medium derived from ^{3}H-valine-labeled fetal melanocytes. SDS-PAGE analysis of indirect immunoprecipitates, obtained with polyclonal antisera to melanoma cells, revealed two major components of 200K and 90K (lane 1). The 200K component was identified as fibronectin by indirect immunoprecipitation with monospecific antiserum to plasma fibronectin. The 90K component in the spent medium of melanocytes was found serologically identical to the 94K molecule detected in the spent medium of melanoma cells since it was immunoprecipitated with hybridoma antibody 250/165, specific for this 94K antigen (lane 2). Both fibronectin and the 90K component of spent medium of melanocytes had apparent molecular weights that were lower than the equivalent molecules detected in spent medium of melanoma cells (lane 3). Furthermore, shedding of the 90K glycoprotein of melanocytes was selectively inhibited by tunicamycin, an inhibitor of N-asparagine-linked glycosylation, in a manner similar to that observed for the 94K antigen of melanoma cells [4]. The 90K glycoprotein was not found in spent medium of fetal fibroblasts or teratocarcinoma cells. In contrast to the 94K MAA, the 240K MAA was not detected in spent medium or cell extracts of fetal melanocytes. Thus, the 94K, but not the 240K MAA appears to be an oncofetal antigen expressed by cells of neural crest origin.

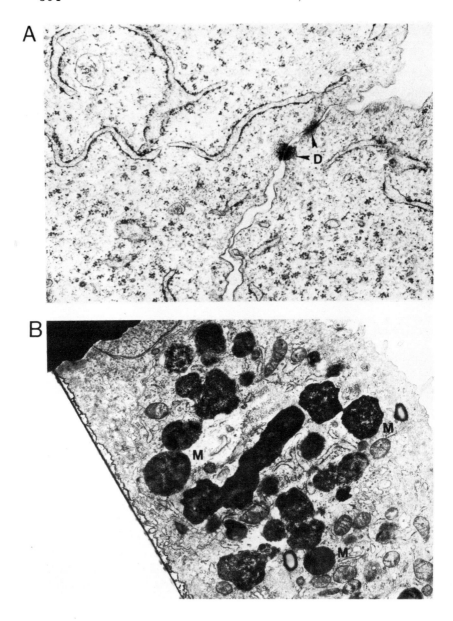

FIG. 3. Electromicrographs of FeMEL 79-4. Cells were examined three to four days after reaching confluence. Numerous desmosomes (A) (× 15,000) and melanosomes (B) (× 7000) were visible.

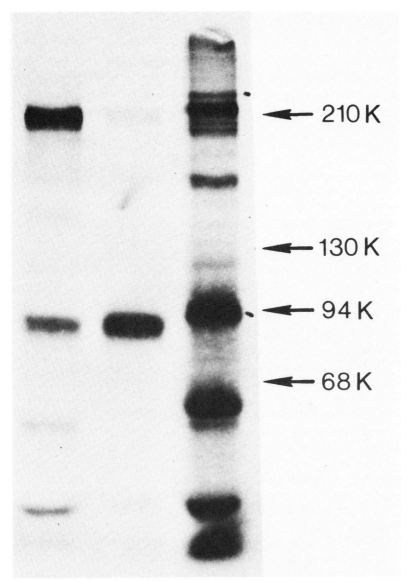

FIG. 4. Shedding of MAA by fetal melanocytes. SDS-PAGE autoradiograph of
³H-valine-labeled spent culture medium from FeMEL 79-4 (lanes 1 and 2) and
M14 melanoma cells (lane 3), immunoprecipitated with rabbit xenoantiserum to
melanoma cells #6522 (lanes 1 and 3) and hybridoma antibody 250/165 (lane 2).
Molecular weight markers used were human plasma fibronectin, β-galactosidase,
phosphorylase B, human serum albumin.

Changes in MAA Shedding Induced
by Tumor Promoters

As part of an investigation to establish the relation of MAA expression and shedding to transformation and differentiation, we studied the effects of tumor promoters on the shedding of glycoprotein from melanoma cells into their spent medium. Tumor promoters have a variety of effects on cells in vitro, including induction of ornithine decarboxylase [20, 21] and plasminogen activator [22], and can either induce or repress differentiation, depending on the type of cells studied [23]. Melanoma cells, when treated with phorbol esters, undergo differentiation with development of neurite-like processes and enhanced melanin production [24].

As a model system, we chose two melanoma cell lines, CAR #1 and CAR #2, derived from the same patient but at different stages of tumor progression [25]. These cell lines are practically identical in morphology and in expression of HLA-A,B and HLA-DR antigens. The antigen profile of spent media derived from intrinsically labeled (^{3}H-valine) melanoma cells was examined by subjecting it to indirect immunoprecipitation with anti-MAA antisera and subsequent analysis by SDS-PAGE (Fig. 5). The CAR #2 profile (B) was identical to that of CAR #1 (A) except for a reduction in a 285K dalton component and the absence of the 240K dalton component. We treated CAR #2 cells with 0.01 to 0.1 μg/ml of 12-0-tetradecanoylphorbol-13-acetate (TPA) or with phorbol, its nonpromoter analog. Within 24 hours after exposure to TPA, the 240K antigen was detected in the spent culture medium of the formerly deficient CAR #2 cells (Fig. 6). Shedding of 240K was not induced by treatment with phorbol. In addition, shedding of a 180K component always detected in the spent medium of untreated CAR #2 cells was blocked in TPA-treated cultures.

TPA treatment in other systems has been shown to induce morphological changes consistent with a transformed phenotype [26] and to increase shedding of fibronectin from normal cells [27]. We therefore exposed normal human fetal melanocytes to varying doses of TPA or phorbol (0.005 to 0.2 μg/ml). TPA treatment resulted in biphasic changes not observed with phorbol treatment: at low doses, neurite-like processes were formed and the production of melanin was increased; at higher dose levels

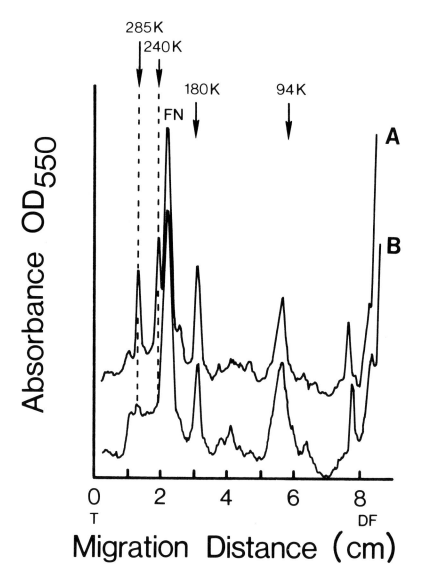

FIG. 5. SDS-PAGE profiles of spent medium of CAR #1 and CAR #2 melanoma cell lines. Cultures of CAR #1 (A) and CAR #2 (B) were intrinsically labeled with ³H-leucine and indirectly immunoprecipitated with rabbit xenoantiserum to melanoma cells (#6522).

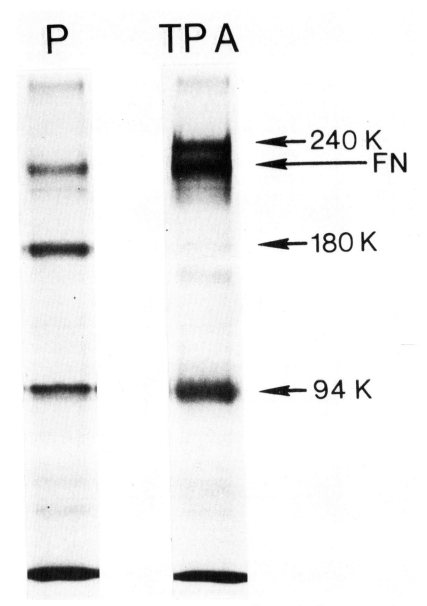

FIG. 6. Induction of 240K MAA on CAR #2 cells treated with tumor promoter. CAR #2 cells were exposed to 0.05 μg/ml of TPA or phorbol [8]. ³H-leucine was added after the first 24 hours of exposure and spent culture medium was harvested after an additional two days of exposure. Labeled spent culture medium was subsequently examined by indirect immunoprecipitation with polyclonal antiserum to melanoma cells.

there was an absence of the differentiation effect, but cells became increasingly refractile and changed to a more epithelial morphology. An increase in shedding of fibronectin also occurred, as judged by indirect immunoprecipitation of spent culture medium and analysis by SDS-PAGE. Although this evidence indicated a transformed phenotype, there was no detectable shedding of the 240K antigen. However, in recent experiments, fetal melanocytes, transformed by SV-40 and passaged more than 12 times after lytic crisis, synthesized and shed a molecule immunologically similar to 240K.

Thus, data from these experiments suggest that the 240K glycoprotein, shed by most melanoma cells, may be a marker of tumorigenicity. This marker seems to be synthesized by cells which are "initiated" like the CAR #2 cells or the SV-40-transformed fetal melanocytes; however, "promotion" without initiation is apparently insufficient to induce synthesis of the 240K antigen.

Discussion and Speculation

Our experience in the production of monoclonal antibodies indicates that MAA were effective immunogens when insolubilized on lentil lectin coupled to Sepharose 4B. Such immunosorbents may effectively induce a humoral response because of their mode of antigen presentation and increased tissue retention time, or because of the adjuvant effect of dextran polymers that are present in Sepharose. A primary consideration in the use of immunosorbent-purified MAA is the removal of competing, immunodominant antigens. This is readily accomplished by our approach since both urea extracts and spent medium from melanoma cells lack detectable amounts of HLA-A,B or HLA-DR antigens that are usually present as competing immunogens on intact melanoma cells [12]. Hybridomas secreting antibodies to these immunogenic histocompatibility antigens, are commonly produced when mice are immunized with intact melanoma cells [28]. In addition, fibronectin, another competing immunogen present in urea extracts and spent medium of melanoma cells, can be effectively removed by affinity chromatography [5]. Under these experimental conditions antibodies to MAA that recognize multiple determinants on these molecules can be optimally elicited. Monoclonal antibodies produced in this manner should be particularly useful to assess whether proteolytically derived fragments of MAA are antigenically reactive and also to make comparisons with epitopes recognized by antibody in patient sera.

Hybridoma antibodies raised to MAA which are shed from cells may be particularly useful in radioimmunodetection of cancer. Current imaging technology indicates the lowest threshold of detection of tumor nodules as 1 cm^2 [29]. It is conceivable that this threshold can be lowered by better imaging techniques [30] or by increasing the effective size of the nodule. The latter possibility may be attained if the antigen to which a hybridoma is directed is a membrane-derived, shed antigen. Assuming vascular integrity of the capillary networks around the tumor, an antigen shed from the tumor is likely to be trapped in extracellular tissue spaces, creating an antigen "halo" of indeterminate size around the tumor nodule. Thus, labeled hybridoma antibody binding to this shed antigen may give an apparently larger image and increase the detection limit of the tumor nodule. If vascular integrity is not maintained, then circulating antigen could block the binding of labeled antibody to tumor nodules in the tissue [31]. To test these hypotheses our laboratory is currently developing collaborative efforts aimed at evaluating the usefulness of hybridoma antibody to shed tumor antigen in the radioimmunodetection of tumors.

In preliminary experiments we found that MAA, as defined by xenogenic antibodies in our laboratory, may elicit an antibody response in humans. Both normal human sera and melanoma patient sera, adsorbed with pooled human IgG-Sepharose 4B, bind to MAA on solid phase, chemically defined spent medium from melanoma cells. In contrast, this type of antibody was not detected in unabsorbed human serum.

These findings are similar to previous observations which indicated that naturally occurring circulating immune complexes of tumor-specific antibody and anti-idiotypic antiglobulin can be disassociated by adsorption on Cohn Fraction II IgG-Sepharose [32]. The induction of this "masked" antibody response may be due to oncofetal antigens shared by melanoma and carcinoma cells and present on normal epithelial cells during cell division. In this regard, numerous findings have indicated that differentiated adult tissues will reexpress antigens associated with their fetal development during cell division [14]. This transient fetal antigen expression could thus induce antibody responses which are perpetuated by anti-idiotypic regulation [32]. The 94K glycoprotein, shed by both melanoma and carcinoma cells and present on fetal melanocytes, may represent the stimulus for this natural antibody response. Evidence for this postulate is the presence of the 94K glycoprotein in spent medium of melanoma cells to which we have demonstrated binding of this natural antibody as well as its presence on dividing but not terminally differentiated melanocytes in the dermis (Natali, personal communication). Further investigations are required to determine the possible role of this component in spent medium of melanoma cells in induction of this antibody response.

It is commonly known that normal cells, transformed by oncogenic viruses and chemical carcinogens, exhibit profound changes in antigen expression and shedding, glucose transport and metabolism, enzyme activities, cytoskeleton arrangement, synthesis of glycolipids and growth characteristics. Many of these characteristics may only be an indirect result of primary transformation-dependent events. For example, induction of specific membrane glycoproteins was observed after transformation of avian, murine, hamster and human cells [33-36]. Induction of these glycoproteins is not a direct consequence of transformation, but is caused by enhanced glucose uptake and subsequent glucose depletion of the culture medium. In this regard, we have observed that extracellular glucose levels can modulate glycosylation and shedding of both the 240K and 94K MAA [6]. In our studies with normal human fetal melanocytes the 240K glycoprotein is synthesized only after transformation by SV-40 and prolonged passaging. Further studies will determine whether this 240K synthesis is a direct consequence of transformation or indirectly related.

In summary, these studies, although preliminary, point to a vital role of these immunochemically defined 240K and 94K MAA in elicitation of host immune responses, and suggest that changes in expression and glycosylation of these tumor markers may be associated with transformation events. Furthermore, these immunochemically defined MAA may eventually be of practical use in immunodiagnostics and in immunodetection of melanoma and other forms of cancers.

Acknowledgements

The authors wish to acknowledge the technical assistance of Mr. John Brock and Mr. Charles Hockman and the secretarial assistance of Ms. Barbara Dodson.

References

1. Woodbury, R.G., Brown, J.P., Yeh, M.-Y. et al: Identification of a cell surface protein, p97, in human melanomas and certain other neoplasms. Proc. Natl. Acad. Sci. U.S.A. 77:2183-2187, 1980.
2. Brown, J.P., Wright, P.W., Hart, C.E. et al: Protein antigens of normal and malignant human cells identified by immunoprecipitation with monoclonal antibodies. J. Biol. Chem. 255:4980-4983, 1980.
3. Steplewski, Z.: Monoclonal antibodies to human tumor antigens. Transplant. Proc. 12:384-387, 1980.
4. Morgan, A.C., Jr., Galloway, D.R., Imai, K. and Reisfeld, R.A.: Human melanoma associated antigens: Role of carbohydrate in shedding and cell surface expression. J. Immunol. 126:365-370, 1981.
5. Galloway, D.R., McCabe, R.P., Pellegrino, M.A. et al: Tumor associated antigens in spent medium of human melanoma cells: Immunochemical characterization with xenoantisera. J. Immunol. 126:62-66, 1981.
6. Morgan, A.C., Jr., Galloway, D.R. and Reisfeld, R.A.: Carbohydrate regulated shedding of immunochemically defined human melanoma antigens. In Saunders, J.P. and Daniels, J.D. (eds.): Fundamental Mechanisms in Cancer Immunology. New York: Elsevier North Holland. (In press.)
7. Gold, P. and Shuster, J.: Historical development and potential uses of tumor antigens as markers of human cancer growth. Cancer Res. 40:2973-2976, 1980.
8. Houston, L.L., Nowinski, R.C. and Bernstein, I.D.: Specific in vivo localization of monoclonal antibodies directed against the Thy 1.1 antigen. J. Immunol. 125:837-843, 1980.
9. Nadler, L.M., Stashenko, P., Hardy, R. et al: Serotherapy of a patient with a monoclonal antibody directed against a human lymphoid-associated antigen. Cancer Res. 40:3147-3154, 1980.
10. McCabe, R.P., Galloway, D.R., Ferrone, S. and Reisfeld, R.A.: Human melanoma associated antigens (MAA): Serological and structural characterization. In Reisfeld, R.A. and Ferrone, S. (eds.): Current Trends in Tumor Immunology. New York:Garland STPM Press, pp. 114-120, 1979.
11. Ruoslahti, E. and Engvall, E.: Immunochemical and collagen-binding properties of fibronectin. Ann. N.Y. Acad. Sci. 312:178-191, 1978.
12. Morgan, A.C., Jr., Galloway, D.R., Wilson, B.S. and Reisfeld, R.A.: Human melanoma associated antigen: A solid phase assay for detection of specific antibody. J. Immunol. Meth. 39:233-246, 1980.
13. Liu, F.T., Bohn, J.W., Ferry, E.L. et al: Monoclonal dinitrophenyl-specific murine IgE antibody: Preparation, isolation, and characterization. J. Immunol. 124:2728-2737, 1980.

14. Jerry, L.M. Lewis, M.G., Rowden, G. et al: Fetal antigens in non-neoplastic conditions. Cancer Res. 36:3446-3452, 1976.

15. Burtin, P.: The carcinoembryonic antigen of the digestive system (CEA) and the antigens cross-reacting with it. Ann. Immunol. (Paris) 129C:185-198, 1978.

16. Chism, S.E., Burton, R.C. and Warner, N.L.: Immunogenicity of oncofetal antigens: A review. Clin. Immunol. Immunopathol. 11:346-373, 1978.

17. Gold, P.: Antigenic reversion in human cancer. Annu. Rev. Med. 22:85-94, 1971.

18. Morgan, A.C., Jr., Galloway, D.R., Jensen, F.C. et al: Immunochemical delineation of an oncofetal antigen on normal and SV-40 transformed human fetal melanocytes. Proc. Natl. Acad. Sci. U.S.A. (In press.)

19. Morgan, A.C., Jr., Galloway, D.R., Imai, K. and Reisfeld, R.A.: Human melanoma associated antigens: Role of carbohydrate in shedding and cell surface expression. J. Immunol. (In press.)

20. Goldberg, A.R., Wolf, B.A. and Lefebure, P.A.: Plasminogen activators of transformed and normal cells. In Reich, E., Riflein, D.B. and Shaw, E. (eds.): Proteases and Biological Control. New York:Cold Spring Harbor, 1975, pp. 857-868.

21. Wigler, M. and Weinstein, I.B.: Tumor promoter induces plasminogen activator. Nature 259:232-233, 1976.

22. O'Brien, T.B., Lewis, M.A. and Diamond, L.: Ornithine decarboxylase activity and DNA synthesis after treatment of cells in culture with 12-0 tetradecanoylphorbol-13-acetate. Cancer Res. 39:4477-4480, 1979.

23. Lotem, J. and Sachs, L.: Regulation of normal differentiation in mouse and human myeloid leukemic cells by phorbol esters and the mechanism of tumor promotion. Proc. Natl. Acad. Sci. U.S.A. 76:5158-5162, 1979.

24. Huberman, E., Heckman, C. and Langenbach, R.: Stimulation of differentiated functions in human melanoma cells by tumor-promoting agents and dimethyl sulfoxide. Cancer Res. 39:2618-2624, 1979.

25. Giovanella, B.C., Stehlin, J.S., Santamaria, C. et al: Human neoplastic cells in tissue culture. I. Cell lines derived from malignant melanomas and normal melanocytes. JNCI 56:1131-1142, 1976.

26. Diamond, L., O'Brien, T.G. and Baird, W.M.: Tumor promoters and the mechanism of tumor promotion. Adv. Cancer Res. 32:1-74, 1980.

27. Keski-Oja, J., Shoyab, M., DeLarco, J.E. and Todero, G.J.: Rapid release of fibronectin from human lung fibroblasts by biologically active phorbol esters. Int. J. Cancer 24:218-224, 1979.

28. Koprowski, H. Steplewski, Z., Herlyn, D. and Herlyn, M.: Study of antibodies against human melanoma produced by somatic cell hybrids. Proc. Natl. Acad. Sci. U.S.A. 75:3405-3409, 1978.

29. Rockoff, S.D., Goodenough, D.J. and McIntire, K.R.: Theoretical limitations in the immunodiagnostic imaging of cancer with computed tomography and nuclear scanning. Cancer Res. 40:3054-3058, 1980.

30. Rollo, F.D. and Patton, J.A.: Imaging techniques for the radioimmunodetection of cancer. Cancer Res. 40:3050-3053, 1980.

31. Primus, F.J., Bennett, S.J., Kim, E.E. et al: Circulating immune complexes in cancer patients receiving goat radiolocalizing antibodies to carcinoembryonic antigen. Cancer Res. 40:497-501, 1980.

32. Morgan, A.C., Jr., Rossen, R.D. and Twomey, J.J.: Naturally occurring circulating immune complexes: Normal human serum contains idiotype-anti-idiotype complexes dissociable by certain IgG antiglobulins. J. Immunol. 122:1672-1680, 1979.

33 Shiu, R.P.C. Pouyssegur, J. and Pastan, I.: Glucose depletion accounts for the induction of two transformation-sensitive membrane proteins in Rous sarcoma virus-transformed chick embryo fibroblasts. Proc. Natl. Acad. Sci. U.S.A. 74:3840-3844, 1977.

34. Pouyssegur, J. and Yamada, K.M.: Isolation and immunological characterization of a glucose-regulated fibroblast cell surface glycoprotein and its non-glycosylated precursor. Cell 13:139-150, 1978.

35. Daviler, A.-L., Hofmann-Clerc, F., Torpier, G. and Montagnier, L.: Glucose-regulated membrane properties of untransformed and virus-transformed BHK 21 cells. Exp. Cell Res. 120:181-189, 1979.

36. McCormick, P.J., Keys, B.J., Pucci, C. and Millis, A.J.T.: Human fibroblast-conditioned medium contains a 100K dalton glucose-regulated cell surface protein. Cell 15:173-182, 1979.

Immunotherapy of Tumors In Vivo with Effector Cells Generated In Vitro

Joseph D. Feldman, M.D. and
Eduardo Fernandez-Cruz, M.D.

Introduction

In this presentation, we describe some recent results of successful immunotherapy of two rat syngeneic sarcomas: one a viral-induced neoplasm, MST, and the other a methylcholanthrene-induced malignancy, BC5. The essence of the treatment was to generate in vitro a large number of effector cells with specificity for the tumors and to infuse these effector cells into syngeneic BN rats bearing an established malignancy with a blood supply.

Materials and Methods

First, let us describe some details of the MST model. A Moloney sarcoma was induced in a neonatal BN rat with an injection of Moloney sarcoma virus. The tumor that formed, MST, has been carried by in vivo passage for six years in our laboratory and has been adapted to in vitro culture, both as suspensions and as spread monolayers. MST displays on its cellular surface virus and viral antigens, p30 and gp70 chiefly; BN histocompatibility antigens; and tumor-associated antigens,

Joseph D. Feldman, M.D., Member; and Eduardo Fernandez-Cruz, M.D., Visiting Scientist, Department of Immunopathology, Scripps Clinic and Research Foundation, La Jolla, Calif.

This is publication No. 2388 from the Department of Immunopathology, Scripps Clinic and Research Foundation. This work was supported by USPHS grants AI 7007, AI/CA 16205 and NIA 924.

different from viral antigens. There were no detectable fetal antigens and these antigens did not play any role in protection or in inducing significant immunologic responses. In syngeneic x-rayed BN rats (400 rads, total body irradiation) a subcutaneous inoculum of 5×10^4 to 1×10^5 cultured MST was fatal in 30 to 40 days; in intact nonirradiated BN rats a fatal dose varied from 10^5 to 10^6 cells, within 40 to 50 days. Metastases were infrequent and were only found late in growth of the tumor, usually in regional and pulmonary hilar lymph nodes [1, 2].

Another tumor line, BM2, has been derived from MST and was used in the experiments to be described later to induce immunity in donor rats and to generate effector T cells in vivo. BM2 was more immunogenic than MST and was a progressive neoplasm only at very large inocula. Immunity to BM2 in vivo protects against fatal doses of MST and vice versa. The same surface antigens, tumor-specific and viral, were detectable in both lines, differing only in quantity. MST was used in all experiments in which effector cells were tested in assay rats bearing an established MST.

Effector cells were generated in vitro as follows [3]: In 40 ml of medium, 5×10^7 donor spleen cells were cultured with 1×10^7 mitomycin-treated MST (MST_{mit}) for five to seven days. Donor spleen cells were derived from rats immunized with an inoculum of BM2 at doses of tumor that would regress; from control rats immunized with BC5, a chemically induced BN tumor that expressed no virus and was antigenically unrelated to MST; from control rats that were unmanipulated. In culture, the tumor cells were more immunogenic after brief trypsinization; i.e., the mixed lymphocyte tumor reaction (MLTR) yielded more, and more effective, effector cells than if MLTR was prepared with nontrypsinized cells. Macrophages were required for effective generation of effector cells, and the concentration was less than 1% of the cultured cells. In both in vitro and in vivo tests, only donor immune spleen cells incubated with MST_{mit} generated effector elements that were specific for MST. Cells reactive with MST could not be generated in seven-day MLTR from nonimmune control spleens, from control spleens immune to BC5 or from spleens immune to MST and incubated with BC5. Only immune spleen cells from donors with regressed BM2, at least 14 days after regression, yielded effector cells in MLTR. Immune spleen cells from donors with progressive tumor not only did not generate effector cells but exhibited evidence of suppressor cell activity.

The yield and composition of cultures at seven days of MLTR are presented in Table 1.

The in vivo assay rat was a 150-gm BN host, either x-rayed with 400 rads or unmanipulated, bearing a subcutaneous tumor of MST of six to eight days' duration, with a blood supply, measuring 0.8 to 1.5 cm in diameter. Into this host, a varying number of effector cells from seven-day MLTR were infused intravenously via a tail vein. Growth of tumor was recorded as the product of the two largest perpendicular measurements of the tumor, every two to three days during the period of observation, up to 100 days. Control assay rats included groups that received no MLTR cells, or MLTR cells from control spleens.

Results

In Figure 1A, results of in vivo immunotherapy are shown. Infusion of 7-day MLTR cultures of immune cells and MST_{mit} eliminated completely all established tumors within 33 days. Assay rats infused with control spleen cells, i.e. spleen cells from nonimmune donors or spleen cells from donors immune to

Table 1. Percentage of Cell Types in MLTR:
Donor Spleen Cells and Mitomycin-Treated MST

Cell Type	Normal		Progressor		Regressor	
	Day 0	Day 7	Day 0	Day 7	Day 0	Day 7
W3/13$^+$ T cells	44	39	44	37	45	57
W3/25$^+$ T cells	38	35	32	35	38	50
Ig$^+$ cells	46	31	42	39	45	24
Macrophages	5-7	1-2	11-14	1-2	5-7	1
Ig$^-$, T$^-$ cells (null)	3-5	28	0-3	22	3-5	18
Total yield (% of original culture)	5%-15%		5%-11%		35%-40%	

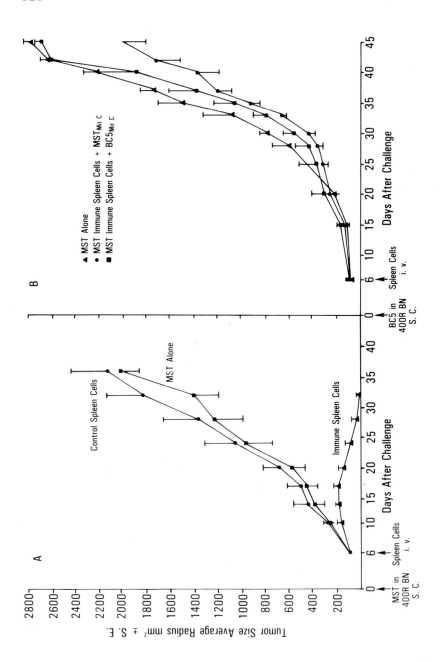

FIG. 1. (A) Irradiated recipients. Elimination in vivo of challenge MST tumor by spleen cells from donor rats immunized with MST, and restimulated in vitro for seven days with MSTmit. Preirradiated BN rats (400 rads, total body irradiation) were injected subcutaneously with 10^5 MST and bore by day 6 an established Moloney sarcoma, 1.0 to 1.5 cm in diameter. Groups of five assay rats were infused IV with 2×10^7 effector cells. Immune spleen cells (▲————▲); control spleen cells from normal, nonimmunized donors, incubated for seven days with MSTmit (●————●); growth of MST tumor cells alone (■————■). The data represent pooled results from four separate experiments; i.e., each point is the mean of 20 experimental rats or 40 control rats. (B) Specificity in vivo of MST-immune lymphocytes restimulated in vitro. Failure to eliminate challenge of BC5 tumors. Recipients were preirradiated (400 rads) and bore a tumor 1.0 to 1.5 cm in diameter. At six days postinoculum in each experiment, groups of five experimental and ten control rats were infused IV with immune spleen cells incubated in MLTR with MSTmit (●————●) or BC5mit (■————■). Three experiments are shown. (Reprinted from Fernandez-Cruz et al [3], © 1979 The Williams & Wilkins Co., Baltimore.)

BC5, were dead at day 35, as were controls that had received tumor alone, without spleen cell infusion.

The successful elimination of MST by effector cells was specific (Fig. 1B). An inoculum of BC5, a chemically induced tumor that is both progressive and fatal, grew without inhibition or regression in host rats that were infused with spleen cells specific for MST. Similarly, infusion of BC5 effector cells into rats bearing MST did not affect growth of the tumor.

Up to this point we have shown elimination of MST in x-rayed hosts. In Figure 2, similar results are shown for non-x-rayed assay rats. In ten intact rats bearing an established tumor and infused with immune effector cells, eight tumors were eliminated within 40 days and two within 60 days. As before, in control rats growth of MST occurred rapidly in the non-x-rayed host and was lethal.

A minimal number of effector cells, 5×10^7, was required to eliminate an established tumor; i.e., there was a dose-response relationship [4]. When effector cells at ratios of 400:1 to tumor cells were infused into assay rats, MST were eliminated completely within 36 days; at 200:1 ratios, growth continued for 8 to 10 days after infusion of effector cells and then MST were eliminated within 50 days; at 100:1 ratios, i.e. 2.5×10^7 effector cells and 2.5×10^5 inocula of tumor, MST grew almost as rapidly and were eventually as fatal as they were in controls. Effector cell to tumor cell ratios were calculated on the basis of the dose of MST given at day 0 to assay rats. For example, if 10^5 MST were inoculated on day 0, 1×10^7 effector MLTR cells were infused on day 6 or 8, for an E/T ratio of 100:1. These results showed that there was an inverse relationship between the growth of constant tumor inoculum and the number of effector spleen cells administered: the larger the number of effector cells, the less the growth and the earlier the elimination of MST.

We were interested to determine the efficacy of cell transfer in assay rats bearing large tumors. We treated rats with neoplasms that had been growing for 12 days (about 3.5 cm in diameter) and for 18 days (about 5 to 6 cm in diameter) with varying numbers of effector spleen cells. Large neoplasms of relatively long duration were eliminated completely after a single infusion or repeated infusions of effector cells in large numbers, up to 1.5×10^9 [4]. The elimination of the largest

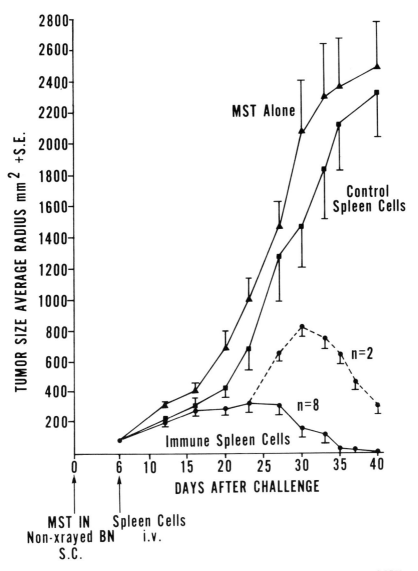

FIG. 2. Nonirradiated recipients. Elimination in vivo of challenge MST tumor with spleen cells from donor rats immunized with MST and restimulated in vitro for seven days. Recipients were nonirradiated BN rats and bore a tumor 1.0 to 1.5 cm in diameter, with a blood supply. At six days postinoculum, groups of five experimental and ten control rats were infused IV with 5×10^7 spleen cells. Immune spleen cells (●———●); normal spleen cells (■———■); growth of MST tumor alone (▲———▲). Two experiments are shown. The dotted line (●— — — —●) represents growth of tumor in 2/10 recipients in which elimination of tumor was delayed. (Reprinted from Fernandez-Cruz et al [3], © 1979 The Williams & Wilkins Co., Baltimore.

neoplasms took up to 100 days after effector cell infusion. One might expect that the digestion and resorption of 5 or more grams of tissue would require this period of time.

We might consider here the magnitude of these results. The assay rats averaged 165 gm in body weight and were 150 to 200 days old at the time of death. Some had neoplasms of 5 to 6 cm in diameter, or 5 to 6 gm. This would be over 3% of the body weight of the tumor-bearing host. In a 70-kg person, a tumor that is 3% of the host's body weight would be greater than 2 kg and would have been growing for 15% of the patient's life. Figure 3 (upper panel) shows a rat with a tumor over 6 cm in diameter that had been expanding for 18 days before infusion of specific effector cells. In the lower panel is the same rat 100 days after treatment, displaying no evidence of tumor.

We have followed a number of "cured" rats for two years and, in all, there have been no recurrences and there was active and potent immunity to inoculation of high, fatal doses of MST. The spleen cells of the cured rats did not display any greater in vitro cytotoxicity to MST than did donor spleen cells of rats with regressed tumors. Furthermore, to transfer successfully effector cells that would eliminate MST in an assay rat, the spleen cells of the cured rat had to be cultured in a seven-day MLTR to yield appropriate numbers and kinds of effector cells.

What are the effector cells? In cultures of spleen cells from an immune donor rat with regressed tumor incubated for seven days with MST_{mit} there were numerous blast cells, and an absence of tumor cells. In control cultures, i.e. spleen cells of immune donor rats incubated with $BC5_{mit}$, there was a paucity of cells, three- to four-fold less than in MLTR with MST_{mit}; some small lymphocytes; many tumor cells; and very few blast cells. This cultural morphology was characteristic of cultures containing nonimmune spleen cells and MST_{mit} and of cultures of spleen cells immune to BC5 but incubated with MST_{mit}. Cultures of immune spleen cells without antigen (MST_{mit}) contained 5% to 10% of the original number of cells and these were small lymphocytes [3]. Let me reiterate the results shown in Table 1, which offers the composition and yield of the culture contents. The significant changes in cellular composition occurred in seven-day MLTR of regressor spleens. Percentage of T cells was increased, percentage of Ig^+ cells was decreased, and null cells, i.e. Ig^-, T^- cells, were increased by comparison with

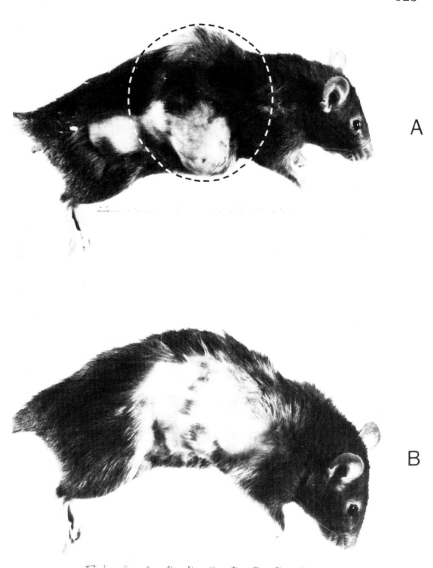

FIG. 3. (A) An assay rat bearing a lethal subcutaneous MST sarcoma, 6 cm in diameter, on day 27 after tumor inoculation. The test rat was treated with repeated intravenous infusions of effector spleen cells (total = 1.5×10^9), beginning on day 18 after inoculation of tumor. (B) Elimination of the tumor 98 days after tumor inoculation and 80 days after infusion of effector cells. (Reprinted from Fernandez-Cruz et al [4], © 1980 The Rockefeller University Press.)

the composition of day 0 culture. A comparison with MLTR of normal spleens and progressor spleens also revealed a significant relative increase of T cells, a decrease of Ig^+ cells and fewer null cells. The yield of viable cells in MLTR of regressor spleens was three- to six-fold greater than the yield of viable cells in MLTR of normal and progressor spleens. The kinetics of cell proliferation, blastogenesis and cell death was such that the total number of T cells in seven-day MLTR of regressor spleens was about 50% of the absolute number of T cells present on day 0, but about fivefold greater than the number of T cells in MLTR of normal and progressor spleens.

We have tried to delineate morphologically and functionally the effector cell generated in MLTR that eliminated an established tumor in vivo. With suitable fluorescent antibodies specific for certain membrane protein markers, we found that the most likely candidate for effector cells in vivo was a T cell blast with the following phenotypic markers: $W3/13^+$; $W3/25^+$; $Ia^{\pm}$; Ig^-; $RT1^+$. W3/13 and W3/25 are T antigens detected on rat lymphocytes by mouse monoclonal antibodies developed by Alan Williams and colleagues [5]. W3/13 is present on all T cells, circulating and sessile, and also on a fraction of immature B lymphocytes resident in bone marrow. W3/25 is a specificity of T antigens, present on circulating mature T cells, presumably T helper cells [6, 7], and is found on 80% of $W3/13^+$ cells [5]. Ia antigens were detected by fluorescein-conjugated mouse antibodies to rat Ia, generously supplied by Dr. David Sachs [8, 9]. Surface Ig was detected with our own polyspecific goat antibodies to rat Ig [10]. In Table 2 are presented some data on the phenotypic markers of day 0 and day 7 cultures from MLTR of normal, progressor and regressor spleens.

We isolated in the FACS several fractions of seven-day MLTR to assay their efficacy in eliminating tumors in vivo. Ig^+ cells, 92% to 96% Ig^+, from MLTR of immune regressor spleens, did not affect the fatal growth of MST in assay rats. Neither did null cells, i.e. cells freed of Ig^+ cells and $W3/25^+$ cells. With infusion of $W3/25^+$ cells, approximately 95% enriched, MST was eliminated quickly (Fig. 4). Note that the number of $W3/25^+$ T cells associated with successful elimination of MST in vivo was 5×10^6 or some 20 times less than the number of unfractionated MLTR cells needed to accomplish the same result. The data show that $W3/25^-$ cells enhance the growth of

Table 2. Surface Markers on Uncultured and Day 7 MLTC Cells*

	T (W3/13+) %	T (W3/25+) %	Ig+ %	Ia+ %	T (W3/13+) Ia+ %	T (W3/25+) Ia+ %	T− Ig−† %
Uncultured Spleen Cells (Day 0)							
Normal spleens	45 ± 1 (4)‡	38 ± 1 (4)	48 ± 2 (4)	27 ± 1 (12)	3 ± 1 (7)	2 ± 1 (7)	7
Progressor spleens	46 ± 2 (4)	34 ± 2 (4)	46 ± 1 (4)	28 ± 1 (2)	4 ± 1 (2)	4 ± 1 (2)	8
Regressor spleens	46 ± 1 (4)	38 ± 1 (4)	45 ± 1 (4)	29 ± 1 (2)	5 ± 1 (2)	4 ± 1 (2)	9
Day 7 MLTC Cells							
Normal spleens	39 ± 3 (3)	35 ± 3 (3)	31 ± 1 (2)	18 (1)	1 (1)	2 (1)	30
Progressor spleens	37 ± 6 (3)	35 ± 3 (3)	39 ± 2 (2)	21 ± 2 (2)	5 ± 1 (2)	4 ± 2 (2)	24
Regressor spleens	57 ± 3 (6)	50 ± 3 (6)	24 ± 6 (4)	58 ± 4 (5)	54 ± 7 (4)	55 ± 7 (4)	19
P§	P = 0.02	P < 0.02	P < 0.02	P < 0.01	P < 0.01	P < 0.01	

*Data shown are the mean percentage of stained cells ± SEM. 3×10^6 uncultured and day 7 MLTC spleen cells were stained with Fl-GARG, anti-W3/13 or anti-W3/25 followed by Fl-GAMG. 1×10^5 viable cells were analyzed for fluorescence intensity in a FACS. For the determination of Ia+ cells and Ia+ T cells, 3×10^6 cells were stained with anti-W3/13 or anti-W3/25 and Rh-GAMG followed by Fl-anti-Ia. The percentage of Ia+ lymphoid cells and Ia+ T cells was determined by fluorescence microscopy.

†Determined by subtracting from 100% the total number of T cells (W3/13+) and B cells (Ig+).

‡Number of trials in parentheses.

§P value was calculated by Student's t test and compared uncultured (day 0) regressor spleen cells and day 7 MLTC regressor spleen cells.

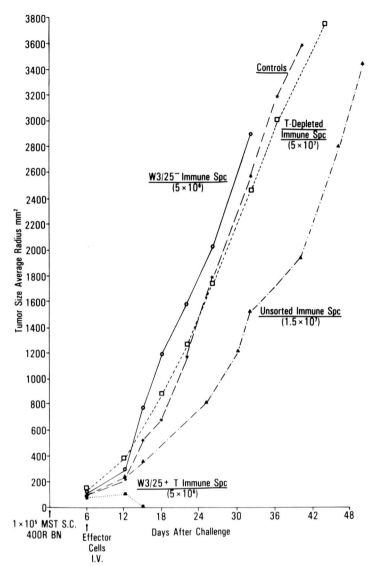

FIG. 4. Effect of W3/25$^+$ and W3/25$^-$ immune spleen cells on tumor growth in vivo. Each curve represents one trial. Similar results were obtained in four different experiments (total = four assay rats) with W3/25$^+$ and W3/25$^-$ cell fractions, but these data are not pooled because different numbers of sorted cells and different doses of tumor challenge were used in each experiment. The growth curves of tumors treated with unfractionated cells, of controls and of tumors treated with T-depleted immune spleen cells represent the mean of three different experiments with three assay rats per group (nine observations per point). (Reprinted from Fernandez-Cruz et al [4], © 1980 The Rockefeller University Press.)

established MST or have no effect. W3/25⁻ cells are a melange of cellular elements consisting of W3/13⁺-W3/25⁻ cells (about 8%), Ig⁺ cells, 1% to 2% macrophages, null cells (18%) and a few unidentified elements. We have not been able to isolate sufficient numbers of viable W3/13⁺-W3/25⁻ cells in the cell sorter to use the in vivo assays. Also, day 0 cultures are ineffective in vivo.

The morphologic association of T cells and tumor cells in vitro is presented in Figure 5. Rosettes consisting of a tumor cell with one or more contiguous lymphoblasts were first observed on day 3 of MLTR, increased in number by day 4, and began to exhibit by day 5 evidence of target cell destruction manifested by a decrease in the number of rosettes and by morphologic signs of cell damage, irregular cell surface, breaks in cell membrane, inhibition of fluid into cytoplasm, alterations of nucleus, etc. When rosettes were examined with fluorescent reagents, some lymphoblasts were both W3/25⁺ and Ia⁺, about 50% to 70% of all cells attached to tumor targets. The remaining cells attached to the tumor target were W3/25⁻, Ig⁻ (about 1% to 2% of all lymphoblasts forming rosettes showed surface Ig molecules) and Ia⁻. We have not yet been able to determine whether these latter cells are null elements, NK cells or even atypical small macrophages. The fluorescent antibody detecting W3/25 was distributed peripherally around the cell surface, usually exhibiting a beaded appearance. There was no capping or concentration of T antigens at the site of contact between lymphoblast and tumor target. When *Ia* was present on rosette-forming cells, it presented a variable pattern of a few small dots, or a labeled small segment of the surface with no discernible relation to tumor or to W3/25 antigen.

These observations suggested that the effector cell generated in vitro for successful therapy in vivo was a T cell that was W3/25⁺. However, there was a disparity between the in vivo and in vitro functions of W3/25⁺ cells [3, 4]. Cytotoxicity of W3/25⁺ cells in ⁵¹Cr release assays against labeled MST ranged from 10% to 15% of specific release at E/T ratios of 20:1 to 50:1. Cytotoxicity of unfractionated seven-day MLTR immune spleen cells ranged from 30% to 60% specific chromium release; and cytotoxicity of W3/25⁻ cells ranged from 15% to 50% at 20:1 and 50:1 E/T ratios [4].

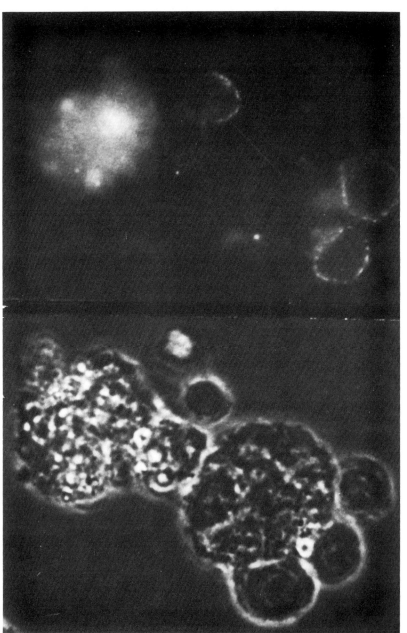

FIG. 5. Immune spleen cell-tumor rosettes in three-day MLTR. The left panel displays two tumor cells, with three lymphoblasts contiguous with one and two lymphoblasts associated with the second (phase micrograph). The right panel (fluorescence micrograph) depicts the same rosettes after reaction with W3/25 antibody. Note the peripheral distribution of W3/25 antigen, beaded in form, on three of five lymphoblasts. There is no capping or increased density of stain at points of contact with targets. The W3/25$^+$ cells were also Ia$^+$. The W3/25$^-$ lymphoblasts were Ia$^-$ and Ig$^-$.

There was a good correlation between the levels of in vitro cytotoxicity and the successful elimination of established tumors in vivo. Only seven-day MLTR cells from regressor spleens were cytotoxic in vitro, and cytotoxicity was specific for MST and not for an unrelated tumor. MLTR cells from control and normal spleens did not yield cytotoxic cells; i.e., there was no primary induction in vitro of cytotoxic elements [3].

We concluded from these observations the following: (a) established syngeneic viral tumors can be eliminated completely and permanently by infusion of T lymphocytes taken from donor spleens that have been immunized to MST and have been cultured in MLTR; (b) the lymphocyte was $W3/13^+$, $W3/25^+$, Ia^+, Ig^-, $RT1^+$; (c) it is probably a helper or amplifier cell, since it exhibited poor cytotoxic activity in vitro and this subset $W3/25^+$ has been shown to contain helper cells in other systems [6, 7]; (d) there was specificity in the model system; and (e) the cytotoxic effector cell was unknown. It may have been $W3/13^+$-$W3/25^-$ T cell, or $W3/25^+$ cells converted from helper to killer cells, or a recruited element from the tumor-bearing host.

We have carried out several studies to ascertain which antigen or antigens were targets for the T cell. Our first trials were directed to viral antigens. Donor rats were immunized with 25 μg of Moloney murine leukemia virus (M-MuLV), injected SC and IV three times, ten days apart. When rats were removed from this group and challenged with 10^7 MST, a fatal dose, 10 to 30 days after the last injection of M-MuLV, MST were eliminated in 28 to 42 days. In brief, immunization with whole virus produced immunity to the tumor.

Donor spleens were removed from rats immunized with M-MuLV, cultured in MLTR with MST_{mit} for seven days and infused into tumor-bearing rats (Fig. 6). MST were eliminated in 35 days (eight rats). There was no effect on the growth of BC5. Spleen cells removed from donors immune to M-MuLV and infused immediately into assay rats, without in vitro cultures, failed to eliminate MST. We also inoculated donor rats with disrupted virus, 25 μg, three times, ten days apart, etc. Cells from these donor spleens did not generate effector cells in seven-day MLTR that were associated with elimination of MST

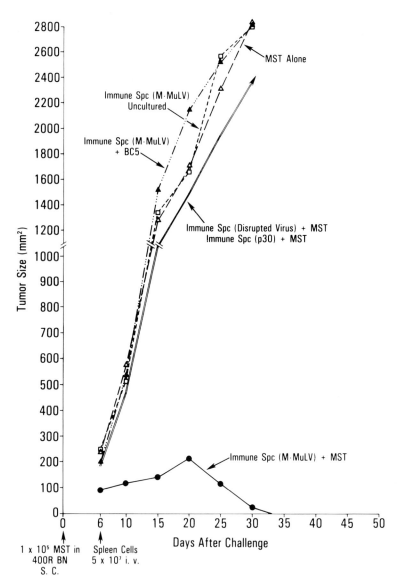

FIG. 6. Irradiated recipients. Elimination in vivo of challenge MST tumor by spleen cells from donor rats immunized with whole M-MuLV and restimulated in vitro for seven days with MST_{mit}. BN rats were irradiated with 400 rads total body radiation and were injected subcutaneously with 10^5 MST on day 0. Tumors averaged 1.0 to 1.8 cm in diameter by day 6. Groups of six assay rats were infused IV with 5×10^7 effector cells. Immune spleen cells to M-MuLV (●———●); immune spleen cells to disrupted virus and to p30, pooled results (▲———▲); immune spleen cells to M-MuLV, uncultured (□— — —□); immune spleen cells to M-MuLV, challenged with BC5 (▲··· ———▲); MST alone, no effector cells (△— — —△).

in vivo. These observations were different from those reported by Bernstein et al [11], and we have no explanation for the disparity. We noted a close correlation between the appearance of blastogenesis in vitro and the successful therapy of tumors in vivo.

The same regimen was repeated for the core polypeptide, p30, of M-MuLV. P30 was selected because there was always an antibody response to p30 when rats were inoculated with MST. Donor rats were inoculated intradermally with 25 μg of homogeneous p30, 25 μg subcutaneously ten days later, and 25 μg intravenously ten days later. When rats were so immunized and challenged with 10^7 MST, tumor growth was enhanced, as was reported by us previously [12].

Donor spleen cells, immune to p30, were placed in MLTR for seven days with MST_{mit}, and the seven-day-cultured cells were transferred to assay rats bearing a tumor. In six rats there was no effect on MST growth, which did not differ from growth in control rats. All died between days 31 and 40. There was also no in vitro cytotoxicity or blastogenesis in MLTR. There was, however, antibody to p30 in seven-day MLTR and in assay rats bearing a tumor. We do not know from this study whether any T cells with specificity were generated in donor spleens or in MLTR. Nor have we determined whether insoluble p30 or p30 on a membrane might be a more effective immunogen and expand a T cell clone in a seven-day culture. One conclusion, however, was that viral antigen(s) was the target for specific cells in this model.

In the second tumor model, BC5, the tumor is one induced by methylcholanthrene in a BN rat. The tumor grows slowly and progressively and is lethal in both x-rayed and non-x-rayed BN recipients at a dose inoculum of 5×10^4. BC5 does not express virus nor are p30, gp70 or any M-MuLV antigens detectable on its surface. RT1 is expressed on cell surfaces. Immunity to BC5 in BN rats was achieved by the following regimen.

BN rats, 100 to 110 days of age were injected subcutaneously with 10^7 BC5 cells treated with mitomycin ($BC5_{mit}$). Ten days later a second subcutaneous inoculum of 2×10^7 $BC5_{mit}$ was administered. One month later a booster of 10^7 $BC5_{mit}$ was given. When rats so immunized were challenged with 10^7 BC5 (not mitomycin-treated) they promptly rejected the tumor. To obtain an established tumor of 0.5 to 1.0 cm in diameter, BN rats were given a subcutaneous inoculum of 5×10^4 to 1×10^5 cells; at eight to ten days a subcutaneous neoplasm was palpable and measurable.

The procedures to generate effector cells in vitro for in vivo use were the same as those for MST. However, the results of therapy with seven-day MLTR cells and with $W3/25^+$ T cells were not as striking. Curves of BC5 growth in assay rats infused with effector cells showed that there was inhibition of growth but no elimination (Fig. 7A). Similarly, infusion of $6-8 \times 10^6$ $W3/25^+$ cells of seven-day MLTR significantly increased survival times to 80 or more days.

We surmised that there was suppression in this system since depletion of adherent cells from immune spleen populations yielded more, and more effective, effector cells (Fig. 7B). Similar observations were noted earlier when spleen cells of rats with progressive MST were placed in MLTR. We first suspected the macrophage and examined a number of culture preparations with and without macrophages. The data of some of these studies are presented in Table 3 and represent results obtained by manipulations of spleen cells from rats with progressive and regressive MST. Similar results have been obtained with spleen cells from rats with progressive BC5 and immune to BC5. We have not yet accumulated sufficient data in this latter model, however, to offer the results with BC5.

As shown in Table 3, recovery of cells after seven-day MLTR with progressor spleen cells ranged from 6% to 15%, and recovery with spleens of regressed donors was 45% to 55%. In the latter culture there was proliferation and blastogenesis, plus loss of tumor cells; in the former, the density of cells was diminished, blastogenesis was limited or absent, and many tumor cells persisted. Correlated with this were the in vitro cytotoxicity assays and in vivo assays. Spleen cells of progressor donors displayed little or no ability to release ^{51}Cr from tumor targets and were not associated with tumor elimination. Spleen cells from regressed donors exhibited 70% to 80% ^{51}Cr release in vitro and complete elimination of tumors within 30 to 40 days.

If spleen cells of progressor donors were depleted of macrophages (1% or less), there was a 30% to 35% recovery of

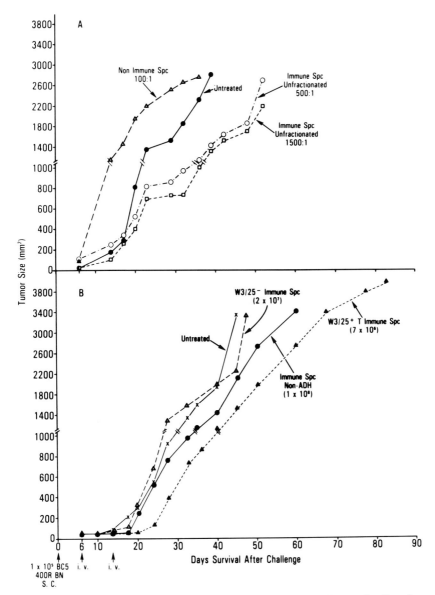

FIG. 7. Inhibition of BC5 in vivo by infusion of unfractionated cells of seven-day MLTR (A) and of fractionated (W3/25+ and W3/25−) cells of seven-day MLTR (B). At effector cell to target cell ratios of 1500:1, growth of BC5 was inhibited and rats survived for 46 days. Controls survived less than 35 days. With infusion of 7 × 10^6 W3/25+ cells, growth of BC5 was inhibited and rats survived to 85 days; with infusion of 2 × 10^7 W3/25− cells, rats survived less than 35 days. Each point on the curves represents five to eight assay rats.

Table 3. Suppressive Activity by Adherent Cells
from Spleens of Progressor Donors

	Recovery of Cells at 7 Days' MLTR	In Vitro Cytotoxicity: 7-Day MLTR Specific ^{51}Cr Release %	In Vivo Assay after Infusion of 7-Day MLTR Cells: Survival Time in Days
Spleen cells, progressor donors	6-15	0-10	30-35
Spleen cells, progressor donors, depleted of macrophages	30-35	20-30	50-80
Spleen cells, regressed donors	45-55	70-80	Elimination of tumors, 30-40 days
Spleen cells, regressed donors, macrophages added	7-12	0-10	30-40

cells after 7 days of MLTR, 20% to 30% in vitro cytotoxicity and survival of test rats for 50 to 80 days. If spleen cells of regressed rats were mixed 2:1 with macrophages from progressor donors, up to 10%, recovery, in vitro cytotoxicity and in vivo survival returned to the same levels as were found with spleen cells of progressor donors.

We may summarize this aspect of our studies by stating that macrophages seemed to play a double role. They were needed in order to generate effector cells in seven-day MLTR, generally at a concentration of 1% or less of the total number of cells placed in culture. They suppressed proliferation, blastogenesis and generation of effector cells at concentrations of 5% or higher. We suspected that there were additional suppressor elements in this system, and our suspicions were directed to the $W3/13^+$-$W3/25^-$ T cell and the null cell. We are currently exploring the activities of these cell types.

Inhibition of tumor growth with infusion of effector cells (Fig. 7A) and survival times were increased by increasing the number of infused effector cells. It was extremely tedious and time-consuming to harvest 1.5×10^8 effector or $5\text{-}10 \times 10^6$ $W3/25^+$ cells. We therefore initiated several T cell lines with specificity for MST and BC5. With antigen (MST_{mit} or $BC5_{mit}$), TCGF and accessory cells we have now in continuous culture several T cell lines. These lines have not yet been cloned or subjected to limiting dilution procedures, nor have they been tested for activity and specificity in vivo or in vitro against tumor targets. It is quite likely that T cell lines can be developed with specificity for MST and BC5 and with specific phenotypic characteristics. Such continuously growing lines will provide sufficient effector cells to eliminate in vivo established tumors, either viral-induced or chemically induced.

In conclusion, do these tumor models have any significance for the human situation? We are all aware of the great technical advances achieved recently in various kinds of cell cultures, of developing permanent and immortal lymphocyte lines, and finally T cell lymphocyte lines with specificities for known antigens [13-16]. It is not outside the realm of biologic reality to consider that what can be accomplished in rodent systems and with rodent cells, can also be achieved in the treatment of spontaneous autochthonous human neoplasms. Lymphoid cells can be removed from the circulation or from lymph nodes of patients with a neoplasm by surgery. The tumor itself can be excised and grown in culture. We are carrying out new experiments in which specific T lymphocytes, with specificity for the host's own tumor or specificities for tumors of one class and origin, may be cultivated and selected, perhaps cloned, for permanent growth. Such cell lines can provide limitless numbers of helper, recruiting or cytotoxic T cells that can be given back to the host afflicted with the tumor. The results should be as dramatic and as happy in the human as they have been in rats, mice and guinea pigs.

References

1. Jones, J.M., Jensen, T., Veit, B.C. and Feldman, J.D.: *In vivo* growth and antigenic properties of a rat sarcoma induced by Moloney sarcoma virus. JNCI 52:1771-1777, 1974.
2. Veit, B.C., Jones, J.M., Miller, G.A. and Feldman, J.D.: Genetic association of the humoral and cellular immune responses of rats to Moloney sarcomas. Int. J. Cancer 19:97-100, 1977.

3. Fernandez-Cruz, E., Halliburton, B. and Feldman, J.D.: *In vivo* elimination by specific effector cells of an established syngeneic rat Moloney virus-induced sarcoma. J. Immunol. 123:1772-1777, 1979.

4. Fernandez-Cruz, E., Woda, B.A. and Feldman, J.D.: Elimination of syngeneic sarcomas in rats by a subset of T lymphocytes. J. Exp. Med. 152:823-841, 1980.

5. Williams, A.F., Calfré, G. and Milstein, C.: Analysis of cell surfaces by xenogeneic myeloma-hybrid antibodies: Differentiation antigens of rat lymphocytes. Cell 12:663-673, 1977.

6. White, R.A.H., Mason, D.W., Williams, A.F. et al: T lymphocyte heterogeneity in the rat. Separation of functional subpopulations with a monoclonal antibody. J. Exp. Med. 148:664-673, 1978.

7. Loop, S.M., Bernstein, I.D. and Wright, P.W.: T cell synergy in the rat: Serologic characterization of T cell subsets. J. Immunol. 125:1237-1239, 1980.

8. Shinohara, N., Cullen, S.E. and Sachs, D.H.: Ag-B-linked analogue of a antigen in the rat. J. Immunol. 118:2083-2087, 1977.

9. Sachs, D.H., Humphrey, G.W. and Lunney, J.K.: Sharing of Ia antigens between species. I. Detection of Ia specificities shared by rats and mice. J. Exp. Med. 146:381-393, 1977.

10. Woda, B.A. and Feldman, J.D.: Density of surface immunoglobulin and capping on rat B lymphocytes. J. Exp. Med. 149:416-423, 1979.

11. Bernstein, I.D., Nowinski, R.C. and Stiefel, J.: The role of viral and cell-associated antigens in the cell-mediated immune response of rats to virus-induced lymphoma cells. J. Immunol. 124:1727-1732, 1980.

12. Jones, J.M., Kennel, S.J. and Feldman, J.D.: Immunization with P30 enhances the growth of a rat Moloney sarcoma. J. Immunol. 118:371-373, 1977.

13. Gillis, S. and Smith, K.A.: Long-term culture of tumor-specific cytotoxic T cells. Nature 268:154-156, 1977.

14. Nabholz, M., Engers, H.D., Collavo, D. and North, M.: Cloned T-cell lines with specific cytolytic activity. Curr. Top. Microbiol. Immunol. 81:176-187, 1978.

15. Baker, P.E., Gillis, S. and Smith, K.A.: Monoclonal cytolytic T-cell lines. J. Exp. Med. 149:273-278, 1979.

16. Von Boehmer, H., Hengartner, H., Nabholz, M. et al: Fine specificity of a continuously growing killer cell clone specific for H-Y antigen. Eur. J. Immunol. 9:592-597, 1979.

Indexes

Author Index

Subject Index

341